Clinician's Guide to
Holistic Medicine

Notice

Medicine is an ever-changing science. As new research and clinical experience broaden our knowledge, changes in treatment and drug therapy are required. The authors and the publisher of this work have checked with sources believed to be reliable in their efforts to provide information that is complete and generally in accord with the standards accepted at the time of publication. However, in view of the possibility of human error or changes in medical sciences, neither the authors nor the publisher nor any other party who has been involved in the preparation or publication of this work warrants that the information contained herein is in every respect accurate or complete, and they disclaim all responsibility for any errors or omissions or for the results obtained from use of the information contained in this work. Readers are encouraged to confirm the information contained herein with other sources. For example and in particular, readers are advised to check the product information sheet included in the package of each drug they plan to administer to be certain that the information contained in this work is accurate and that changes have not been made in the recommended dose or in the contraindications for administration. This recommendation is of particular importance in connection with new or infrequently used drugs.

Clinician's Guide to
Holistic Medicine

Robert A. Anderson, M.D.

Founding Member and Past President,
American Holistic Medical Association

President, American Board of Holistic Medicine

McGraw-Hill
Medical Publishing Division

New York   Chicago   San Francisco   Lisbon   London   Madrid   Mexico City
Milan   New Delhi   San Juan   Singapore   Sydney   Tokyo   Toronto

McGraw-Hill

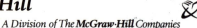

A Division of The McGraw·Hill Companies

Clinician's Guide to Holistic Medicine
Copyright © 2001 by The **McGraw-Hill** Companies, Inc. All rights reserved. Printed in the United States of America. Except as permitted under the United States Copyright Act of 1976, no part of this publication may be reproduced or distributed in any form or by any means, or stored in a data base or retrieval system, without the prior written permission of the publisher.

1 2 3 4 5 6 7 8 9 0 DOC DOC 0 9 8 7 6 5 4 3 2 1

ISBN 0-07-134714-3

This book was set in Korinna by Keyword Publishing Services.
The editor was Martin Wonsiewicz.
The production supervisor was Catherine Saggese.
Project management was provided by Keyword Publishing Services.
The cover design was by Aimee Nordin.
R.R. Donnelley & Sons was the printer and binder.

This book is printed on acid-free paper.

Library of Congress Cataloging-in-Publication Data
Anderson, Robert A. (Robert Arthur), 1932–
   Clinician's guide to holistic medicine / author, Robert A. Anderson.
     p. ; cm.
   Includes bibliographical references and index.
   ISBN 0-07-134714-3
     1. Holistic medicine. 2. Alternative medicine. I. Title
     [DNLM: 1. Holistic Health. W61 A549c 2001]
   R733.A56 2001
   615.5—dc21   00-050016

Contents

Preface

For physicians trained in the conventional schools of allopathic medicine, the rise of variations of medical practice called
"alternative," "complementary," and "holistic" engenders all
responses from antagonism to curiosity to enthusiastic acceptance. Editorialists and defenders of conventional medicine insist
"there is no proof" that any but a very few alternative options
have any merit whatsoever. And further, the fact that twenty-eight
persons died in the early 1990s from contaminated tryptophan-
induced eosinophilia myalgia, and that about six patients died several years ago from adverse liver effects of the herb chaparral,
brought dire warnings of the inherent dangers in the trend toward
increasing interest in unconventional medicine. But never mind
the 1998 estimate, by Lazarou et al.,[1] of 106,000 deaths and 2.5
million injuries each year from the appropriate conventional medical in-hospital use of pharmaceuticals.

Most physicians are quite aware of the two Eisenberg et al.
surveys of over one thousand randomly selected consumers in
1991 and 1997, concluding that 32 and 41 percent, respectively,
used some form of alternative healthcare services or products.[2,3]
Termed "unconventional" in their first survey, Eisenberg et al.
defined "alternative" as embracing those products, services, and
practices related to interventions not taught widely in medical
schools and not generally available in US hospitals. Consumers in
1997 were estimated to have spent $26 billion of largely unreim-
bursed, out of pocket, discretionary income. And further, 75 percent did not inform their physicians of what they were doing. The
depth of this shift incorporating medically unrecommended alter-

native initiatives intended to prevent or treat common chronic conditions should not be underestimated.

The motivations of users of alternative options appear to be deeply rooted in a paradigmatic shift of values. Astin's randomized survey of 1,000 adults confirmed the Eisenberg estimate of incidence of use exceeding 40 percent of US consumers.[4] The significance of the study could be summarized in the following conclusions. Those responding affirmatively to using alternative services and products:

1. were not especially disenchanted with conventional medical care;
2. were generally more educated than those not using alternative services;
3. were generally sicker that those seeking conventional care;
4. sought alternative care most often for chronic pain, anxiety, urinary tract problems, and back problems;
5. were inclined to use both alternative and conventional resources;
6. were prone not to tell their conventional practitioners what they were doing;
7. were significantly more likely to come from a segment of people within society who could be described as cultural creatives, with intense commitment to (1) environmental concerns with earth ecology, (2) feminism and feminine values, (3) personal growth psychology, and (4) spirituality;
8. were also significantly more likely to have had a "transformational" experience which motivated them to choose to have their medical care congruently aligned with their altered and newly found worldview;
9. expressed a holistic orientation in regard to health;
10. made up 41 percent of all respondents, totally consistent with the findings in the second Eisenberg survey.

The significant trend in which only a small percentage of users used alternatives exclusively without conventional resources is notable. This, combined with the tendency for them not to inform their conventional physicians about their alternative interests, means they were assertively making their own decisions about how to combine available treatment options, mixing and matching their conventional and alternative choices as they saw fit. Users of alternatives in this study were not generally dissatisfied with conventional care, but motivated by poorer health status, commitment to environmentalism, feminism, spirituality, and personal growth psychology. They were generally more highly educated, espoused a holistic orientation to health and life, and *many had had a transformational experience that shifted their worldview*. These aspects of users of alternative medicine describe a significant pattern which heralds a paradigmatic shift in society, including the means by which healthcare services are used and delivered. Many individual comments of respondents in the Astin survey expressed the opinion that their interest was in part due to the fact that alternative practitioners "promote health rather than just focusing on illness." This underscores the need to respond with a greater emphasis on health promotion and make such services available to the segment of society that considers this a priority.

Although public interest in alternative medicine had been building slowly from the 1960s, little professional attention or interest was elicited until the 1990s. The only professional membership organization addressing the entire spectrum of complementary topics was initiated with the founding meeting of the American Holistic Medical Association in 1978. Widespread interest in the field awaited the publication of Eisenberg's "Unconventional Medicine in the United States" in the *New England Journal of Medicine* in 1993.[2] Public interest has continued to expand, playing some role in the formation of the Office of Alternative Medicine within the National Institutes of Health by an Act of Congress in 1993. That office has recently been upgraded to the status of a separate office within the National Institutes of Health with an eight-fold increase in funding to $60 million in the 1999–2000 federal budget.

The changes occurring in professional medical circles in relation to holistic and complementary medicine reflect to some degree the previously mentioned consumer interest, but also burgeoning interest on the part of students, residents, and practicing physicians. Over one hundred medical schools now have at least one course devoted to alternative, complementary, or holistic medicine.[5] Affiliated institutes, or full-fledged departments devoted to these topics, have been established as well in a small number of institutions.

In the mid-1990s, three medical journals devoted to peer-reviewed publishing of alternative studies began publication. In November 1999 the journals of the AMA, including *JAMA*, devoted an issue to alternative and complementary medicine, publishing studies demonstrating both positive effects and lack of effectiveness of alternative treatments. Reactions to the choice of the AMA journals to publish in this field were, expectedly, mixed.

One of the steps leading to the establishment of a specialty within the framework of American medical practice is the assembling of a database of research information which permits an area of medical interest to clearly distinguish itself from other fields of medical interest. Over the last ten years that has been accomplished, as witness the publishing of a number of alternative books and compilations of data.[6–8]

A further step in marking the evolution of the holistic paradigm was the initiation of a certifying examination by the American Board of Holistic Medicine in December 2000.[9] Establishing minimum standards through a peer-developed written examination began to give greater definition to the development of complementary approaches as a specialty within the medical community.

Clinician's Guide to Holistic Medicine is offered as an additional resource emphasizing the shift from the duality of either–or thinking of conventional vs. alternative approaches to the unity of one holistic medicine, incorporating the best of both.

REFERENCES

1. Lazarou J et al. Incidence of adverse drug reactions in hospitalized patients. *JAMA* 1998; 279(15):1200–5
2. Eisenberg DM et al. Unconventional medicine in the United States. *N Engl J Med* 1993; 328(4):246–52

3. Eisenberg DM, Davis RB, Ettner SL et al. Trends in alternative medicine use in the United States, 1990–1997: results of a follow-up national survey. *JAMA* 1998; 280(18):1569–75

4. Astin JA. Why patients use alternative medicine. *JAMA* 1998; 279(19):1548–53

5. Bhattacharya B. M.D. programs in the United States with complementary and alternative medicine education opportunities: an ongoing listing. *J Altern Complement Med* 2000; 6(1):77–90

6. Anderson R. *The Scientific Basis for Holistic Medicine*, 4th edn. Box 5388, Lynnwood, WA: American Health Press, 2000

7. Micozzi M, ed. *Fundamentals of Complementary and Alternative Medicine*. London: Churchill Livingstone, 1996

8. Novey D, ed. *Clinician's Complete Reference to Complementary and Alternative Medicine*. New York: Mosby, 2000

9. Anderson R. American Board of Holistic Medicine to offer first certification examination in December 2000. *Altern Ther Health Med* 2000; 6(4):34

Clinician's Guide to
Holistic Medicine

1

Chapter One

Introduction

In recent years, four terms have come to be used to describe "non-conventional," "unconventional" or "non-traditional" forms of medical practice in nations where the dominant medical practice model is "allopathic." The terms are: alternative; complementary; integrative; and holistic.

In common usage, the term alternative medicine has come to mean the spectrum of treatment approaches whose theoretical or historical derivations are either culturally or developmentally quite distinct from the tenets of conventional medical practice in the United States. Another way of describing the content of alternative medicine is the spectrum of medical knowledge which is not officially taught in required courses in the medical schools of the United States. The list, not intended to be complete, would include nutritional medicine; environmental medicine; clinical ecology; biomolecular medicine; exercise medicine; psychoneuroimmunology; biofeedback and relaxation training; psychological medicine; social medicine; energy medicine; spiritual medicine; ethnomedicine (Ayurvedic medicine; traditional Chinese medicine and acupuncture; and Native American medicine); botanical medicine; manual medicine; and homeopathic medicine.

Complementary medicine incorporates the concept of moving beyond the either–or thinking that has tended to separate conventional and alternative medicine. It implies a synthesis of the two bodies of knowledge by combining the best that is available from both.

Integrative medicine implies a higher-level amalgamation of conventional medical practice and the many disciplines mentioned above into some orderly aspect of theories, practices and options. One of its principal advocates has been Andrew Weil, MD, whose books and appearances on the subject have met with resounding acceptance and popularity with the lay public. Weil, with an academic faculty post at the University of Arizona School of Medicine, has pioneered the establishment of a 2-year post-residency Fellowship in Integrative Medicine at the University of Arizona in Tucson.

Holistic Medicine is the descriptor for the utilization of the integration of the techniques mentioned above, with the addition of a strong emphasis on a *philosophy of medical practice* beyond the espousal of the alternative disciplines and techniques mentioned earlier. There is also a major emphasis on the creation of optimal health, and special attention to "Energy medicine," and what might be called "Spiritual Medicine."

It is of interest to note that, while there are separate professional organizations for many of the disciplines mentioned earlier, only one organization involving the integral or holistic approach embracing them all is known to exist. The American Holistic Medical Association (AHMA) was organized in 1978 to bring together physicians with an interest in holistic concepts.

Citing the principles of practice of the AHMA will afford some insight into the philosophy espoused by many in the whole field of complementary medicine.

1. Holistic physicians embrace a variety of safe, effective options in diagnosis and treatment, including: education for lifestyle changes and self-care; complementary approaches; and conventional drugs and surgery.

2. Optimal health is much more than the absence of sickness. It is the conscious pursuit of the highest qualities of the spiritual, mental, emotional, physical, environmental, and social aspects of the human experience.

3. It is imperative to expend as much effort in establishing what kind of patient has a disease as establishing what kind of disease a patient has.*

4. It is preferable to diagnose and treat patients as unique individuals rather than as members of a disease category; illness is viewed as a manifestation of a dysfunction of the whole person, rather than an isolated event.

5. When possible, lifestyle modifications are preferable to drugs and surgery as initial therapeutic options.

6. Prevention is preferable to treatment and is usually *more* cost-effective. The *most* cost-effective approach evokes the patient's own innate healing capabilities.

7. In most situations encouragement of patient autonomy is preferable to decisions imposed by physicians.

8. The ideal physician–patient relationship considers the needs, desires, awareness, and insight of the patient as well as those of the physician.

9. The quality of the relationship established between physician and patient is a major determinant of healing outcomes, and physicians significantly influence patients by their example.

10. Illness, pain, and the dying process can be learning opportunities for patients and physicians.

11. Holistic physicians encourage patients to evoke the healing power of love, hope, humor, and enthusiasm and to release the toxic consequences of hostility, shame, greed, depression and prolonged fear, anger, and grief.

12. Unconditional love is life's most powerful medicine. Physicians strive to adopt an attitude of unconditional love for patients, themselves, and other practitioners.

The body of knowledge of each of these areas is mentioned, as appropriate, under each disease grouping in the following chapters. The following pages introduce generic principles, to which references are made in the topic chapters ahead.

---

* Quotation from William Osler, one of the "fathers" of medicine on the North American continent.

Alternative Medical Options ....

Nutritional medicine. In 1992, both the American Cancer Society and the National Cancer Institute announced a shift in research funding. Each announcement, in effect, admitted great lack of success in finding the cause and cure for cancer from the spending of several billion research dollars over the span of 25 years following the declaration of "war on cancer" by a sitting president of the United States. Each announcement indicated a future emphasis on prevention of cancer, with a strong emphasis on nutritional research.

Numerous studies have found that the intake of nutrients of most Americans is suboptimal. While a majority of people is overweight or obese by most standards, intake of most micronutrients has been shown to fall below Recommended Dietary Allowances (RDAs) recommended by the Food and Nutrition Committee of the National Academy of Sciences. Magnesium appears to be deficient in 70–85 percent of many subgroups of Americans;[1] calcium intake is below RDAs in 65 percent of adult men and 85 percent of adult women;[1] elderly patients in France were found deficient in every micronutrient except vitamins C and A;[2] serum levels, too, are frequently found deficient in healthy elderly people.[3] Malnourishment occurs commonly in hospitalized patients,[4] and serum levels of vital nutrients are even lower in those with specific illnesses compared to the healthy population.[5]

Better nutrition begins with a generous endorsement of better intake of fruits, vegetables, whole grains, fish, truly unsaturated fat (from nuts, seeds, vegetables, and whole grains), and decreased intake of total fat, saturated fat, hydrogenated trans fats, animal meats, and sugars. Even with optimal macronutrient intake, supplementation with substantial doses of micronutrients appears to be necessary. Table 1-1 shows the chart based on amounts of individual micronutrients (vitamins and minerals) which a very large number of studies have been shown to be of preventive or therapeutic benefit in a variety of disease processes.

TABLE 1-1. MICRONUTRIENT SUPPLEMENTATION

Micronutrient	Suggested intake
A/Beta carotene	2.0–5.0 mg (10–25,000 IU)
B_1	50–100 mg
B_2	25–50 mg
B_3	100 mg
B_5	500 mg
B_6	75–100 mg
B_{12}	400 µg
Folic acid	800 µg
Biotin	400 µg
Inositol	100–1,000 mg
PABA	100–500 mg
Choline	100 mg
C	1,000 mg
D	1.25 µg (50 IU)
E	267 mg (400 IU)
Boron	3 mg
Calcium	200–1,500 mg
Chromium	200 µg
Copper	0–2 mg
Iodine	200 µg
Iron	0–18 mg
Magnesium	400 mg
Manganese	15 mg
Molybdenum	100 µg
Phosphorus	0–1,000 mg
Potassium	100 mg
Selenium	200 µg
Vanadium	100 µg
Zinc	15 mg

Many of the suggested daily intakes are several-fold greater than the RDAs. Reports of toxic effects of these levels of intake are extremely rare to non-existent. For convenience, many reputable nutrition companies with excellent quality controls provide multivitamin–mineral high-dose preparations with these approximate included amounts. In the text, reference is often made to the availability of these products.

Environmental medicine deals with the impact of toxic agents in the physical environment of human beings. The rapid multiplication of a myriad of chemicals used in industry, and the results of exposure to those agents that are potentially toxic, both to those who work in those industries, and those who use the manufactured products. Chief classes of toxic agents include petrochemical solvents, pesticides and herbicides, halogenated hydrocarbons, heavy metals, ionizing radiation, excessive ultraviolet radiation, noise exceeding 80 dB, air pollution, and personal toxins of tobacco products, and excess alcohol. These agents extract an enormous assault on health, and play a prominent role in the multiplication of oxygen-free radicals, the common thread in the etiology of most degenerative disease. Generic responses to toxins include avoidance, selective use of less-toxic products, filtering of drinking water, air cleaners and negative air ion generators, and abatement of smoking (primary and second hand), and moderation in alcohol intake.

Clinical ecology. This is the descriptor for the awareness of the impact on health of reactivity to inhalants and ingestants including food. These may be true allergic reactions, of clinically important sensitivities not technically definable as IgE or IgG reactions. Not accepted by most of their conventional colleagues, clinical ecologists include food sensitivities as a potential cause of disease of nearly every organ system in the body, beyond the conventionally accepted target organs of lungs, nose, and skin; these include the heart, central nervous system, renal, intestinal, joints, circulatory vessels, genital tract, and gall bladder. A substantial body of research, as well as the results of decades of utilizing clinically successful protocols, supports this approach.

The food elimination protocols, repeatedly mentioned in the following topic chapters, can be described as follows.

If food sensitivities are suspected or are a possibility for consideration resulting from a process of elimination, the nutritional elimination period extends for five days; in testing for joint problems such as arthritis, the elimination period must be 2 weeks.[6]

Three different approaches can be used, from the simple to the rigorous. The simplest approach is the elimination of the few most commonly found culprits, including cow's milk and all derivatives, wheat, corn, sugar, eggs, peanuts, citrus fruits, and chocolate. This group of foods, with the addition to the list of the non-foods coffee, tea, alcohol, and any foods with additives, including artificial coloring, texturing, and flavoring agents, fillers, and preservatives, includes about 85 percent of potential offenders. The next choice in the elimination phase is the limitation of intake to four foods: rice, carrots, lamb, and pears. These four foods are at the extreme low end of the list of potential food sensitizers. The third, and most rigorous elimination protocol, requires a 5-day total fast except for water. While this approach is theoretically the most thoroughgoing, many patients are not ready to take this extreme step.

With any of these approaches, symptoms typically get worse on the first to third days of the elimination diet. This is thought to be a rebound phenomenon resulting from sudden elimination of the targets of reaction in the adapted immune state, similar to a withdrawal phenomenon. By the fifth day, symptoms typically improve, often dramatically. If this improvement is noted, each of the eliminated foods then needs to be reintroduced in a pure form, one new food every 3 days. If the reintroduced food is one of the culprits, symptoms recur within hours of the first ingestion. If the reaction to the identified culprits is powerful, permanent elimination may be necessary. If the reactions are mild to moderate, those foods can usually be tolerated in a moderate amount in rotation fashion, once in every 4, 5, or 6 days.

The following actual history will help to clarify this procedure. A 40-year-old woman reported that she was extremely tired because of insomnia of many years' duration. The cause of the sleep disorder was a nocturia of 5 times nightly. Her urinary urgency and frequency required her to void her bladder about every hour and a half while awake. She had had two extensive urological work-ups with no established diagnosis. She agreed to go on a food elimination trial for 5 days, totally avoiding the eight foods listed earlier, plus coffee, tea, alcohol, and additives. In 48 hours, her nocturia was reduced to twice nightly, and her voiding pattern was totally normal in 5 days. On re-challenge with her foods, she reactivated the nocturia and daytime frequency within hours of introducing both wheat and chocolate. Avoiding these permanently, her elimination pattern remained normal indefinitely.

Biomolecular medicine. This term describes the use of endogenous hormones and other biosynthetic agents used in pharmacological amounts, such as coenzyme Q_{10}, melatonin, dehydroepiandrosterone, and non-essential amino acids that are not contained in significant amounts in food. Many of these agents synthesized in the body are produced in decreasing amounts with age. "Biomolecular" also refers to the use of exogenous agents and drugs in off-label ways and circumstances, and unconventional procedures such as chelation, bio-oxidative therapy and spa hydrotherapy.

Exercise medicine is commonly utilized in conventional practice, especially in suggestions made to patients with cardiovascular disease and diabetes. It is also employed in alternative ways, with applications in cancer prevention and treatment, sports performance, and as a stress management option.

Behavioral medicine alternatives include *biofeedback and relaxation* procedures, psychoneuroimmunology, and psychological medicine. Biofeedback and allied relaxation procedures such as progressive relaxation, autogenics, and hypnosis, share in common the induction of an altered state of consciousness. These patient-oriented approaches involve the learning of the techniques to enter the alpha and theta states of consciousness, as opposed to the beta state in which most people find themselves during most of their waking hours. In alpha and theta states, the basic brain-wave frequency is much slower, the autonomic nervous system operates at a much lower baseline, and a total state of general and muscular relaxation ensues. Hypnosis involves the use of suggestions given in this altered state of consciousness. Affirmations are also utilized in relaxation processes. Any suggestion or affirmation presented in an altered state of consciousness is incorporated with greater acceptance and less resistance. Benefits of these procedures are widely applicable in a variety of disease processes. The results of these therapies are often striking, resulting in a reduction in the intensity of autonomic nervous system responses, and less costly emotional and chemical reactions on the part of the body during the experience of stress.

"Behavioral medicine—and one of its progenitors, bio-feedback—are expanding as the Third Therapeutic Revolution, supplementing surgery and pharmacology in treating human illnesses. Parallel development of non-science-based therapies is a part of the same revolution. Labeling their positive results as "placebo effects" hides a greater truth: faith and trust play an enormous role in therapy. The successes of both behavioral medicine and unorthodox complementary medicine are the result of the de bonafide effect (...latin for 'from good faith'). Readers are urged to adopt this better definition of the 'inexplicable' and substantial good results of both the placebos in research and the ministration of unorthodox treatments."[7]

Psychoneuroimmunology describes the field of mind–brain–body connections which has gained great impetus following Dr. Robert Ader's demonstration of the conditioning of immune cells of animals in the mid-1970s.[8] Effects of thoughts, images, concepts and ideas have far-reaching effects, not only on the functions of the central nervous system, but also on the immune and endocrine systems, as well. The devastating effects of stress on immunity are mediated through these systems,[9] and hormone levels are equally susceptible to stress effects.[10] These interactions have enormous effects on degenerative disease, longevity, and sudden unexpected death.

Psychological medicine includes a number of techniques that could be described as proactive and interactive approaches to cognitive therapy. Psychiatry, centered for several decades in the more passive psychoanalysis approach, has largely given way in the last 15 years to psychopharmacology and the use of psychotropic pharmacological agents as therapeutic tools. Proactive interpersonal counseling techniques, utilized principally by non-medically trained practitioners, includes Transactional Analysis, Psychosynthesis, Brief Therapy, Guided Imagery, Family Therapy, and Jungian approaches. Many of these approaches are also utilized in group work, and are more proactive in the sense that practitioners often give prescriptions for assigned behavioral tasks to be tried by clients.

Social medicine is based on research of the last several decades in which the risk of adverse outcomes in a variety of degenerative diseases has been shown to be greatly exaggerated in those who are socially isolated. Outcomes in prevention and treatment of cancer, cardiovascular disease, autoimmune disease, and diabetes are consistently and sometimes strikingly better in patients who have a strong support system, who are in relationship with a spouse or confidant, and those who participate extensively in the life of the community. While medical practitioners do not control these social factors, an awareness of their importance can influence the nature of non-pharmacological prescriptions and suggestions given to patients.

Energy medicine includes the application of in-vitro and in-vivo research published in the past couple of decades regarding human influence on plants, microbiological organisms, deionization of water, and enzyme systems. The use of noncontact techniques including healing touch, Reiki, and Therapeutic Touch has been supported by substantial amounts of credible research.[11-13] Other pejorative studies have been criticized for methodological problems.[14]

Spiritual medicine, practiced in the non-medical community for centuries, includes prayer, meditation, distance healing, laying-on of hands, and the effects of belief systems, which for many have a religious or spiritual connotation. Two well-controlled studies on prayer with positive conclusions have recently been published, supplementing the 1988 Byrd study.[15-17]

Belief systems clearly have an impact on outcomes. The evidence is supported in hundreds of published placebo studies, in which the result of treatment is clearly dependent on the belief system of the patient.[18] A recent meta-analysis of 80 studies in ulcer treatment found a 44 percent cure rate in the placebo arms of those studies when the placebo was administered q.i.d.[19] and a 3-year Australian study in hypertension found marked falls in systolic and diastolic blood pressures in 1,900 hypertensive control patients taking a placebo.[20]

The importance of positive attitudes and beliefs and the poisonous nature of pervasive negative emotions, repeatedly emphasized, has been the cumulative experience of many practitioners of complementary medicine since early research by Dr. Harold Wolff. "For every patient, his[/her] prompt and full appreciation of the truly poisonous and destructive nature of hate, resentment, jealousy, envy and fear is of crucial importance. . . . Discussions should emphasize an alteration of attitudes and the development of a way of life within which the patient can pursue his[/her] day-to-day activities, with less and less costly emotional and bodily reactions."[21]

Ethnomedical systems include healing traditions used for thousands and hundreds of years in India (Ayurveda), the Orient (Traditional Chinese Medicine and Acupuncture) and North America (Native American Medicine). Many other ethnic healing systems are also in use around the globe. Ayurveda emphasizes treatment with diet, herbs, detoxification, breathing exercises, meditation, and yoga to achieve a healthy balance of the life force called prana. Traditional Chinese Medicine utilizes concepts of vital energy (Chi or Qi), the roles of attitudes and diet, and employs herbs, acupuncture, meditation, exercise (Qi gong) to achieve healthy functioning and balance. Acupuncture has attracted the most interest in the United States, and is now practiced by thousands of trained physicians, Chinese medical doctors, and licensed acupuncturists, and used for a wide variety of pathological conditions. Native American Medicine traditions of healing practiced by shamans include herbs, mental practices, exercise, laying-on of hands, and healing ceremonies. A large collection of research in acupuncture has been published in the Orient, and increasingly, in Western literature as well. Chinese and Ayurvedic herbs have been the subject of increasing research interest with a burgeoning body of published literature.

Manual medicine includes the use of manipulative therapies, Osteopathy and Chiropractic, both in use in the United States for over a hundred years. Other manual methods, classified as body-work therapies, include a wide variety of massage techniques, Shiatsu, Rolfing, Alexander, Trager, Feldenkrais, Hellerwork, reflexology, and polarity therapy. The research documentation of benefit in these therapies varies from one discipline to the next, but a few excellent controlled studies have shown significant benefit.

Botanical medicine (herbs) have enjoyed rapidly increasing degrees of attention and use by the American consumer in the last ten years. Allopathic and Naturopathic literature sources have published controlled studies documenting the effectiveness of botanical remedies in treatment of numerous pathological conditions. Interest in Naturopathy has also accelerated in recent years. This discipline emphasizes extensive training in the use of natural healing methods including diet and nutritional supplements, exercise, counseling, physical therapies, and botanical and homeopathic remedies.

Homeopathic medicine has been practiced in Europe and the United States for 200 years. The effectiveness has only begun to be the subject of extensive research in the last 20 years. Controlled studies in certain disease states and extensive reviews have recently been published, giving testimony to its effectiveness.[22,23] The effects of homeopathic treatment can only be explained by invoking theories of quantum energy application. Theoretically incompatible with allopathic concepts of pharmaceutical treatment, the concept of homeopathy has met with great resistance in the conventional medical community.

It is the objective of physicians practicing complementary or holistic medicine to synthesize the best resources of conventional allopathic and alternative traditions in the process of addressing disease treatment and prevention, and the promotion of optimal health for all patients.

REFERENCES

1. Morgan KJ et al. Magnesium and calcium dietary intakes of the U.S. population. *J Am Coll Nutr* 1985; 4(2):195–206.
2. de Carvalho MJ et al. Vitamin status of healthy subjects in Burgundy (France). *Ann Nutr Metab* 1996; 40(1):24–51.
3. Joosten E et al. Metabolic evidence that deficiencies of vitamin B-12 (cobalamin), folate, and vitamin B-6 occur commonly in elderly people. *Am J Clin Nutr* 1993; 58(4):468–76.

4. Lipkin EW et al. Assessment of nutritional status. The clinician's perspective. *Clin Lab Med* 1993; 13(2):329–52.
5. Shaw DM et al. Senile dementia and nutrition. *Br Med J* 1984; 288(6419):792–3.
6. Rapp, D. *Allergies and the Hyperactive Child.* New York: Simon and Schuster, 1979.
7. Basmajian JV. The third therapeutic revolution: behavioral medicine. *Appl Psychophysiol Biofeedback* 1999; 24(2):107–16.
8. Ader R et al. Behaviorally conditioned immunosuppression. *Psychosom Med* 1975; 37(4):333–40.
9. Palmblad J et al. Lymphocyte and granulocyte reactions during sleep deprivation. *Psychosom Med* 1979; 41(4):273–8.
10. Malarky WB et al. Influence of academic stress and season on 24-hour mean concentrations of ACTH, cortisol, and beta-endorphin. *Psychoneuroendocrinology* 1995; 20(5):499–508.
11. Winstead-Fry P et al. An integrative review and meta-analysis of therapeutic touch research. *Altern Ther Health Med* 1999; 5(6):58–67.
12. Gordon A et al. The effects of therapeutic touch on patients with osteoarthritis of the knee. *J Fam Pract* 1998; 47(4):271–7.
13. Wirth DP. Full thickness dermal wounds treated by non-contact therapeutic touch: a replication and estension. *Complement Ther Med* 1993; 1:127–32.
14. Rosa L et al. A close look at therapeutic touch. *JAMA* 1998; 279(13):1005–10.
15. Sicher F et al. A randomized double-blind study of the effect of distant healing in a population with advanced ADIS. *West J Med* 1998; 169(6):356–63.
16. Harris WS et al. A randomized, controlled trial of the effects of remote, intercessory prayer on outcomes in patients admitted to the coronary care unit. *Arch Intern Med* 1999 Oct 25; 159(19):2273–8.
17. Byrd RC. Positive therapeutic effects of intercessory prayer in a coronary care unit population. *South Med J* 1988; 81(7): 826–9.
18. Benson H et al. Angina pectoris and the placebo effect. *N Engl J Med* 1979; 300(25):1424–9.
19. De Craen AJ et al. Placebo effect in the treatment of duodenal ulcer. *Br J Clin Pharmacol* 1999; 48(6):853–60.

20. Anonymous. Untreated mild hypertension. A report by the Management Committee of the Australian Therapeutic Trial in Mild Hypertension. *Lancet* 1982; 1(8265):185–91.

21. Wolff H et al. *Stress and Disease.* Springfield, IL: C. C. Thomas. 1968:231.

22. Jacobs J et al. Treatment of acute childhood diarrhea with homeopathic medicine: a randomized clinical trial in Nicaragua. *Pediatrics* 1994; 93(5):719–25.

23. Linde K et al. Are the clinical effects of homeopathy placebo effects? A meta-analysis of placebo-controlled trials. *Lancet* 1997; 350(9081):834–43.

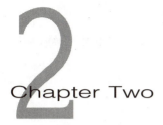

Chapter Two

Cardiovascular Diseases

Coronary Artery Disease

■ DESCRIPTION

Coronary artery disease is a condition of restricted coronary blood supply, resulting from gradual atherosclerotic changes, or sudden, severe arterial vasospasm. It gives no symptoms in early stages. The underlying atherosclerosis, the basis for most coronary disease, may begin in childhood or adulthood, triggered by a combination of many factors. A significant fraction of heart disease patients become aware of their disease with the sudden chest pain of a myocardial infarction. The pain is typically severe, centered in the front of the chest and slightly to the left of the mid-line, and often radiated to the left arm, neck, chin, or upper left side of the back. The sudden rupture of an athero-sclerotic plaque in a diseased artery is currently thought to best explain the pathogenesis of the classical myocardial infarction. When coronary disease announces its presence less dramati-cally, the pain, usually related to exertion and occasionally to stress, is called angina·pectoris. Severe vasospasm triggered by stressful environmental and emotional events can also trigger angina, ischemia, and even precipitate an infarction in the pre-sence of relatively little atherosclerotic plaque. The diagnosis of an acute heart attack is confirmed by history, physical examina-tion, and tests in a hospital emergency room, including chemistry battery, hemogram, cardiac enzymes, electrocardiograms, and angiography. Thallium stress tests may also be helpful in supplying valuable diagnostic information.

■ PREVALENCE

All cardiovascular diseases combined account for 30 percent of all deaths in the United States. The presence of elevated blood lipids, a major risk factor for vascular disease, is estimated at about 15 percent of the adult population. Atherosclerosis, the primary cause of myocardial infarctions and strokes, increased steadily in America from 1900 to the 1960s. It has, however, been on the decline since 1968, with a 50 percent fall in the incidence and death from myocardial infarctions and a 60 percent decrease in strokes. Both major improvements in lifestyle and better medical care of those with atherosclerotic vascular disease have contributed to the decline.

Myocardial infarctions, rare before 1920, now cause 20 percent of all deaths to lead the causes of mortality in the United States. Sixty million Americans are thought to be living with some degree of coronary artery disease, with angina pectoris occurring as a warning of CAD in 50–60 percent of patients.

■ ETIOLOGY AND RISK FACTORS

A higher incidence of coronary artery disease is found in people with a prominent diagonal earlobe crease.[1] Another associated marker for risk of coronary artery disease is short stature.[2] Men below 6 ft 1 in. in height have a 35 percent excess risk for myocardial infarction compared to taller men. The explanations for these two associations are unclear. Magnesium depletion, nicotine from tobacco (smoked or chewed), and hypoglycemia contribute to stress-related, severe coronary arterial spasm, which can lead to significant ischemia.

Coronary artery disease, which can lead to myocardial infarction, is usually the result of a combination of risk factors. The *classical risk factors* for atherosclerotic events are:

1. genetic predisposition
2. hyperlipidemias
3. hypertension
4. smoking
5. diabetes.

The Frederickson phenotype classification highlights five genetic patterns of predisposition to hyperlipidemias, and other less common patterns have been described. In some of these groups, males can have myocardial infarctions in their 20s. Perhaps the most common genetic pattern found to date is hyperhomocysteinemia, involving a mishandling of the conversion of methionine to cysteine.[3] Some authorities believe this may explain up to 30 percent of the incidence of cardiovascular disease. Elevated fibrinogen, a strong, independent risk factor for atherosclerosis, is also genetically influenced, with contributions as well from stress, obesity, diabetes, hypertension, high triglycerides, low HDL-C, high LDL-C, and renal disease.[4]

Authorities with no exception accept hypertension as a significant risk factor contributing to the damage to arterial intimal surfaces. Hyperlipidemia patterns which make their contribution include an elevated ratio of cholesterol to HDL cholesterol; low HDL cholesterol; elevated apolipoprotein [a];[5] and hypertriglyceridemia, all related to the incidence of myocardial infarctions and strokes. The rapid increase in the number of adults smoking cigarettes from 1920 to 1950 paralleled the rapid increase in the incidence of the cardiovascular diseases. Beginning in the 1960s, the portion of adults smoking regularly fell from 46 to 24 percent in recent years. This is believed to have been a strong contributor to the decreasing incidence of heart disease and strokes in the same period of time. Passive exposure to smoke in the environment also carries a significant risk for cardiovascular disease. The presence of diabetes accelerates premature degeneration of the intimal lining of arteries, hastening atherosclerotic complications. Type II diabetes, with a strong genetic component, insulin resistance, and elevated insulin levels, leads to biochemical changes including higher compensating levels of corticosteroids, increased biochemical stress, and production of elevated levels of oxygen free radicals.

Some studies have shown that up to 50 percent of men having myocardial infarctions have none or only one of the classical risk factors.[6] "The best combinations of standard risk factors fail to identify most new cases of coronary heart disease."[7] Additional risk factors therefore need to be considered. These include the following nutritional, environmental, psychological, spiritual, and social issues.

Increased Oxidant Stress

Elevated free radical populations, which overwhelm antioxidant defenses, are now recognized to play critical roles in oxidation of low-density lipoprotein cholesterol (LDL-C), triggering the alteration in monocyte/macrophage function, deposition of endothelial cholesterol, and initiation of atherosclerosis. And, compared to healthy adults, oxidative stress markers are much higher in those with ischemic cardiac disease and severely affected, unstable angina patients, and only moderately higher in stable angina patients.[8,9]

Nutrition

Factors include deficient fiber, fruits, vegetables, antioxidants, omega-3 oils, and water; and excess sugar, and saturated, oxidized, and hydrogenated *trans* fats.[10–12]

Nutritional changes which have a major impact on heart disease and stroke incidence include the decreased consumption of fruits, vegetables, and whole grains, and the enormous increase in use of refined and bleached wheat flour occurring about 100–125 years ago. These nutritional shifts in society are recognized to have created deficiencies or lower intakes of essential nutrients that prevent atherosclerosis—vitamins C, E, B_6, B_{12}, beta carotene, folic acid, zinc, magnesium, chromium, and selenium, all associated with increased risk.[13–15] Copper deficiency predisposes to arterial aneurysms.[16] Data from the Seven Countries Study found coronary disease significantly inversely related to dietary intake of bioflavonoids.[17] Intake of fruits, vegetables, and whole grains improved steadily since 1980; this trend was perhaps the most important positive sign in nutrition in the United States as the decade closed. Accompanying the shift to refined flour was an increase in the intake of fat from greater consumption of animal meats and cow's milk derivatives high in saturated fats. This is thought to have significantly contributed to the rapid increase in atherosclerosis between 1920 and 1970. Since the 1970s, per capita intake of these caloric sources has declined. It was also thought that substituting vegetable sources of polyunsaturated fats would not contribute to heart disease and strokes. However, most of these derivatives were hydrogenated to be solid at room temperature (hydrogenated cooking fats, margarines, and peanut butter). These foods contain *trans* fats, ultimately found to make greater contributions to atherosclerosis than saturated fats. And, experience with Greenland Eskimos taught us that in spite of consuming a diet very high in animal fat, intake of high quantities of omega-3 fatty acids from fish offered protection against a high incidence of heart disease.[18]

Since the 1980s, sugars have been found to be a significant risk factor for heart disease. In spite of little conventional interest in this topic, a 1992 editorial from the *Journal of the Royal Society of Medicine* asserted that there "is more evidence of sugar as a cause [of coronary artery disease] than there is for dietary fat and cholesterol."[19] The intake of excess loads of sugar promotes hyperinsulinemia, leading to a cascade of compensatory shifts in hormones and chemical factors, spawning a variety of problems including adverse shifts in lipids, diabetes, coronary artery disease, myocardial infarctions, gout, and hypertension.[20] This condition has been called "syndrome X" by some authorities. Fat intake has fallen modestly since the 1970s, but sugar intake has increased.

A 1998 study found that men drinking two or fewer glasses of water daily had twice the risk of mortality from myocardial infarctions compared to those drinking 5 or more glasses daily. Women drinking 2 glasses or less per day experienced half again the fatality rate.[21] Regular and excessive alcohol consumption contributes to hypertension and caffeine and coffee intake appear to contribute to myocardial infarctions, although studies disagree.[22,23]

Biomolecular Factors

Deficiencies of biosynthesized intrinsic compounds appear to contribute to risk of myocardial infarctions. These include coenzyme Q_{10}, an essential enzyme in the mitochondrial electron transport chain, and L-carnitine, a "non-essential" amino acid. Heart disease patients have lower coenzyme Q_{10} levels than healthy subjects.[24] L-carnitine is essential in cellular energy production and is rapidly lost from cardiac myocytes in the presence of coronary artery disease.[25]

Other Physical Factors

Obesity. Particularly with increase in abdominal girth in both men and women, excessive weight is a risk factor for heart disease. Risk for women is twice as great in those with a waist circumference over 38 in or whose ratio of waist to hip measurement is 0.76 or greater.[26]

Sleep deficiency. The risk of myocardial infarction is greater in men with sleep deficiency, including sleep apnea.[27]

Air pollution in major cities is a risk factor. The risk is highest in industries that require workers to be exposed to petrochemicals and solvents.[28]

Previous infection with Chlamydia pneumoniae. This organism has been recovered from biopsies of coronary atherosclerotic plaque, and anti-Chlamydial antibody levels are higher in patients with coronary artery disease.[29] Periodontal disease, too, has been associated with coronary artery disease risk.[30] Other infections and inflammatory conditions are now seen as possible risk factors.[31]

The deconditioning syndrome, the lack of physical fitness that comes with sedentary lifestyle, is a major consideration. Men with the least exercise have an incidence of atherosclerosis and mortality which is twice that of men who exercise the most.[32] The increase in the numbers of exercising Americans has been a major factor in the decrease in the incidence of myocardial infarctions in the last 30 years.[33] On the other hand, extreme exertion in the totally sedentary patient is hazardous; the risk of mycordial infarction (MI) in these circumstances goes up 100-fold.[34]

Mental and Emotional Factors

Stress is a risk factor for heart disease and strokes as well as for most degenerative diseases.[35] Compared to other times of the week, the incidence of MI, strokes and sudden cardiac deaths is higher on Monday mornings—the time when many people are unhappily returning to work.[36] Stress accelerates atherosclerosis and accelerates blood coagulation. In primates, accumulation of intimal plaque occurred more than twice as fast in stressed versus unstressed monkeys on a high fat diet, and 5 times as fast in those on a low-fat diet.[37] Stress erodes magnesium levels by at least two biochemical mechanisms involving catecholamines and corticosteroids.[38] Chronic stress also elevates the fundamental threshold of corticosteroid production, leading to increased insulin resistance, in turn evoking increased insulin secretion to counteract the resistance. This favors hyperlipidemia and accelerated atherogenesis.[39]

Hostility and the negative emotions of depression, grief, anger, and anxiety are risk factors.[40] Medical students exhibiting high levels of hostility were found in the next 25 years as physicians to have a 4-fold higher incidence of myocardial infarctions compared to those with low hostility as students.[41] Depression increases by *6-fold* the risk of dying in the first $1\frac{1}{2}$ years after surviving a myocardial infarction and increases the incidence of angina during recovery 3-fold.[42] When grieving the loss of a loved family member, the risk for MI is 14-fold greater than normal for the first 24 hours following the death, subsiding slowly to a 2-fold higher risk after a month.[43] Higher levels of anger also contribute to increased incidence of myocardial infarctions, angina and cardiac complications.[44] Within 2 hours after an intense flare-up of anger, the risk for having a MI increases by $2\frac{1}{2}$-fold.[45] Higher anxiety in college students is related to a $2\frac{1}{2}$-fold higher incidence of coronary artery disease as adults.[46] So-called Type D behavior—the experiencing of intense emotions in the face of inability to express them—has also been shown to be a risk factor.[47]

Loneliness and social isolation magnify all risks for heart disease and negatively influence post-MI prognosis. Men are much more vulnerable than women; widowed, separated, and divorced men have lost many opportunities for experiencing unconditional love, caring, and intimacy.[48] Women appear to be protected from this risk due to more involvement in a social network. The self-criticism frequently found in men can leave feelings of fear and vulnerability, with secondary feelings of anger about being powerless. Dr. James Lynch in *The Broken Heart* has observed that there is reflected in the physical heart a biological basis for the need to form loving human relationships. Failing to fulfill this need imperils health. This has been described by some as "the hardened heart."

Experience teaches that people who have positive belief systems, a sense of purpose and an awareness of a transpersonal cosmic connection with a universal higher power often overcome a variety of genetic, physical, and biochemical predispositions to heart disease. This is usually associated with an attitude of optimism, which has been shown to significantly improve prognosis after cardiac events.[49] The miniscule experience of many people in this arena is a risk factor for cardiovascular problems.

■ CONVENTIONAL MEDICAL TREATMENT

Because heart attacks are the leading cause of death in this country, identifying people at risk is high priority. All of the classical risk factors are considered and a careful family history is essential. When a history of exertional chest pain, rhythm disturbances, or shortness of breath is elicited, coronary heart disease can be confirmed by finding abnormalities in exercise electrocardiograms (stress tests), angiograms, and radioisotope heart scans. Laboratory blood tests can confirm evidence of increased risk from lipid abnormalities (see above).

Preventive measures include, if appropriate, smoking cessation; improving nutrition with decreased intake of saturated fat and cholesterol; increased consumption of fruits, vegetables, and whole grains; bringing blood pressure under control; and improving cholesterol levels with drug treatment.

The wide array of commonly used drugs to lower cholesterol includes the following: Colestid, Questran, Atromid-S, Lopid, Lorelco, and niacin (vitamin B_3) derivatives (Niaspan, Nicobid, Nicolar). HMG-CoA-reductase inhibitors, the newest class of pharmaceuticals and now widely used, include Mevacor, Pravachol, Zocor, Lipitor, Baycol, and Lescol. After a decade of lowering cholesterol with the first generation of hypolipidemic drugs, research showed only mildly improved prognosis in heart disease but *increased* total mortality from all causes. A 1992 review of 19 studies in *Circulation* revealed that 18 of them found the use of cholesterol-lowering agents associated with an increased incidence of chronic lung disease, pneumonia, influenza, hemorrhagic strokes, cirrhosis of the liver, digestive diseases, alcohol dependence, suicide, leukemias, lymphomas, and cancers of the liver and lung,[50] though this remains hotly disputed. In the widely known MRFIT study, cardiac risk factors were reduced 46 percent in the cohort intensively treated with hypolipidemics and antihypertensives, but 10 years later, there were 45 percent more deaths in the intensively treated drug group compared to more casually treated controls.[51] Another potential side effect is found in the manufacturer's literature for the widely prescribed drug gemfibrozil: "There was no difference in mortality between the clofibrate-treated subjects and . . . placebo-treated subjects, but twice as many clofibrate-treated subjects developed cholelithiasis requiring surgery." Powerful drugs must always be cautiously used.

Use of the newer "statin" drugs to lower cholesterol has shown a lowered incidence of myocardial infarctions *and* overall mortality rate, even in those whose cholesterols were normal at the outset. Long-term results deserve careful monitoring. A 1996 review of research in laboratory rodents found a pattern of carcinogenicity for clofibrate and the "statin" drugs in concentrations comparable to blood levels achieved in humans at standard doses.[52] Statin drug makers recommend blood tests every 6 months to monitor the patient for possible elevations in liver enzymes, and exhort physicians to be very cautious in use in patients with any degree of renal failure.

At the onset of early symptoms of MI, thrombolytic drugs including streptokinase, tissue plasminogen activator (t-PA), hirudin, and alteplase are used to restore coronary artery luminal patency. Aspirin is given to inhibit platelet aggregation, reducing the incidence of initial and second myocardial infarctions; again, the extent of this effect is disputed.[53] Anticoagulation, used in the 1960–1970 era, is again coming into more common use, employing low doses of heparin and Coumadin.

Vasodilators commonly prescribed for treatment and prevention of angina include nitroglycerin tablets taken sublingually for quick relief and long-acting oral nitrates (Isordil, Sorbitrate), patches (Nitrodur, Transderm-Nitro), and ointment (Nitrobid). Other drugs used in angina include beta-blockers (Tenormin, Inderal, Lopressor) and calcium channel blockers (Calan, Cardizem, Procardia, Isoptin, Norvasc, Adalat). The calcium channel blockers, particularly short-acting forms, appear to reduce beta thromboglobulin, potentially increasing rates of gastrointestinal hemorrhage,[54] and cardiac mortality compared to placebo controls.[55]

Very recent reports have tentatively concluded that the risks for complications of coronary disease, apparently resulting from previous experience with a Chlamydia infection, can be reduced with appropriate antibiotic treatment for an assumed continuing low-grade infection.[56] This development in the understanding of the infectious aspect of this disease bears close watching.

Surgery

Angioplasty is utilized to dilate constricted segments of coronary arteries, sometimes leaving a stent in place to prevent the recurrence of narrowing which often occurs. Some observers think cardiac invasive procedures are overused. Thomas Graboys, a controversial cardiologist, published in *JAMA* in 1992 a study in which non-invasive tests found that 134 of 168 patients for whom angiography had been recommended did not actually need it. Four years later, the annualized mortality in this group was 1.1 percent, much lower than the mortality rate of bypass surgery (5–30 percent) or angioplasty (1–2 percent). Only 15 percent of the patients in this study eventually needed angioplasty or coronary bypass.[57]

Coronary bypass operations have become commonplace, recently modified by minimally invasive techniques resulting in swifter recovery and greatly reduced post-operative morbidity. Up to one-third of the bypasses, however, are found to be thrombosed in a matter of months or years, and atherosclerosis in bypass segments appears quickly, being found in 1 out of 3 patients within a year. A last surgical option in end-stage coronary heart disease is a heart transplant. The average cost approaches $350,000 dollars. A *Medical Tribune* citation from 1992 highlighted a study in which 40 percent of those initially qualified to be on a waiting list for a donor heart no longer met the criteria for a transplant by the time a heart became available after they had undergone vigorous medical treatment while waiting. *Operative procedures do not halt the progression of the atherosclerosis.*

■ HOLISTIC TREATMENT

Complementing conventional management principles is an emphasis on the risk factors beyond the classical ones—proliferating free radical levels, nutritional factors including sugar, deficiency of biosynthetic compounds, sleep deficiency, physical deconditioning, air pollution, stress, hostility and negative emotions, lack of forgiveness, and social isolation.

An often overlooked simple clinical measure of atherosclerosis used by many physicians utilizing complementary approaches is the ankle–arm index, the ratio of systolic blood pressure at the ankle divided by the brachial systolic pressure. A ratio of less than 0.9 confers a 4.5-fold higher suspicion for the presence of significant atherosclerosis.[58]

The complementary approach includes challenging all patients to modify their lifestyle to minimize identified risk factors.

Even in those rare persons who have a genetically determined progressive cholesterol buildup, lifestyle modifications can neutralize part of the risk.

Nutrition

Increasing the intake of whole foods (including fruits, vegetables, whole unrefined grains, legumes, beans, nuts, and seeds), vitamins, minerals, and essential fatty/amino acids is an important step in prevention and treatment. Only 8 percent of Americans meet the nutritional daily standard of at least 2 fruit and 3 vegetable servings. Increasing fiber, found in the same whole foods, to a reasonable level of 15 g daily requires most patients to double or triple their intake. While increased fiber intake decreases both HDL-C and LDL-C, its effect on LDL-C is much greater, with an impact of decreasing coronary events by one-third.[59]

Omega-3 fatty acids are increased with greater consumption of fish and fish oils. Men eating at least an ounce of fish daily have been shown to have a 20-year mortality below that of non-fish-eaters. If 2–3 fish servings per week are not feasible, fish oil capsules can supply omega-3 oils (see supplements, below). Flaxseed oil, containing 50 percent omega-3 oils is a good vegetable source and can be used as a salad dressing. Onions and garlic contain active ingredients which tend to lower cholesterol and blood pressure and decrease platelet aggregation. A drink of purple grape juice daily has recently been shown to reduce susceptibility of LDL cholesterol to oxidation, and improve endothelial relaxation.[60]

If body stores of the carotenoid lycopene are at highest levels, risk of myocardial infarction is reduced 50 percent compared to people with low levels.[61] Lycopene is found in watermelon, guava, pink grapefruit, tomatoes, tomato juice, catsup, and dried apricots.

Reduction of saturated fats (meats, whole milk products), and hydrogenated polyunsaturated fats (margarines), refined and bleached white flour products, sugar, caffeine-containing beverages, and alcohol are also priorities. Reduction of oxidized fats—those becoming pre-rancid—is high priority. Rancidification is well under way before becoming detectable by the human olfactory apparatus. While many authorities have recommended reduction of high-cholesterol foods such as egg yolks, the evidence for any benefit is marginal. Reduction may be important in families with a high genetic predisposition; otherwise, reasonable egg consumption is not a problem.[62] Consumption of walnuts 5 days a week has been shown to reduce the risk of fatal infarctions 50 percent.[63] Reducing sucrose intake is more important than many authorities believe. Substituting iso-caloric amounts of starch in place of sugar in the diet significantly lowers triglycerides and raises HDL-C.[64] Sugar intake in the United States has risen steadily since 1940.

Nutritional Supplements

As a result of intake of more whole, less processed foods, the intake of antioxidant micronutrients has greatly increased. Unrestrained proliferation of oxygen free radicals exceeding the capacity for antioxidant neutralization is very detrimental. Scores of studies have found that few Americans meet all the Recommended Dietary Allowances for vitamins and minerals. In many instances, intakes are up to 50–70 percent below RDAs, which themselves may be low in some instances; children, teenagers, and the elderly have the worst records.[65]

The evidence for the helpful role of antioxidant supplements in managing ischemic heart disease is persuasive.

In healthy volunteers consuming vitamin E 1,600 mg daily, markers of free radical activity decreased 66 to 530 percent.[66] In an extensive study of 12 European male populations, low levels of vitamin E explained 62 percent of the risk of mortality from myocardial infarction compared to high cholesterol which explained only 17 percent of the risk.[15] In another study, a 50 percent reduction in non-fatal myocardial infarctions was achieved in a 6 month period in men taking vitamin E 400–800 IU daily compared to those taking a placebo.[67] In several intervention trials with beta-carotene and vitamin E showing no benefit, the dosages used have been substantially below those used in trials showing benefit.

Subjects with a higher intake of β-carotene supplements turned out to have a 45 percent lower incidence of myocardial infarction compared to those with lower supplementation and dietary intake.[68] If the intake of lycopene-containing foods is low, supplements are available; a reasonable dose is 75 mg daily.

The typical vasoconstrictive spasm resulting from a high-fat meal is prevented by ingestion of 1 g of vitamin C plus 800 IU of vitamin E before the meal; vitamin C prevents vasoconstriction in smokers, accelerates circulation,[69] and, given with mannitol during a MI, has been shown to *double* 1-year survival.[70] The rate of restenosis after angioplasty is reduced 50 percent with intake of vitamin C 500 mg daily.[71]

Niacin (vitamin B_3) in pharmacological doses of 0.5–1.5 g daily and occasionally up to 3–4.5 g daily, decreases serum cholesterol about 20 percent, triglycerides 40 percent, and increases HDL-C 30 percent.[72] Flushing of the skin 20 minutes after ingestion is a bothersome side effect. It is attenuated by taking niacin with food and preceding each dose with an aspirin. Time-release forms have led to liver toxicity in some cases. Inositol hexaniacinate, an ester of niacin, is essentially free of the flushing reaction and achieves substantial results with very few other side effects. The dosage is 500 mg t.i.d. with meals, increased after 2 weeks to 1 g t.i.d.[73]

Pantethine, a form of pantothenic acid (vitamin B_5), is rapidly depleted in ischemic hearts: 300 mg t.i.d. has been shown to very significantly lower total cholesterol and triglycerides while increasing HDL-C.[74]

The homocysteinemia genetic risk factor (see Etiology and Risk Factors) is largely neutralized with daily intake of adequate folic acid (400–800 µg), vitamin B_6 (100 mg) and vitamin B_{12} (1,000 µg). Every additional 100 µg of daily folic acid intake cuts the MI risk by 6 percent. Betaine, another biosynthetic substance derived from the B-vitamin choline, is also therapeutic in doses of 3 g b.i.d. Levels of vitamin B_6 (pyridoxine) are significantly lower in MI patients compared to healthy people. The relative risk for MIs in those with the lowest levels of pyridoxine is estimated to be 5-fold higher.[75] The MI risk was calculated to be reduced 6 percent for every additional milligram of daily vitamin B_6 intake.[76] Doses of 25–100 mg daily are sufficient to negate homocysteinemia effects along with B_{12} and folic acid.

Magnesium, in doses up to 500 mg daily, raises HDL-C by up to 30 percent and reduces total cholesterol up to 14 percent, substantially improving the cholesterol/HDL-C ratio.[77] Intravenous magnesium treatment as early as possible during a myocardial infarction improves survival 25 percent.[78] The large ISIS study that showed no benefit did not use a placebo group, was not double-blinded, and inordinately delayed the initial bolus of magnesium. Crescendo, unstable, and Prinzmetal's angina respond well to 1–2 g of magnesium given intravenously over 10–20 minutes. There is evidence for the importance of selenium and chromium as well. Iron is important in the free radical promotion of atherosclerosis, and excessively high ferritin levels are associated with significant increase in risk.[79] Not all studies have confirmed this finding. Nonetheless, donating blood 1–3 times a year and taking supplements without iron to reduce excess iron stores seems reasonable, and is supported by recent studies.

Many disease states, as well as stress and powerful emotional experiences, stimulate increased release of epinephrine, in turn accelerating platelet adhesiveness. Certain nutrients, including vitamins C, E, B_6, magnesium, garlic and omega-3 oils, as well as physical exercise, reduce excessive platelet adhesion which initiates the clotting cascade, the precipitating event in many MIs and strokes. Some studies have suggested that vitamin E functions better than aspirin for this purpose.

A non-essential amino acid, L-arginine, 0.5–1.0 g t.i.d. is beneficial in angina and peripheral circulation problems.[80] Arginine is the substrate for synthesis of nitric oxide, a potent vasodilator.

Botanicals

Commiphora mukul (gugulipids), an Ayurvedic herb, reduces platelet adhesiveness and increases thrombolysis. Published studies have documented 20 percent reductions in cholesterol, 30 percent reductions in triglycerides and 35 percent increases in HDL-C in

16 weeks with a dose of 2.25 g b.i.d.[81] Purified derivatives of gugu-lipids have few side effects.

Garlic powder, 600 mg daily, reduced susceptibility of apoli-poprotein-B to oxidation by 34 percent in 2 weeks.[82] Another study documented a 12 percent reduction of total cholesterol in 3 months on 800 mg of concentrated garlic powder daily.[83,84] Other studies show little benefit. One important difference may be the age of the preparation used: garlic must be fresh.

Ginger, using 1 g of powdered product daily, has been shown to lower cholesterol and decrease platelet aggregation in ani-mals.[85] Hawthorn berry (*Crataegus*) extract, 3–5 g of the dried powder daily, acts to protect arterial walls, has vasodilating prop-erties and is helpful in angina.[86] *Ginkgo biloba*, 250 mg t.i.d. improves circulation and exerts powerful free radical scavenging activity.[87]

Khellin, an *Ammi visnaga* derivative, 40 mg q.i.d. and at h.s. for several months was highly effective in decreasing frequency and severity of angina, improving exercise tolerance and appear-ance of the electrocardiogram. Khellin possesses outstanding vasodilating properties.[88] Artichoke (*Cynara scolymus*) given in controlled fashion to hyperlipidemic patients lowered cholesterol and improved lipid ratios.[89]

Serum cholesterol fell over 12 percent in a month with doses of 50 g daily of the Ayurvedic herb amla (Indian gooseberry).[90] Substantial hypolipidemic effects and increased HDL-C have been shown with administration of a traditional Chinese herb, Ba-wei-wan.[91]

Biomolecular Options

One year survival after myocardial infarction was 10-fold greater than placebo in those receiving pharmacological doses of 4 g daily of L-carnitine. L-carnitine is rapidly depleted in hearts that are ischemic. It substantially increases maximal cardiac work-load, delays onset of anginal pain, improves the EKG and workload in treadmill testing, and greatly reduces the need for and doses of conventional drugs.[92] Usual dosage: 0.5–1.0 g b.i.d.

The antioxidant properties of coenzyme Q_{10} are more powerful than those of vitamins C, E and beta-carotene. Co-Q_{10} is reported to improve treadmill exercise performance up to 40 percent in patients with ischemic heart disease, reduces the frequency of anginal attacks by up to 50 percent, decreases nitroglycerine use by one-third, improves arteriolar and capillary circulation, reduces blood viscosity, markedly improves symptoms in mitral valve prolapse, and protects against the free radical injury occurring during reperfusion in an organ that has been rendered ischemic during experimental surgery in animals.[93-96]

Glycosaminoglycans, compounds composed of protein and sugar molecules synthesized by the body, help maintain integrity of collagen, and moderate the progression of atherosclerotic intimal thickening. Mesoglycan, a glycosaminoglycan derivative, is found in high amounts in alfalfa. The dosage as a supplement is 100 mg daily.[97]

Dehydroepiandrosterone (DHEA) is available in health and nutrition stores without prescription. DHEA blood levels should be determined before contemplating any treatment. In research, mortality from atherosclerosis complications in men with a low DHEA was 3 times more likely over a 12-year period of observation than those whose levels were high.[98] Studies generally demonstrate benefits, especially in those where deficient levels have been found. Appropriate dosages are usually in the 15–25 mg daily range.

Low testosterone levels have also been found in men who later develop coronary heart problems. Cautious doses of 200 mg weekly by injection have been shown to increase treadmill performance and electrocardiographic abnormalities.[99] Since testosterone may increase prostate cancer risk, this decision must be carefully weighed.

Chelation treatment involves the IV injection of agents that chelate and remove from the body heavy metals (lead, mercury, cadmium) and intermediate metals (iron and copper). It is standard conventional medical treatment for acute and chronic heavy metal poisoning. For the last 25 years, chelation with ethylenediamine tetra-acetic acid (EDTA, an amino acid-like compound) has been offered by a small number of physicians in the United States for the treatment of atherosclerotic disease. Considered unscientific and unproven by conventional authorities, numerous case histories and before/after treatment studies have shown benefit, especially in advanced disease.[100] Since the inception of formalized guidelines adopted in 1972, no deaths in several hundred thousand chelation treatments have been recorded. Although the mechanisms of action are not well understood, one of the likely possibilities was emphasized in a 1989 review published in the *New England Journal* which pointed out that the degenerative processes occurring with atherosclerosis "depend on a common initiating step—the peroxidation of polyunsaturated fatty acids in the LDL lipids. The modification of LDL by cells is totally inhibited by antioxidants," and the "oxidative modification is absolutely dependent on the concentrations of iron and copper in the medium and is therefore completely inhibited by EDTA or other metal chelators."[101] No large placebo-controlled studies have demonstrated unequivocal benefit. .

Homeopathy

Comprehensive constitutional prescribing is a function of experienced homeopaths. Symptomatic remedies which may be helpful in 12X to 30C potencies include Aconite for anxiety and tachycardia, Glonoine for tachycardia, pain and palpitations, and Cactus for chest constriction and left-arm pain.

Exercise

Physical exercise is an initiative in prevention and treatment fully as important as the nutritional choices emphasized above. Patients who were raised in families where exercise was valued are fortunate. Consistent aerobic exercise raises HDL-C about 10 percent and substantially decreases triglycerides, and numerous studies confirm a 15 percent reduction in cholesterol/HDL-C ratios.[102] Participants in an experimental calisthenic exercise group for a year increased time-to-onset of angina 70 percent compared 30 percent in a group treated with drugs alone.[103]

In those with advanced disease, the prescription for exercise must be very cautiously and gradually increased. For sedentary persons who have several other risk factors for heart disease, sudden heavy exercise carries a 100-fold increased risk of myocardial infarction.[104] Beside improving cholesterol ratios and lowering blood pressure, exercise decreases platelet aggregation and reduces fibrinogen levels by 10 percent.[105] Mortality rates from myocardial infarctions and strokes are 60 percent diminished in the most fit patients compared to the least fit.[106] Yoga and Tai Chi, gentle traditional Asian forms of exercise, have been shown in research to increase fibrinolysis.[107]

Mental and Emotional Treatment Options

The ubiquitous nature of stress and its profound effects on cardiovascular function need to be addressed by providing opportunities for patients to acquire skills to manage it appropriately. Biofeedback, meditation, and progressive relaxation are all highly successful in making gradual, substantial, and permanent changes in autonomic nervous system function.[108] Levels of catecholamines, corticosteroids, and cholesterol all diminish substantially with the practice of these skills. Meditation, besides its physical benefits enumerated above, often leads to remarkable and sometimes dramatic insights, creative answers, shifts in belief and a sense of equanimity about life which is as effective as any medication or nutrient. Meditation has been shown to actually reverse carotid intimal-medial thickening over 9 months compared to non-meditating controls.[109]

The time required for relaxation practice varies upwards from 10 minutes daily; nearly all patients who regularly practice their skills make substantial progress. Disturbed moods of anger, anxiety, and depression, all of which contribute to cardiovascular disease risk, tend to be greatly attenuated with regular relaxation practice.[110] Preoperative hypnosis has been shown to substantially improve relaxation states after coronary bypass surgery, with significant decrease in use of post-operative narcotics.[111]

Personal growth counseling is also highly successful in dealing with toxic levels of emotions and modifying hostility in the positive direction of greater unconditional love. A *75 percent reduction* in risk for cardiac "events" in a group of coronary artery disease patients resulted from comprehensive stress management training.[112] Dr. Dean Ornish utilized daily meditation practice with positive imagery and twice weekly group counseling sessions as part of his program which accomplished actual reversal of the atherosclerotic process within a year.[113] A paramount issue in counseling is a shift in attitude toward a willingness to honor others and themselves by investing in forgiveness which restores the flow of unconditional love and reduces the demands on others and themselves—demands which define the stress they experience. The energy of the heart in the spiritual sense is related to all the negative emotional and attitudinal issues known to be important in genesis of heart disease including hostility, resentment, cynical distrust, anger, grief, anxiety, and loneliness.[114,115] It encompasses as well the positive energies of forgiveness, unconditional love, compassion, hope and trust.[116]

A major 1988 study, authored by Dr. Randolph Byrd, found that the death rate, complication rate, incidence of congestive heart failure, and need for mechanical respiration were all substantially reduced in hospitalized myocardial infarction patients for whom regular organized prayers were offered in comparison to those for whom organized prayers were not offered.[117] A recent study confirmed the significant benefit during coronary care unit hospitalization.[118]

Studies of the placebo effect have shown 82 percent relief of angina from drugs and procedures which were later shown to have *no therapeutic effect whatsoever*.[119] Placebos are powerful because of belief in their effectiveness. Beliefs are a central factor in the spiritual life of patients and have enormous effects on worldview and real-time experience. The intrinsic healing value of prescriptions given and suggestions made to patients is enhanced through the placebo effect by the equanimity, enthusiasm, positivity, certainty, and communication style of the physician or counselor. Astute holistic physicians and knowledgeable counselors utilize this potential for benefit.

Social Health

Ongoing support of family and friends shortens hospitalization time with an MI and improves subsequent survival.[120] The odds of dying within 6 months after an MI is one-third as great among patients with many social contacts and an intimate relationship to a spouse or small circle of significant others compared to patients who are lonely, isolated and devoid of this kind of community connection.[121] Group support also improves prognosis. Education about the nature of angina and practical relevant advice given in a regular supportive group setting for angina patients had far better outcomes than those handled with "routine" conventional care.[122] The greatest lifestyle differences came in greater exercise and substantial nutritional improvements in the support group. Social isolation has an enormous detrimental effect on prognosis in chronic illness, and on cardiovascular disease in particular.[123]

Strokes

■ DESCRIPTION

Strokes are the presentation of sensory or motor neurological deficits resulting from ischemic or hemorrhagic damage to the brain. Thrombotic strokes occur when blood flow to a segment of the brain is interrupted as the result of a thrombus formation, an embolus, or rupture of an atheromatous plaque. Hemorrhagic strokes result from rupture or an aneurysm or a weakened atherosclerotic arterial wall.

Transient ischemic attacks (TIAs) involve a temporary loss of blood supply to a small area of brain tissue, thought to be due to transient spasm in an already partly compromised arteriole, or to tiny thrombi which form and then undergo lysis. Since there is no permanent damage resulting from TIAs, they are not threatening in and of themselves, but warn of more serious problems. Severe vasoconstriction of the vasoconstrictive phase of a migraine episode can also predispose to risk for ischemic stroke.[124] Profound hypoglycemia with transient paralysis can occasionally be mistaken for a TIA.

Classical stroke symptoms present with a hemi-paralysis or hemi-paresis which may involve the upper or lower limbs, face and neck, or any combination of the three. If the brain damage is left-sided, loss of speech often accompanies the loss of motor function. Strokes may also be manifested in loss of consciousness, loss of sensation, or death, which occurs in about 30 percent of cases. Stroke is the greatest cause of long-term disability in the nation.

■ **PREVALENCE**

Strokes are the third leading cause of death in the United States after heart attacks and cancer. The 550,000 strokes occurring each year are responsible for 6 percent of the annual mortality toll. Major improvements in lifestyle and better care of those with arteriosclerotic problems have contributed to a 60 percent decline in stroke mortality since the late 1960s. Barring significant interventions, risk for a second stroke within 5 years is 40–60 percent.

■ **ETIOLOGY AND RISK FACTORS**

The most important risk factors for stroke are hypertension and arteriosclerosis. All the risk factors for these two problems, discussed elsewhere in this chapter, are also risk factors for stroke. Certain factors deserve special emphasis.

There is a strong positive correlation between alcohol intake over three drinks daily and the risk for stroke. A British study found that alcohol intoxication was 3 times more common prior to a stroke than it was in healthy people. The greatest association was in those below the age of 40.[125] A recent study found no relationship of consumption of spirits and beer with stroke, but, compared to non-drinkers, did find a 30 percent reduced risk for stroke in those drinking wine on a daily or weekly basis.[126] The proanthocyanidins and polyphenols in wine may be the beneficial factor.

Smoking increases stroke risk little above the age of 65, but it is very strong risk factor in those under that age. Males smoking 2 packs-a-day double their risk of stroke and women increase it $2\frac{1}{2}$-fold over non-smokers.[127]

High levels of catecholamines are associated with stroke risk and higher death rate in strokes. Exaggerated catecholamine synthesis is triggered by high levels of tension secondary to poorly managed physiological and psychological stress.[128] High catecholamines trigger quickened platelet adhesion, increased blood viscosity, and acceleration of carotid atherogenesis, all risk factors for stroke.[129]

Hyperglycemia is also a risk factor for strokes, even in stages before diabetes can be recognized.[130] There is also a relationship with obesity.[131] Marginal deficiencies of vitamin C and other antioxidant vitamins are also contributing risk factors.[132]

High levels of leptin, a hormone produced by adipocytes, important in regulation of body weight, is apparently a strong risk marker for first-ever stroke. The full significance of this observation remains to be elucidated.[133]

Street drugs including amphetamines increase risks for hemorrhagic stroke. The risk increases several fold in oral contraceptive use; this risk is greatly exaggerated in smokers and increases with the length of time of use. Sedentary lifestyle raises risks for stroke as it does for coronary artery disease.[134]

Increased risk of stroke has been related to psychosocial issues of a need to control, feelings of vulnerability and lack of trust.

■ CONVENTIONAL TREATMENT

The immediate treatment for a stroke includes life support if necessary, followed by extensive rehabilitation to regain all possible function and build compensating strengths and skills for remaining deficits. Recently, acute treatment has begun to include the same fibrinolytic approach used in myocardial infarctions. Great caution and judgment is required: fibrinolytic agents in hemorrhagic strokes will aggravate the damage.

Conventional preventive measures for those with hypertension, hyperlipidemias, and atherosclerosis are carried out as described elsewhere in this chapter. Aspirin is commonly recommended for prevention of strokes and recurrent strokes; there is a small hazard of increasing risks for hemorrhagic strokes.

■ HOLISTIC TREATMENT

All of the elements of prevention and treatment of coronary artery disease and hypertension in other portions of this chapter apply to lowering of risk of stroke and reducing risks for second strokes.

A few measures specifically more applicable to stroke should be mentioned. Research reports credit 5 weekly servings of carrots, and daily ingestion of spinach and at least five servings of fruits and vegetables with substantial lowering of the risk of stroke.[135] Interestingly, such foods increase potassium and magnesium intake.[136] In the 15-year European Zutphen study, stroke risk in men was reduced a striking 75 percent in those with high intake of flavonoids, mainly from black tea. High beta-carotene intake was also substantially protective.[137] The protective benefit of supplements of 400 IU and vitamin C is unsettled, with studies in disagreement,[138] although the use of vitamin E 400 IU daily in preventing recurrent transient ischemic attacks was outstanding.[139] *Ginkgo biloba* may also have a special use in preventing stroke and recurrent stroke in those with high risk factors.[140]

In the intensive rehabilitation work of recovering from a stroke, a unique, gentle variety of body work known as Feldenkrais often works well. The central nervous system retraining aspect of rehabilitation appears to be enhanced with this therapy.

There is strong evidence that persistent use of acupuncture in rehabilitation after stroke has notable long-term benefits for greater recovery and greater functionality in regard to activities of daily living.[141]

In the whole picture of incidence, rehabilitation, adaptation and prevention of recurrence of strokes, a major shift of lifestyle is usually necessary. Central to that process is a shift in beliefs and attitudes which may be assisted by especially understanding complementary medicine health professionals and counselors.

Hypertension

■ DESCRIPTION

Hypertension is the elevated blood pressure generated by the heart to overcome increased vasoconstriction in the peripheral arterial system. Atherosclerosis contributes to this resistance, but the major factor is the constriction of the medial smooth muscle layer of the arterioles. This narrowing occurs normally in vast areas of the body when the arousal (fight or flight) reflex is triggered, in order to shunt more blood to the muscles used in physical activity. Sustained hypertension leads to cardiac hypertrophy, aggravates atherosclerotic damage to the intima of the arteries, and contributes to the risk for myocardial infarction, stroke, and peripheral vascular disease. Chronic elevation of either the systolic or diastolic pressures carries an increased risk of premature death.

Hypertension commonly gives no obvious symptoms, and is discovered unexpectedly at the time of an examination; many patients have the problem without knowing it, although tinnitus and headache may occasionally signal its presence. The latest guidelines for hypertension are as follows: "high-normal" pressure: 130–139/85–89 mmHg; stage one hypertension: 140–159/90–99 mmHg; stage 2 hypertension: 160–179/100–109 mmHg; stage 3 hypertension: 180–209/110–119 mmHg. These levels are based on an average of at least three readings with the patient at rest and free of acute stress.

■ PREVALENCE

Hypertension is very common in advanced nations. An estimated 20 percent of the white population and 30 percent of the African American population have blood pressures above 165/95 mmHg. Thirty percent of the entire population will eventually face hypertension. Hypertension is essentially unknown among members of indigenous peoples and remote tribes of the world.

■ CAUSES AND RISK FACTORS

Ninety-five percent of cases of hypertension have no conventionally recognized cause. A number of factors, however, appear to be related.

Physical Factors

An increased risk of hypertension is incurred by smoking and tobacco use. Nicotine from tobacco chewed or smoked is a vasoconstrictive agent, aggravating the vasoconstriction in the arterial tree. Alcohol in modest or large amounts is strongly related to the risk for hypertension, and coffee and caffeine lead to mild elevations in some but not all studies. Overweight persons have a higher risk of developing hypertension; increased demands on the heart, and changes in hormonal factors are thought to explain this risk.

Familial susceptibility makes those with a family history of hypertension significantly more vulnerable to influences of excess sodium and loss of potassium. The genetic factor is relatively small compared to conditioning and other lifestyle factors.

Nutritional Factors

Since vegetarians have consistently lower blood pressures than omnivores who also eat meat, the latter practice probably makes its contribution. Even utilizing the balance of foods in the USDA food pyramid nudges people toward a more vegetarian diet.

Sugar. In laboratory rats, groups consuming 10, 15, and 20 percent of total calories as sucrose for 14 weeks had significantly higher systolic pressures than rats consuming no sucrose.[142]

Sucrose in Western diets averages >20 percent of calories. Studies in humans also suggest that increased salt retention and elevated blood pressure occur with higher intake of sugars.[143]

Mineral deficiencies. Deficiency in calcium, magnesium, potassium, and zinc from the diet is known to contribute to high blood pressure.[144,145] Excess sodium appears to be more of a problem in women. Only about 15–20 percent of the population are thought to be salt-sensitive. Some investigators have found a much greater risk for cardiovascular "events" in men with a low sodium intake and renal excretion.[146] In hypertension there tends to be a deficiency of taurine, an amino acid obtained in small amounts in food and synthesized in the body.[147]

Food sensitization. Hypertension can be a response to food sensitivity. The probability that food sensitivities will play a role is increased in persons with a family history of allergies, those with food cravings or habitual caloric dependence on a small number of foods, and those whose hypertension is noticeably intermittent. A carefully taken history and food elimination-and-re-exposure trials can identify offending sensitizing foods. When foods play a role, the most common culprits are milk, wheat, chocolate, corn, nuts (especially peanuts), pork, coffee, rice, beef, shrimp, seafood, chicken and apples.[148]

Environmental Factors

Hypertensive patients have higher blood levels of lead (from gasoline, paint, drinking water) and 3-fold higher amounts of cadmium (batteries and cigarettes) than non-hypertensive persons.[149,150] All toxins including heavy metals increase oxidative stress in the detoxification process, and hypertension is on the long list of diseases linked to free radical problems. Hypertension is more common in persons exposed to inhalant sensitizing agents including chemical odors (natural gas, gasoline fumes, chlorine), air pollution, auto exhaust, soft plastic, cleaning chemicals (Lysol, phenol), perfume, polyurethane, tobacco smoke, polyesters, fiberglass, Naugahyde, new carpeting, formaldehyde, pesticides, pest strips, and foam rubber.[151]

Physical Deconditioning

Being sedentary increases risks of hypertension about 50 percent.[152] Since tension accruing from stressful experiences is dissipated during physical exercise, sedentary patients miss one opportunity to wind themselves down. The elevated blood pressure that occurs with athletic or vigorous physical exertion is much less damaging because it does not remain sustained after the exertion is terminated. The gradual rise in blood pressure that accompanies aging is attenuated in people who remain physically fit.

Mental Factors

Stress. The arousal response (fight or flight) is triggered by all stressful phenomena which are perceived to be threatening and requiring adaptation. Documented stresses related to elevation of blood pressure include public speaking and performance tasks, reading aloud in a group, worksite pressures including critical time-related requirements (air-traffic controllers), little opportunity for promotion at work and uncertain job futures, mental arithmetic calculations, and ongoing family conflicts.[115] Other research-confirmed chronic factors include increased life dissatisfactions, impatience, and "type A" behavior which includes increased hostility and anger, and a high degree of defensiveness.[153] Imagined stresses, also, can raise blood pressure equivalent to those experienced in reality. Elevated blood pressures also develop in subjects who suppress or repress emotions while maintaining a calm exterior appearance (Type D behavior).[47] A study within the black community found that the risk of hypertension among African Americans is aggravated by experiences of racial discrimination and unwillingness to challenge unfair treatment.[154]

Attitude and emotional states. Elevated blood pressure reactions have been identified in persons whose sympathetic nervous system overreacts to stressful stimuli with overt, visible emotional disturbance, and in persons who suppress or repress strong emotions and maintain a calm exterior appearance. Hypertensive surges under stress are very much greater in emotionally defensive personalities than those with low defensiveness.[153] Persons prone to more anger have significantly higher blood pressures at night than persons who are predominantly happy and pleasant.[155] Anxiety-prone men and women carry a higher risk for hypertension.[46] Counselors frequently link hypertension to states of frustration and anger, often with underlying inflexibility.

■ CONVENTIONAL TREATMENT

Certain people elevate their blood pressure only in the presence of a doctor or nurse—the so-called "white coat" effect. The taking of repeated blood pressures at home by patients themselves or by family members will usually bring this discrepancy to awareness. In one carefully done study, when treatment was based on ambulatory pressures, patients stopped antihypertensive medications 26 percent of the time versus 7 percent of those whose treatment was based on office-recorded pressures.[156] A blood pressure that is elevated only in the doctor's office should not be treated by drugs. Blood pressures also rise when people speak; recorded pressures should reflect the non-verbal state.

The conventional approach to the treatment of hypertension includes suggestions to reduce dietary salt, lose weight, begin or increase exercise, and cease smoking. Conventional treatment also usually involves prescription medications. The classes of drugs used, with the more commonly used drugs in each category, include:

- alpha adrenergic blockers (Dibenzyaline, Regitine);
- alpha-1 adrenergic blockers (Cardura, Hytrin, Minipress);
- central alpha agonists (Aldomet, Catapres);
- central alpha-2 agonists (Tenex, Wytensin);
- beta adrenergic blockers (Inderal, Tenormin, Blocadren, Corgard, Coreg);
- cardioselective beta-adrenergic blockers (Lopressor, Toprol, Kerlone);
- angiotensin-converting enzyme inhibitors (Zestril, Capoten, Vasotec, Monopril, Prinivil, Accupril, Lotensin);

- angiotensin II receptor blockers (Cozaar, Diovan, Atacand);
- diuretics (Enduron, Lasix, Edecrin, hydrochlorothiazide, Lozol, Zaroxolyn);
- potassium-sparing diuretics (Dyrenium, Aldactone);
- calcium channel blockers (Cardizem, Calan, Norvasc, Isoptin, Procardia);
- rauwolfia derivatives (reserpine);
- vasodilators (minoxidil, Hydralazine).

Combinations of drugs from two different classes are available in many fixed combinations, or two or more agents can be given separately with a lower dosage of both to minimize side effects.

When should mild to moderate hypertension be treated? All authorities agree that in mild to moderate hypertension lifestyle modifications are in order. The question of when to use drugs continues to be a matter of disagreement. The majority of physicians start drug treatment for readings at 150/90 mmHg, with a few authorities concluding that drug treatment is not justified until levels are much higher, citing studies showing (1) lack of effectiveness in reducing cardiac mortality;[157] (2) higher cardiac mortality rates in drug-treated patients;[51,158] and (3) higher total mortality in drug-treated patients.[159] There is apparently no reduction in mortality with drug treatment of mild to moderate hypertension.

Side effects of potent drugs are varied. Diuretics have long been known to have downside effects with increased renal potassium loss; less well known but no less important is the fact that diuretics also remove magnesium and zinc.[160] Recently, calcium channel blockers have been shown to increase thromboglobulin, and significantly increase the incidence of gastrointestinal hemorrhage.[161]

Other side effects impacting quality of life are persistent cough with ACE inhibitors and impotence and decreased libido reported in nearly all classes of drugs mentioned above. The side effects are the most common reason patients fail to take their antihypertensive medications at all, or fail to take them regularly.

The American Heart Association insists that an antihypertensive drug, once started, must be continued for life. Experience teaches otherwise. Many persons on drugs, having made important lifestyle changes as outlined below, can safely go off their medications.

■ HOLISTIC PREVENTION

Lifestyle modifications—maintaining proper weight, participating in a regular aerobic exercise plan, and engaging in some form of regular relaxation or meditation practice—are the paramount issues in reducing the risk of developing hypertension. Avoiding exposure to sources of lead and cadmium can be important. Abatement of or reduction in smoking decreases blood vessel constriction and reduces intake of cadmium.

In this instance, perhaps more than in any other, the ability of the prescribing physician to communicate wisely and advocate for change is essential. In the era of myriad possible choices, merely telling the patient what to do is unlikely to be successful. Reason, shared decision making, stories of success, setting an appropriate objective, canvassing possibilities for practical steps, asking for commitment to given incremental changes, positive reinforcement, and unconditional acceptance are elements of a "style" with enhanced possibility for success.

Improvement in nutritional habits including maintaining a modest intake of sodium 1.5–3 g daily, and consuming adequate potassium, magnesium, calcium, and antioxidant vitamins[162] are also important steps in prevention. Higher intakes of polyunsaturated fatty acids are associated with decreased blood pressure and better cardiac output.[163]

Management of stress, which increases blood pressure, involves relaxation training, reduction in hostile, negative attitudes, and modulation of anger. All appropriate steps in hypertension treatment that follow are part of a program for prevention.

■ HOLISTIC TREATMENT

Conventional authorities think that careful attention to lifestyle changes can control blood pressure 40 percent of the time to the point that prescription medications can be eliminated.[164] The holistic perspective is even more enthusiastic. Broad experience has shown that optimizing an even broader combination of all lifestyle factors can achieve a normal blood pressure, while eliminating drugs, 85 percent of the time.

Physical Factors

Stabilizing weight to within 5–10 percent of ideal is often strikingly helpful in persons with hypertension (see Chapter 13). Blood pressures usually fall promptly as weight loss ensues. Ideal weights can be determined by normal tables, measurements of abdominal girth, body mass index charts, and calculations based on measurement of fat layers. Percentage of body fat should be below 18 for men and 24 for women. Limiting alcohol to one drink or less per day is also important, since excess alcohol is a major contributor to hypertension.[165] Smoking independently raises blood pressure by increasing blood viscosity and arterial wall rigidity.[166] Reduction or elimination of smoking is an obvious necessity. Acupuncture, cognitive therapy, biofeedback, imagery, and aerobic exercise appear to offer the highest rates of success.

Nutritional initiatives

Healthy options include increasing the intake of whole foods, including vegetables, fruits, whole unrefined grains, legumes, beans, nuts, seeds, fiber, vitamins, minerals and essential fatty acids. Such a diet lowers systolic pressure 12 mmHg and diastolic 6 mmHg.[167] Vegetarians have lower blood pressures than omnivores.[168]

- *Reducing sugar.* Sucrose, glucose, fructose, and lactose exert an anti-natiuretic effect on sodium excretion that is unrelated to aldosterone.[169] In animals in whom sugar is substituted for starch intake, significant increases in blood pressure follow.

- *Increasing linoleic acid intake lowers blood pressure.*[170] Sources high in linoleic acid include sunflower seeds, sesame seeds, wheat germ, corn, soybeans, rice bran, peanuts, brazil nuts, walnuts, and their oils.
- Doubling intake of fiber from 12 to 24 g daily decreased the incidence of hypertension 57 percent in a study of 30,000 men.[171] Examples of therapeutic fiber include psyllium seeds, guar gum, apple pectin, and oat bran.

Nutritional Supplements

Including adequate daily amounts of the following supplements, if macronutrient intake is questionably adequate, gives assurance that requirements are subscribed:

- Vitamin C. Mean blood pressure fall of 7 mmHg was associated with each incremental increase of 50 μmol of plasma vitamin C.[172] Vitamin C acts to oppose the arterial vasoconstriction triggered by smoking and high fat meals, consequently promoting arterial flexibility and dilation.
- Vitamin E 600 mg.[162]
- β-Carotene 30 mg.[162]
- Zinc 45 mg.[162]
- Vitamin B_1 10–20 mg.[173]
- Vitamin B_6, given for a month in doses of 5 mg per kg body weight significantly lowered systolic and diastolic pressures in hypertensives.[174]
- Men consuming more than 1 g of calcium daily compared to those ingesting less than 0.5 g daily have a 20 percent lower incidence of hypertension; those consuming more than 400 mg of magnesium compared to those taking in less than 250 mg have a 50 percent lower incidence; and men consuming more than 3.5 g of potassium daily compared to those ingesting less than 2.5 g have a 55 percent lower incidence.[171]

- Avoiding extremes of sodium ingestion appears wise. Appropriate intake appears to be between 1.5 and 3 g daily for most people. This range can be achieved with minimal to modest salting of foods and by avoiding many highly salted and brined foods including pickles, canned foods, preserved meats and fast foods.
- Nine grams of fish oil (high in omega-3 fatty acids) daily for 6 weeks has been shown to reduce diastolic pressures an average of 5 mmHg.[175]
- Taurine supplements lower blood pressure: six grams daily has been shown to drop systolic pressure 10 mmHg and diastolic 5 mmHg in 7 days, with no effects seen in subjects with normal blood pressures.[176] Taurine indirectly decreases sympathetic vasoconstriction, the primary cause of hypertension. Reasonable doses are 1–1.5 g daily.
- Coenzyme Q_{10} 50 mg b.i.d. in one group of men reduced average systolic blood pressure 18 mmHg and diastolic pressure 12 mmHg.[177]

Exercise

Blood pressure responds well to physical activity, including walking, running, gardening, and other steady-state activities. Medication can usually be reduced or eliminated with long-term commitment to an exercise program. Low- and moderate-intensity exercise is as good as high-intensity exercise and is especially effective in mild to moderate hypertension. In severe hypertension, exercise is effective but higher intensity is required. Results emerge within a few weeks of initiating a regular program. A meta-analysis of 30 exercise/hypertension studies found a mean fall of 7 mmHg in both systolic and diastolic pressures in patients incorporating some kind of regular exercise into their schedules.[178] The factors that enhance compliance are designing a program that is enjoyable, is imminently practicable, and offers some aspects of sociability such as exercising in a group or with a friend. *Any amount of exercise begins to reduce risk.*

Environmental Factors

Since water supplies can carry heavy metal toxins, including small amounts of lead from soldered copper pipes, using a filter for cooking and drinking water should be considered an important initiative.

When other measures do not yield improvement in blood pressure control, review of possible environmental and food sensitivity causes of hypertension is warranted. Once offensive foods have been identified, strict avoidance of the most sensitizing foods, rotation diets to permit consumption of mildly or moderately sensitizing foods, and careful environmental controls for inhalant substances mentioned under environmental risk factors can bring noticeable improvement.

Botanical Medicine

Crataegus 80 mg b.i.d. has consistent but mild blood pressure lowering effects.[179] Garlic and onions both have modest blood pressure lowering properties. In some studies, liberal use of fresh garlic has lowered systolic pressure by 20–30 mmHg and diastolic pressure by 10–20 mmHg.[180] Mistletoe (*Viscum album*), as a whole plant 1 : 1 fluid extract, lowers blood pressure in 0.5 ml doses.[180] Extended use and intake of doses exceeding the equivalent of 4 g daily of the crude herb are not recommended. Documented case reports of benefits with homeopathy, acupuncture and massage therapy have been published.

Mental and Emotional Factors

Behavioral initiatives. Biofeedback practice leads to significant and often permanent reduction in systolic and diastolic blood pressures. Systolic readings often reduced 15–20 mmHg from baseline and diastolic 8–12 mmHg.[181] Cortisone levels often fall as much as 20–25 percent, tending to postpone a number of degenerative diseases.[182] Biofeedback does not lower readings in normotensive patients.

Hypnosis. Hypnosis has been found to lower systolic and diastolic pressures an average of 16–20 mmHg, equivalent to the effect of many pharmaceuticals.[183] Results persist through years of followup.

Meditation. Regular meditation consistently lowers systolic and diastolic readings. Hypertensive African-Americans practicing meditation for 3 months were recently shown to achieve reductions of 11 and 7 mmHg in systolic and diastolic pressures compared to no changes in a lifestyle modification education group.[184] Some meditation studies have shown benefits two-fold better than drug treatment in long-term followup. Two great advantages are (1) freedom from the risk of side effects with drug treatment, and (2) the tendency for the improved blood pressure dynamics to be permanent. Regular practice of Qi Gong, a gentle Chinese moving meditation and martial art, has also been shown to lower blood pressure.[185]

Spiritual and Social Factors

Beliefs. A 1982 Australian study reported the reduction of mean blood pressure in 1,100 hypertensives from 158/102 to 144/91 after taking a placebo for 3 years as controls for a comparison group taking drugs. Forty-eight percent had totally normal blood pressures at the close of the study.[186] Placebo effects depend on beliefs that tend to evoke images to which the nervous system responds. What patients believe and expect entrains the central nervous system to elaborate changes in multiple organ systems consistent with the belief. If beliefs and images are positive, arousal–fight–flight responses are minimized, and nervous and hypothalamic–pituitary–adrenal systems function at a lower baseline, thereby reducing blood pressure.

Social health. The presence of a friendly dog is associated with lower systolic and diastolic blood pressures in children while reading aloud. Elderly patients likewise manifest the same reductions with a pet dog present.[187]

Remote Healing

Ninety-six hypertensive patients, age 16–60, were exposed to a series of long-distance treatments by a healer. In double-blind fashion, 48 randomly selected patients received the treatments and the remainder acted as untreated controls, and all 96 continued their usual drug treatment. Each healer engaged in relaxation, attuned him/herself to a Higher Power or Infinite Being, affirmed in images the patient's perfect state of health, and expressed gratitude to the Source of all power and energy. The systolic blood pressures significantly improved in 92 percent of the treated group versus 74 percent of the control group ($p = 0.0144$).[188]

Congestive Heart Failure

■ DESCRIPTION

Congestive heart failure (CHF), or cardiac insufficiency, is a marked, sustained reduction in the intrinsic contractility of the heart in which cardiac output becomes inadequate to meet its workload. Congestive heart failure tends to be progressive, with a very significant shortening of life expectancy. Cardiomegaly is almost inevitably present, most often an attempt on the part of the heart itself to compensate for poor pumping action. A healthy heart increases stroke volume in response to exertion; a sick heart has no reserve to meet this kind of demand. Fifty percent of CHF patients die within 5 years, and 50 percent of patients with advanced disease live less than a year.

Symptoms of congestive heart failure include orthopnea and dyspnea on exertion, the appearance of edema and weight gain, particularly in the lower extremities. The clinical diagnosis made from the typical history is confirmed by physical findings of ankle edema, pulmonary rales, cardiomegaly, more labored respiration and, in advanced conditions, reduced oxygen blood saturation and carbon dioxide retention. Laboratory confirmation can be accomplished with an echocardiogram, and a chest X-ray will show cardiac enlargement. A treadmill test will demonstrate decreased cardiac work capacity with the challenge of walking.

■ PREVALENCE

Two to three million Americans are thought to have congestive heart failure (about 1 percent of the population). It is the most common reason for hospitalization in those aged 65 and older. Slightly under one million new cases are diagnosed each year.

■ CAUSES AND RISK FACTORS

Congestive heart failure is secondary to heart deterioration from:

- arteriosclerotic coronary artery disease,
- hypertension,
- constrictive pericarditis,
- chronic obstructive pulmonary disease,
- cardiomyopathy, a particularly lethal cause of progressive congestive failure, developing from alcohol toxicity, postviral infections, toxic side effects from drugs including chemotherapeutic cancer agents, deficiency of selenium, the presence of potentially toxic amounts of mercury and antimony, and often for reasons unknown,
- unknown factors with none of these recognized contributors.

Nutritional Factors

- Excess intake of sodium, primarily as salt, predisposes susceptible people to congestive heart failure.
- Congestive heart failure patients have significantly lower levels of potassium and magnesium,[189] and deficiency of both is highly suspect in the majority of arrhythmic deaths, the most common cause of the sudden demise of the CHF patient, whether or not their condition has been stable or progressive.[190] Low serum potassium is commonly recog-

nized and treated, but low magnesium levels are not. These electrolytes are lost from the body during times of excess stress,[191] and, along with zinc, are excreted in excess amounts during diuretic drug treatment.[192,193]

- Individuals with subclinical selenium deficiency with no overt signs of cardiomyopathy may nonetheless experience subtle reductions of myocardial contractility and excessive excitability response to normal and abnormal stimuli.
- Congestive heart failure is clearly an oxidative stress-mediated problem. The degree of heart failure is positively and progressively correlated with increasing levels of free radical activity markers and negatively correlated with levels of antioxidant enzymes.[194,195] Deficiency of antioxidants should soon be recognized as a risk factor for congestive heart failure.

Biomolecular Factors

- In heart disease, coenzyme Q_{10} is easily displaced and lost from cardiac myocytes. This leads to depleted inotropic action, tending to lead to heart failure. Low levels of coenzyme Q_{10} are predictive of heart failure; cardiomyopathy patients have levels 20 percent below those in healthy people.[196]
- The serum taurine levels in domestic cats with congestive heart failure is consistently low. Humans with cardiomyopathy are consistently found to have significantly low levels of this non-essential amino acid, which is predominantly synthesized in the body from methionine and cysteine metabolism.[197]
- L-carnitine levels in cardiac muscle of patients in congestive heart failure were 45 percent below those of healthy controls,[198] and free carnitine levels 21 percent lower.[199]
- Hypothyroidism appears to contribute to CHF of cardiomyopathic origin.[200]

Environmental Factors

- Environmental toxins contribute to CHF. In large cities, acute exacerbations requiring hospitalization are related to times of increased air pollution alerts and weather variations.[201]
- In a 1974 study of patients hospitalized for an acute myocardial infarction, the 6 month mortality was 3 times as great as controls if antibodies to milk proteins or egg albumin were present.[202]

Mental and Emotional Factors

- Emotional factors also play contributing roles. The left ventricular ejection fraction has been shown to decrease 7 percent during times when patients with established coronary artery disease recounted incidents in which they had responded with anger. This exceeded the decreases from physical exercise (2 percent), mental arithmetic testing (0 percent) and a speech stressor experience (0 percent).[203]
- Psychological stress induces extra workloads on the heart without physical exertion, with chronically elevated sympathetic nervous system activity in the resting and stressed state.[204]
- Patients with a Type D personality (tendency to suppress negative emotions) were 60 percent more likely to experience an adverse cardiac event after myocardial infarction than the cohort of those with LVEF < 30 percent.[205]

■ **CONVENTIONAL TREATMENT**

Dietary sodium restriction is routinely recommended. Drugs are prescribed primarily from the following classes of pharmaceuticals:

1. Derivatives of digitalis (digoxin, Lanoxin) increase inotropic action of the cardiac myocytes.

2. Diuretics improve renal excretion of water and electrolytes to reduce edema (Hydrochlorothiazide, Dyazide, Zaroxylyn, Lasix, and potassium-sparing Aldactone and Dyrenium).
3. Angiotensin-converting enzyme inhibitors (Zestril, Capoten, Vasotec, Monopril, Prinivil, Lotensin) add another dimension to drug treatment, reducing the load on the heart.
4. Drugs having selective alpha-1 and non-selective beta-adrenergic receptor blocking actions are also used as fourth-line medications (Coreg, Normodyne).
5. A recent report cited promising benefits with Natrecor, a human natriuretic peptide.[206]

Side effects of pharmaceuticals used to treat congestive heart failure are also a consideration. Commonly experienced untoward effects of drugs include toxicity from digitalis, a higher than expected death rate associated with loss of potassium and magnesium from diuretic use,[207] and sexual impotence with many classes of drugs. One loop diuretic, furosemide, tends to deplete thiamin (vitamin B_1), essential for cardiac function.

Conventional treatment also emphasizes the control of predisposing conditions including high blood pressure and coronary artery disease. Anticoagulation may be used to reduce hazards of embolization common in atrial fibrillation often accompanying congestive heart failure.

In terminal cardiac insufficiency associated with cardiomyopathy or ischemic heart disease, patients may qualify as candidates for cardiac transplantation.

■ HOLISTIC PREVENTION

Since coronary artery arteriosclerotic disease and hypertension are significant contributing causes of congestive heart failure, all aspects of prevention and management of those conditions apply here. Aggressive treatment of pericarditis will frequently prevent the heart failure which may follow in the constrictive phase; conventional treatment with cortisone is frequently successful in this condition, and in stubbornly resistant cases, administration of colchicine is strikingly successful.[208]

Prevalence of oxygen free radicals is excessive in a high percentage of patients with congestive heart failure compared to healthy subjects. The supplying of adequate nutrients including antioxidants and minerals, amino acids and biosynthetic agents may be essential in the prevention of congestive heart failure. Further basic research will need to be completed to resolve these questions.

■ HOLISTIC TREATMENT

Nutritional Supplements

1. Antioxidants. Because congestive heart failure is in significant measure a problem of oxidant stress, it is no surprise that antioxidants including vitamins A, C and E as well as biosynthesized agents with antioxidant properties contribute to prevention and control of congestive heart failure. The addition of vitamin E 400 IU daily to treatment of heart failure patients has persuasively shown additional dimensions of improvement.[209]

2. Magnesium and potassium are consistently lower in patients with congestive heart failure, only partially due to diuretics.[191] Consistent replacement is indicated. It may take up to 6 months to restore magnesium body stores with oral doses which should be 400–800 mg daily.[192] In congestive failure, IV magnesium markedly benefits most patients within 3 months, with added improvement continuing to manifest for up to a year in 85 percent of patients.[210] *Magnesium is contraindicated in cerebral hemorrhage and in severe renal failure.* Magnesium is a natural calcium channel blocker. Magnesium also facilitates the repletion of potassium in hypokalemia.

3. Thiamine 200 mg daily for 6 weeks improved indices of cardiac insufficiency 20 percent in a 1995 study. Thiamine is readily depleted by diuretics. There is no risk and the cost is minimal for potentially great benefits.[211]

4. Polyunsaturated fat increases in the diet are associated with cardiac function by its antivasopressor action, reduction of blood viscosity and increasing cardiac beta-adrenergic responsiveness.[212] Omega-3 oils in doses of 1–2 g b.i.d. are appropriate.

Biomolecular Options

1. Forty percent decrease in severity of cardiac insufficiency resulted from 8 weeks of treatment with taurine 2 g b.i.d. in an open research trial.[213] Side effects were very rare.
2. L-carnitine is a "non-essential" amino acid helpful in congestive heart failure. Given as a 4 g intravenous injection, it is even helpful in cardiogenic shock.[214] Oral doses of L-carnitine 2 g daily restore energy metabolism, improve treadmill performance in CHF patients and markedly reduce the need for drugs, with improvement usually appearing within a month of starting treatment.[215] Propionyl-L-carnitine (1 mg/ kg body weight daily) significantly reduced pulmonary artery pressure, peak oxygen consumption, and peak exercise heart rate.[216]
3. Coenzyme Q_{10}. The lower the CoQ_{10} blood levels in patients with cardiac insufficiency, the more severe the failure.[197] Given CoQ_{10} 100–150 mg/day, the inotropic efficiency of far advanced cardiomyopathy patients increases up to 50 percent, manifesting in extraordinary clinical improvement.[217,218] Studies show the 2-year survival on continuous doses of CoQ_{10} to be 85 percent contrasted to the usual experience of 50 percent.[219] Patients in congestive heart failure receiving coenzyme Q_{10} have been shown to require hospitalization only 20 percent of the time compared to 48 percent for those taking a placebo.[220] A 1999 study showing no benefit used abnormally short treatment times with no "washout" time between crossover phases with placebo.[221]
4. Careful attention to appropriate dosing of thyroid replacement in patients with hypothyroidism is necessary; this is particularly critical in patients receiving beta-blockers.[222]

5. Saunas and warm water baths, previously thought to be contraindicated in CHF appear to have therapeutic benefit.
Confirmed by Swan-Ganz catheter measurements in CHF
patients (NYHA classes II, III, and IV) before and after a sauna
or warm water bath at 41°C, left ventricular ejection fraction
and heart size decreased significantly.[223]

Botanical Agents

1. *Astragalus membranaceus.* Left ventricular function significantly improved in patients given *Astragalus membranaceus*
   100–150 mg t.i.d. (0.5 percent 4-hydroxy-3-methoxy isofla-
   vone content) following an MI.[224]
2. *Crataegus oxycantha.* Pressure-rate-product and subjective
   distress in heart failure NYHA class II patients improved
   significantly after 80 mg Crataegus extract b.i.d. for 8
   weeks.[225,226]
3. *Sunitang.* Significant improvement in left ventricular shortening and NYHA class, and reduction in peripheral resistance
   and predilection to rhythm disturbances resulted from treatment with 0.5–1 g daily of *Sunitang*, a traditional Chinese
   herb.[227]
4. *Terminalia arjuna*, a traditional Ayurvedic herb. In 12 patients
   with refractory NYHA class IV disease, deteriorating in spite
   of full pharmacological treatment, 9 of 12 patients moved to
   class II and 3 of 12 to class II after 4 months of treatment with
   500 mg q 8 h of *T. arjuna.*[228]

Other herbs long traditionally used, for which there is less
research available, include Dandelion (*Taraxicum officinalis*)
which has potassium-sparing diuretic properties, and Lily of the
Valley (*Convallaria majalis*), aiding cardiac tonicity in CHF (up to
gtts 30 daily of 1 : 5 extract).

Acupuncture, homeopathy and the use of castor oil packs
(see elsewhere) have also been used.

Exercise

Patients with severe heart failure engaging in appropriate low-grade aerobic exercise with walking and bicycle exercise for a year improved all measures of heart activity, breathing capacity, and quality of life as well.[229] A specific individually designed prescription can be offered to patients as appropriate.

Psychological Initiatives

Congestive failure responds to biofeedback. A single session has been demonstrated to very substantially improve cardiac output 0.3 L/minute.[230] All similar relaxation practices have similar effects on lowering sympathetic tone and improving peripheral vasodilation.

Counselors have observed that issues of congestive heart failure are often symbolic for the emotional congestion of maintaining unfulfilling relationships and situations when one's "heart is not in it," and in failing to resolve overwhelming feelings of grief—the "broken heart."[231]

REFERENCES

1. Alderman EL et al. Ten-year follow-up of survival and myocardial infarction in the randomized Coronary Artery Surgery Study. *Circulation* 1990; 82(5):1629–46.
2. Kannam JP et al. Short stature and risk for mortality and cardiovascular disease events. The Framingham Heart Study. *Circulation* 1994; 90(5):2241–7.
3. Ubbink JB et al. Vitamin B-12, vitamin B-6, and folate nutritional status in men with hyperhomocysteinemia. *Am J Clin Nutr* 1993; 57(1):47–53.
4. Ernst E et al. Fibrinogen as a cardiovascular risk factor: a meta-analysis and review of the literature. *Ann Intern Med* 1993; 118(12):956–63.

5. Babir M et al. Lipoprotein(a) and accelerated coronary artery disease in cardiac transplant recipients. *Lancet* 1992; 340(8834–5):1500–2.
6. Epstein FH. The epidemiology of coronary heart disease. A review. *J Chronic Dis* 1965;18(8):735–74.
7. Jenkins CD. Psychologic and social precursors of coronary disease (first of two parts). *N Engl J Med* 1971; 284(5):244–55.
8. Ferrari R et al. Oxidative stress during myocardial ischaemia and heart failure. *Eur Heart J* 1998; 19 Suppl B:B2–11.
9. Dubois-Rande JL et al. Oxidative stress in patients with unstable angina. *Eur Heart J* 1994; 15(2):179–83.
10. Croft KD et al. Low density lipoprotein composition and oxidizability in coronary disease—apparent favourable effect of beta blockers. *Atherosclerosis* 1992; 97(2–3):123–30.
11. Mancini M et al. Antioxidants in the Mediterranean diet. *Can J Cardiol* 1995; 11 suppl G:105G–109G.
12. Wood R et al. Effect of butter, mono- and polyunsaturated fatty acid-enriched butter, trans fatty acid margarine, and zero trans fatty acid margarine on serum lipids and lipoproteins in healthy men. *J Lipid Res* 1993; 34(1):1–11.
13. Kim SY et al. Serum levels of antioxidant vitamins in relation to coronary artery disease: a case control study of Koreans. *Biomed Environ Sci* 1996; 9(2–3):229–35.
14. Gey KF et al. Poor plasma status of carotene and vitamin C is associated with higher mortality from ischemic heart disease and stroke: Basel Prospective Study. *Clin Investig* 1993; 71(1):3–6.
15. Gey KF et al. Inverse correlation between plasma vitamin E and mortality from ischemic heart disease in cross-cultural epidemiology. *Am J Clin Nutr* 1991; 53(Suppl 1):326S–334S.
16. Tilson MD et al. Decreased hepatic copper levels. A possible chemical marker for the pathogenesis of aortic aneurysms in man. *Arch Surgery* 1982; 117(9):1212–13.
17. Hertog MG et al. Flavonoid intake and long-term risk of coronary heart disease and cancer in the seven countries study. *Arch Intern Med* 1995;155(4):381–6.
18. Dyerberg J et al. Eicosapentaenoic acid and prevention of thrombosis and atherosclerosis? *Lancet* 1978; 2(8081):117–19.
19. Yudkin J. Diet and coronary heart disease: why blame fat? *J R Soc Med* 1992; 85(9):515–16.

20. Feskens EJ et al. Hyperinsulinemia, risk factors, and coronary heart disease. The Zutphen Elderly Study. *Arterioscler Thrombos* 1994; 14(10):1641–7.
21. Chan J. Loma Linda University. Twentieth Congress of the European Society of Cardiology, Oct. 1998. *Fam Pract News* 1998 Oct 15; 28(20):1–2.
22. Rosenberg L et al. Coffee drinking and nonfatal myocardial infarction in men under 55 years of age. *Am J Epidemiol* 1988; 128(3):570–8.
23. Nygard O et al. Coffee consumption and plasma total homocysteine: The Hordaland Homocysteine Study. *Am J Clin Nutr* 1997; 65(1):136–43.
24. Langsjoen PH et al. Overview of the use of CoQ10 in cardiovascular disease. *Biofactors* 1999; 9(204):273–84.
25. Bartels GL et al. Effects of L-propionylcarnitine on ischemia-induced myocardial dysfunction in men with angina pectoris. *Am J Cardiol* 1994; 74(2):125–30.
26. Willett WC et al. Weight, weight change, and coronary heart disease in women. Risk within the 'normal' weight range. *JAMA* 1995; 273(6):461–5.
27. Welin CL et al. Behavioural characteristics in patients with myocardial infarction: a case-control study. *J Cardiovasc Risk* 1995; 2(3):247–54.
28. Ciccone G. SO$_2$ air pollution and hospital admissions in Ravenna: a case-control study. *Epidemiol Prev* 1995; 19(62):99–104.
29. Leinonen M et al. Interaction of *Chlamydia pneumoniae* infection with other risk factors of atherosclerosis. *Am Heart J* 1999; 138(5 Pt 2):504–6.
30. Gillum RF et al. Dental disease and coronary artery disease. *Am Heart J* 1994; 128(6 Pt 1):1267.
31. Danesh J et al. Association of fibrinogen, C-reactive protein, albumin, or leukocyte count with coronary heart disease: meta-analyses of prospective studies. *JAMA* 1998; 279(18):1477–82.
32. Chang-Claude J et al. Dietary and lifestyle determinants of mortality among German vegetarians. *Int J Epidemiol* 1993; 22(2):228–36.
33. Hurley B. Aerobic or strength training for coronary risk factor intervention? *Ann Med* 1994; 26(3):153–5.

34. Toffler GH et al. Physical activity and the triggering of myocardial infarction: the case for regular exercise. *Heart* 1996; 75(4): 323–5.

35. Miche S et al. Overwork can kill. *BMJ* 1996; 312(7036):921–2.

36. Muller JE et al. Circadian variation in the frequency of onset of acute myocardial infarction. *N Engl J Med* 1985; 313(21):1315–22.

37. Manuck SB et al. Effects of stress and the sympathetic nervous system on coronary artery atherosclerosis in the cynomolgus macaque. *Am Heart J* 1988; 116(1 Pt 2):328–33.

38. Seelig MS. Adverse stress reactions and magnesium deficiency: preventive and therapeutic implications. *J Am Coll Nutr* 1992; 11(5):609.

39. Brindley DN et al. Possible connections between stress, diabetes, obesity, hypertension and altered lipoprotein metabolism may result in atherosclerosis. *Clin Sci* 1989; 77(5):453–61.

40. Gutstein WH et al. Increased serum mitogenic activity for arterial smooth muscle cells associated with relaxation and low educational level in human subjects with high but not low hostility traits: implications for atherogenesis. *J Psychosom Res* 1999; 46(1):51–61.

41. Williams RB et al. Type A behavior, hostility, and coronary atherosclerosis. *Psychosom Med* 1980; 42(6):539–49.

42. Barefoot JC et al. Symptoms of depression, acute myocardial infarction, and total mortality in a community sample. *Circulation* 1996; 93(11):19767–80.

43. Mittleman M. Harvard Medical School. American Heart Association Conference: Cardiovascular Disease and Epidemiology, 1996. *Fam Pract News* 1996; 26(8):8.

44. Kawachi I et al. A prospective study of anger and coronary heart disease. The Normative Aging Study. *Circulation* 1996; 94(9):2090–5.

45. Mittleman MA et al. Triggering of acute myocardial infarction onset by episodes of anger. Determinants of Myocardial Infarction Onset Study Investigators. *Circulation* 1995; 92(7):1720–5.

46. Russek LG et al. The Harvard Mastery of Stress Study: 35-year follow-up: Prognostic significance of patterns of psychophysiological arousal and adaptation. *Psychosom Med* 1990; 52(3):271–85.

47. Denollet J et al. Personality and coronary heart disease: the type-D scale-16 (DS16). *Ann Behav Med* 1998; 20(3):209–15.

48. Ruberman W et al. Psychosocial influences on mortality after myocardial infarction. *N Engl J Med* 1984; 311(9):552–9.

49. Scheier MF et al. Dispositional optimism and recovery from coronary artery bypass surgery: the beneficial effects on physical and psychological well being. *J Pers Soc Psychol* 1989; 57(5):1024–40.

50. Jacobs D et al. Report of the Conference on Low Blood Cholesterol: Mortality Associations. *Circulation* 1992; 86(3):1046–60.

51. Strandberg TE et al. Long-term mortality after 5-year multifactorial primary prevention of cardiovascular diseases in middle-aged men. *JAMA* 1991; 266(9):1225–9.

52. Newman TB et al. Carcinogenicity of lipid-lowering drugs. *JAMA* 1996; 275(1):55–60.

53. Chalmers TC, Celano P, Sacks HS, Smith H Jr. Bias in treatment assignment in controlled clinical trials. *N Engl J Med* 1983; 309(22):1358–61.

54. Lichtlen PR et al. Retardation of angiographic progression of coronary artery disease by nifedipine. Results of the International Nifedipine Trial on Antiatherosclerotic Therapy. INTACT Group Investigators. *Thromb Res* 1994; 72(3):257–62.

55. Lichtlen PR et al. Retardation of angiographic progression of coronary artery disease by nifedipine. Results of the International Nifedipine Trial on Antiatherosclerotic Therapy. INTACT Group Investigators. *Lancet* 1990; 335(8690): 1109–13.

56. Muhlestein JB et al. Increased incidence of Chlamydia species within the coronary arteries of patients with symptomatic atherosclerotic versus other forms of cardiovascular disease. *J Am Coll Cardiol* 1996; 27(7):1555–61.

57. Graboys TB et al. Results of a second-opinion trial among patients recommended for coronary angiography. *JAMA* 1992; 268(18): 2537–40.

58. Vogt MT et al. Decreased ankle/arm blood pressure index and mortality in elderly women. *JAMA* 1993; 270(4):465–9.

59. Humble CG et al. Dietary fiber and coronary heart disease in middle-aged hypercholesterolemic men. *Am J Prev Med* 1993; 9(4):197–202.

60. Stein JH et al. Purple grape juice improves endothelial function and reduces the susceptibility of LDL cholesterol to oxidation in patients with coronary artery disease. *Circulation* 1999; 100(10): 1050–5.

61. Kohlmeier L et al. Lycopene and myocardial infarction risk in the EURAMIC Study. AB. *Am J Epidemiol* 1997; 146(8):618–26.

62. Schnohr P et al. Egg consumption and high-density-lipoprotein cholesterol. *J Intern Med* 1994; 235(3):249–51.

63. Sabate J et al. Effects of walnuts on serum lipid levels and blood pressure in normal men. *N Engl J Med* 1993; 328(9):603–7.

64. Yudkin J et al. Effects of high dietary sugar. *Br Med J* 1980; 281(6252):1396.

65. De Carvalho MJ et al. Vitamin status of healthy subjects in Burgundy (France). *Ann Nutr Metab* 1996; 40(1):24–51.

66. Reaven PD et al. Comparison of supplementation of RRR-alpha-tocopherol and racemic alpha-tocopherol in humans. Effects on lipid levels and lipoprotein susceptibility to oxidation. *Arterioscler Thromb* 1993; 13(4):601–8.

67. Stephens NG et al. Randomised controlled trial of vitamin E in patients with coronary disease: Cambridge Heart Antioxidant Study. *Lancet* 1996; 347(9004):781–6.

68. Klipstein-Grobusch K et al. Dietary antioxidants and risk of myocardial infarction in the elderly: the Rotterdam Study. *Am J Clin Nutr* 1999; 69(2):261–6.

69. Williams MJ et al. Impaired endothelial function following a meal rich in used cooking fat. *J Am Coll Cardiol* 1999; 33(4): 1050–5.

70. Laskowski H et al. Mortality and clinical course of patients with acute myocardial infarction treated with streptokinase and antioxidants: mannitol and ascorbic acid. *Int J Cardiol* 1995; 48(3):235–7.

71. Tomoda H et al. Possible prevention of postangioplasty restenosis by ascorbic acid. *Am J Cardiol* 1996; 78(11):1284–6.

72. King JM et al. Evaluation of effects of unmodified niacin on fasting and postprandial plasma lipids in normolipidemic men with hypoalphalipoproteinemia. *Am J Med* 1994; 97(4):323–31.

73. Head KA. Inositol hexaniacinate: safer alternative to niacin. *Alt Med Rev* 1996; 1(3):176–84.

74. Arsenio L et al. Effectiveness of long-term treatment with pantethine in patients with dyslipidemia. *Clin Ther* 1986; 8(5):537–45.
75. Kok FJ et al. Low vitamin B_6 status in patients with acute myocardial infarction. *Am J Cardiol* 1989; 63(9):513–16.
76. Ellis JM et al. Prevention of myocardial infarction by vitamin B_6. *Res Commun Mol Pathol Pharmacol* 1995; 89(2):208–20.
77. Itoh K et al. The effects of high oral magnesium supplementation on blood pressure, serum lipids and related variables in apparently healthy Japanese subjects. *Br J Nutr* 1997; 78(5):737–50.
78. Shechter M et al. Beneficial effect of magnesium sulfate in acute myocardial infarction. *Am J Cardiol* 1990; 66(3):271–4.
79. Salonen JT et al. High stored iron levels are associated with excess risk of myocardial infarction in eastern Finnish men. *Circulation* 1992; 86(3):803–11.
80. Blum A et al. Clinical and inflammatory effects of dietary L-arginine in patients with intractable angina pectoris. *Am J Cardiol* 1999; 83(10):1488–90.
81. Verma SK et al. Effect of Commiphora mukul (gum guggulu) in patients of hyperlipidemia with special reference to HDL-cholesterol. *Indian J Med Res* 1988; 87:356–60.
82. Phelps S et al. Garlic supplementation and lipoprotein oxidation susceptibility. *Lipids* 1993; 28(5):475–7.
83. Silagy C et al. Garlic as a lipid lowering agent—a meta-analysis. *J R Coll Physicians Lond* 1994; 28(1):39–45.
84. Bordia A et al. Effect of garlic (*Allium sativum*) on blood lipids, blood sugar, fibrinogen and fibrinolytic activity in patients with coronary artery disease. *Prostaglandins Leukot Essent Fatty Acids* 1998; 58(4):257–63.
85. Srinivasan K et al. The effect of spices on cholesterol 7 alpha-hydroxylase activity and on serum and hepatic cholesterol levels in the rat. *Int J Vitam Nutr Res* 1991; 61(4):364–9.
86. Blesken R et al. Crataegus in cardiology. *Fortschr Med* 1992; 110(15):290–2.
87. Maitra I et al. Peroxyl radical scavenging activity of Ginkgo biloba extract EGb 761. *Biochem Pharmacol* 1995; 49(11):1649–55.
88. Osher HL et al. Khellin in the treatment of angina pectoris. *N Engl J Med* 1951; 244:315–21.

89. Montini M et al. Controlled application of cynarin in the treatment of hyperlipemic syndrome. Observations in 60 cases. *Arznei-mittelforschung* 1975; 25(8):1311–14.

90. Jacob A et al. Effect of the Indian gooseberry (amla) on serum cholesterol levels in men aged 35–55 years. *Eur J Clin Nutr* 1988; 42(11):939–44.

91. Yoshida H et al. The effects of Ba-wei-wan on plasma levels of high density lipoprotein-cholesterol and lipoperoxide in aged individuals. *Am J Chin Med* 1985; 13(1–4):71–6.

92. Davini P et al. Controlled study on L-carnitine therapeutic efficacy in post-infarction. *Drugs Exp Clin Res* 1992; 18(8):355–65.

93. Kamikawa T et al. Effects of coenzyme Q10 on exercise tolerance in chronic stable angina pectoris. *Am J Cardiol* 1985; 56(4):247–51.

94. Stocker R et al. Ubiquinol-10 protects human low density lipo-protein more efficiently against lipid peroxidation than does alpha-tocopherol. *Proc Natl Acad Sci USA* 1991; 88(5): 1646–50.

95. Kato T et al. Reduction in blood viscosity by treatment with coen-zyme Q10 in patients with ischemic heart disease. *Int J Clin Pharmacol Ther Toxicol* 1990; 28(3):123–6.

96. Chello M et al. Protection by coenzyme Q10 from myocardial reperfusion injury during coronary artery bypass grafting. *Ann Thorac Surg* 1994; 58(5):1427–32.

97. Laurora G et al. Delayed arteriosclerosis progression in high risk subjects treated with mesoglycan. Evaluation of intima-media thickness. *J Cardiovasc Surg (Torino)* 1993; 34(4):313–18.

98. Barrett-Conner E et al. A prospective study of dehydroepiandros-terone sulfate, mortality and cardiovascular disease. *N Engl J Med* 1986; 315(24):1519–24.

99. Jaffe MD. Effect of testosterone cypionate on postexercise ST segment depression. *Br Heart J* 1977; 39(11):1217–22.

100. Cranton EM et al. Current status of EDTA chelation in occlusive arterial disease. *J Adv Med* 1989; 2:107–19.

101. Steinberg D et al. Beyond cholesterol. Modifications of low-den-sity lipoprotein that increase its atherogenicity. *N Engl J Med* 1989; 320(14):915–24.

102. Warner JG et al. Long-term (5-year) changes in HDL cholesterol in cardiac rehabilitation patients. Do sex differences exist? *Circulation* 1995; 92(4):773–7.

103. Todd IC et al. Antianginal efficacy of exercise training: a comparison with beta blockade. *Br Heart J* 1990; 64(1):14–19.
104. Mittleman MA et al. Triggering of myocardial infarction by heavy physical exertion. Protection against triggering by regular exertion. Determinants of Myocardial Infarction Onset Study Investigators. *N Engl J Med* 1993; 329(23):1677–83.
105. Rosengren A et al. Social influences and cardiovascular risk factors as determinants of plasma fibrinogen concentration in a general population sample of middle aged men. *BMJ* 1990; 300(6725):634–8.
106. Blair SN et al. Changes in physical fitness and all-cause mortality. A prospective study of healthy and unhealthy men. *JAMA* 1995; 273(14):1093–8.
107. Chohan IS et al. Influence of yoga on blood coagulation. *Thromb Haemost* 1984; 51(2):196–7.
108. Nelson DV et al. 6 month followup of stress management training versus cardiac education during hospitalization for acute myocardial infarction. *J Cardiopulm Rehabil* 1994; 14(5):384–90.
109. Castillo-Richmond A et al. Effects of stress reduction on carotid atherosclerosis in hypertensive African Americans. *Stroke* 2000; 31(3):568–73.
110. Schwartz GE et al. Patterning of cognitive and somatic processes in the self-regulation of anxiety: effects of meditation versus exercise. *Psychosom Med* 1978; 40(4):321–8.
111. Ashton C Jr et al. Self-hypnosis reduces anxiety following coronary artery bypass surgery. A prospective, randomized trial. *J Cardiovasc Surg (Torino)* 1997; 38(1):69–75.
112. Blumenthal JA et al. Stress management and exercise training in cardiac patients with myocardial ischemia. *Arch Intern Med* 1997; 157(19):2213–23.
113. Ornish D et al. Intensive lifestyle changes for reversal of coronary heart disease. *JAMA* 1998; 280(23):2001–7.
114. Matthews KA et al. Are hostility and anxiety associated with carotid atherosclerosis in healthy postmenopausal women? *Psychosom Med* 1998; 60(5):633–8.
115. Gulette ECD et al. Mental stress during daily life triggers myocardial ischemia. *JAMA* 1997; 277(19):1521–6.
116. Schwartz GE et al. Cardiovascular differentiation of happiness, sadness, anger and fear following imagery and exercise. *Psychosom Med* 1981; 43(4):343–64.

117. Byrd RC. Positive therapeutic effects of intercessory prayer in a coronary care unit population. *Southern Med J* 1988; 81(7):826–9.

118. Harris WS et al. A randomized, controlled trial of the effects of remote, intercessory prayer on outcomes in patients admitted to the coronary care unit. *Arch Intern Med* 1999; 159(19):2273–8.

119. Benson H et al. Angina pectoris and the placebo effect. *N Engl J Med* 1979; 300(25):1424–9.

120. Medalie JH et al. Angina pectoris among 10,000 men: psychological and other risk factors. *Am J Med* 1976; 60(6):910–21.

121. Ruberman W et al. Psychosocial influences on mortality after myocardial infarction. *N Engl J Med* 1984; 311(9):552–9.

122. Cupples ME et al. Randomised controlled trial of health promotion in general practice for patients at high cardiovascular risk. *BMJ* 1994; 309(6960):993–6.

123. Orth-gomér K et al. Social isolation and mortality in ischemic heart disease. *Acta Med Scand* 1988; 224(3):205–13.

124. Buring JE et al. Migraine and subsequent risk of stroke in the Physicians' Health Study. *Arch Neurol* 1995; 52(2):129–34.

125. Hillbom M et al. Does ethanol intoxication promote brain infarction in young adults? *Lancet* 1978; 2(8101):1181–3.

126. Truelsen T et al. Intake of beer, wine, and spirits and risk of stroke: the Copenhagen city heart study. *Stroke* 1998; 29(12): 2467–72.

127. Wolf PA et al. Cigarette smoking as a risk factor for stroke. The Framingham Study. *JAMA* 1988; 259(7):1025–9.

128. Axelrod JJ et al. Stress hormones: their interaction and regulation. *Science* 1984; 224(4648):452–9.

129. Jovanovic Z. Risk factors for stroke in young people. *Srp Arh Celok Lek* 1996; 124(9–10):232–5.

130. Wannamethee SG et al. Nonfasting serum glucose and insulin concentrations and the risk of stroke. *Stroke* 1999; 30(9): 1780–6.

131. Rexrode KM et al. A prospective study of body mass index, weight change, and risk of stroke in women. *JAMA* 1997; 277(19): 1539–45.

132. Daviglus ML et al. Dietary vitamin C, beta-carotene and 30-year risk of stroke: results from the Western Electric Study. *Neuroepidemiology* 1997; 16(2):69–77.

133. Soderberg S et al. Leptin is a risk marker for first-ever hemorrhagic stroke in a population-based cohort. *Stroke* 1999; 30(2): 328–37.

134. Lee IM et al. Physical activity and stroke incidence: the Harvard alumni health study. *Stroke* 1998; 29(10):2049–54.

135. Gillman MW et al. Protective effect of fruits and vegetables on development of stroke in men. *JAMA* 1995; 273(14):1113–17.

136. Ascherio A et al. Intake of potassium, magnesium, calcium, and fiber and risk of stroke among US men. *Circulation* 1998; 98(12):1198–1204.

137. Keli SO et al. Dietary flavonoids, antioxidant vitamins, and incidence of stroke: the Zutphen study. *Arch Intern Med* 1996; 156(6):637–42.

138. Ascherio A et al. Relation of consumption of vitamin E, vitamin C, and carotenoids to risk for stroke among men in the United States. *Ann Intern Med* 1999; 130(12):963–70.

139. Steiner M et al. Vitamin E plus aspirin compared with aspirin alone in patients with transient ischemic attacks. *Am J Clin Nutr* 1995; 62(6 Suppl):1381S–1384S.

140. Eckmann F. Cerebral insufficiency—treatment with *Ginkgo biloba* extract. Time of onset of effect in a double-blind study with 60 inpatients. *Fortschr Med* 1990; 108(29):557–60.

141. Kjendahl A et al. A one-year follow-up study on the effects of acupuncture in the treatment of stroke patients in the subacute stage: a randomized, controlled study. *Clin Rehabil* 1997; 11(3):192–200.

142. Ahrens RA et al. Moderate sucrose ingestion and blood pressure in the rat. *J Nutrition* 1980; 110(4):725–31.

143. Hodges RE et al. Carbohydrates and blood pressure. *Ann Intern Med* 1983; 98(2, part 2):838–41.

144. Krishna GG et al. Increased blood pressure during potassium depletion in normotensive men. *N Engl J Med* 1989; 320(18): 1177–82.

145. Witteman JC et al. A prospective study of nutritional factors and hypertension among US women. *Circulation* 1989; 80(5): 1320–7.

146. Alderman MH et al. Low urinary sodium is associated with greater risk of myocardial infarction among treated hypertensive men. *Hypertension* 1995; 25(6):1144–52.

147. Fujita T et al. Effects of increased adrenomedullary activity and taurine in young patients with borderline hypertension. *Circulation* 1987; 75(3):525–32.

148. Gay LP. Nonreaginic food allergy in the management of essential hypertension. *J Appl Nutr* 1959; 12(2):71–4.

149. Glauser SC et al. Blood-cadmium levels in normotensive and untreated hypertensive humans. *Lancet* 1976; 1(7962):717–18.

150. Pirkle JL et al. The relationship between blood lead levels and blood pressure and its cardiovascular risk implications. *Am J Epidemiol* 1985; 121(2):246–58.

151. Dickey LD. Presenting, reproduced, induced, and relieved symptoms observed with provocative tests. In L D Dickey, ed. *Clinical Ecology*. Springfield, IL: Thomas, 1976; Chapt. 11:152–4.

152. Blair SN et al. Physical fitness and incidence of hypertension in healthy normotensive men and women. *JAMA* 1984; 252(4):487–90.

153. Grossman P et al. Blood pressure responses to mental stress in emotionally defensive patients with stable coronary artery disease. *Am J Cardiol* 1997; 80(3):343–6.

154. Harberg E et al. Socioecological stressor areas and black-white blood pressure: Detroit. *J Chron Dis* 1973; 26(9):595–611.

155. Shapiro D et al. Daily mood states and ambulatory blood pressure. *Psychophysiology* 1997; 34(4):399–405.

156. Staessen JA et al. Antihypertensive treatment based on conventional or ambulatory blood pressure measurement. *JAMA* 1997; 278(13):1065–72.

157. Helgeland A et al. Treatment of mild hypertension: a five year controlled drug trial. The Oslo study. *Am J Med* 1980; 69(5):725–32.

158. Miettinen TA et al. Multifactorial primary prevention of cardiovascular diseases in middle-aged men. Risk factor changes, incidence, and mortality. *JAMA* 1985; 254(15):2097–2102.

159. Anonymous. Multiple Risk Factor Intervention Trial Research Group. Risk factor changes and mortality results. *JAMA* 1982; 248(12):1465–77.

160. Mountokalakis T et al. Diuretic-induced zinc deficiency in mild hypertension. *J Am Coll Nutr* 1985; 4(3):354 abstr # 92.

161. Pahor M et al. Risk of gastrointestinal haemorrhage with calcium antagonists in hypertensive persons over 67 years old. *Lancet* 1996; 347(9008):1061–5.

162. Galley HF et al. Combination oral antioxidant supplementation reduces blood pressure. *Clin Sci (Colch)* 1997; 92(4):361–5.
163. Rao RH et al. Effect of polyunsaturate-rich vegetable oils on blood pressure in essential hypertension. *Clin Exp Hypertens* 1981; 3(1):27–38.
164. Stamler R et al. Nutritional therapy for high blood pressure. Final report of a four-year randomized controlled trial—the Hypertension Control Program. *JAMA* 1987; 257(11):1484–91.
165. Criqui MH et al. Multivariate correlates of adult blood pressures in nine North American populations: The Lipid Research Clinics Prevalence Study. *Prev Med* 1982; 11(4):391–402.
166. Levenson J et al. Cigarette smoking and hypertension. Factors independently associated with blood hyperviscosity and arterial rigidity. *Arteriosclerosis* 1987; 7(6):572–7.
167. Appel LJ et al. A clinical trial of the effects of dietary patterns on blood pressure. DASH Collaborative Research Group. *N Engl J Med* 1997; 336(16):1117–24.
168. Margetts BM et al. Vegetarian diet in mild hypertension: a randomised controlled trial. *Br Med J (Clin Res Ed)* 1986; 293(6560): 1468–71.
169. Hodges RE et al. Carbohydrates and blood pressure. *Ann Intern Med* 1983; 98(2 part 2):838–41.
170. Grimsgaard S, Bonaa KH, Jacobsen BK, Bjerve K. Plasma saturated and linoleic fatty acids are independently associated with blood pressure. *Hypertension* 1999; 34(3):478–83.
171. Ascherio A et al. A prospective study of nutritional factors and hypertension among US men. *Circulation* 1992; 86(5): 1475–84.
172. Bates CJ et al. Does vitamin C reduce blood pressure? Results of a large study of people aged 65 or older. *J Hypertens* 1998; 16(7):925–32.
173. Wynn A, Wynn M. Magnesium and other nutrient deficiencies as possible causes of hypertension and low birthweight. *Nutr Health* 1988; 6(2):69–88.
174. Ayback M et al. Effect of oral pyridoxine hydrochloride supplementation on arterial blood pressure in patients with essential hypertension. *Arzneimittelforschung* 1995; 45:1271–3.
175. Passfall J et al. Different effects of eicosapentaenoic acid and olive oil on blood pressure, intracellular free platelet calcium,

and plasma lipids in patients with essential hypertension. *Clin Investig* 1993; 71(8):628–33.

176. Fujita T et al. Effects of increased adrenomedullary activity and taurine in young patients with borderline hypertension. *Circulation* 1987; 75(3):525–32.

177. Digiesi V et al. Coenzyme Q10 in essential hypertension. *Mol Aspects Med* 1994; 15 Suppl:S257–63.

178. Anonymous. National High Blood Pressure Education Program Working Group report on primary prevention of hypertension. *Arch Intern Med* 1993; 153(2):186–208.

179. Ammon HP et al. *Crataegus*, toxicology and pharmacology. Part III: Pharmacodynamics and pharmacokinetics. *Planta Med* 1981; 43(4):313–22.

180. Petkov V. Plants and hypotensive, antiatheromatous and coronarodilatating action. *Am J Chin Med* 1979; 7(3):197–236.

181. Patel C. 12-month follow-up of yoga and bio-feedback in the management of hypertension. *Lancet* 1975;1(7898):62–4.

182. McGrady A et al. Effect of biofeedback-assisted relaxation on blood pressure and cortisol levels in normotensives and hypertensives. *J Behav Med* 1987; 10(3):301–10.

183. Deabler HL et al. The use of relaxation and hypnosis in lowering high blood pressure. *Am J Clin Hypn* 1973; 16(2):75–83.

184. Schneider RH et al. A randomised controlled trial of stress reduction for hypertension in older African Americans. *Hypertension* 1995; 26(5):820–7.

185. Kuang AK et al. Long-term observation on qigong in prevention of stroke—follow-up of 244 hypertensive patients for 18–22 years. *J Tradit Chin Med* 1986; 6(4):235–8.

186. Anonymous. Untreated mild hypertension. A report by the Management Committee of the Australian Therapeutic Trial in Mild Hypertension. *Lancet* 1982; 1(8265):185–91.

187. Anderson WP, Reid CM, Jennings GL. Pet ownership and risk-factors for cardiovascular disease. *Med J Aust* 1992; 157(5):298–301.

188. Miller RN. Study on the effectiveness of remote mental healing. *Med Hypotheses* 1982; 8(5):481–90.

189. Anderson R. Pharmacologic treatment of congestive heart failure. *JAMA* 1995; 273(19):1491–2.

190. The SOLVD Investigators. Effect of enalapril on survival of patients with reduced left ventricular ejection fractions and congestive heart failure. *N Engl J Med* 1991; 325(5):293–302.

191. Seelig MS. Adverse stress reactions and magnesium deficiency: preventive and therapeutic implications. *J Am Coll Nutr* 1992; 11(5):609 abstr 40.

192. Dorup I et al. Oral magnesium supplementation restores the concentrations of magnesium, potassium and sodium-potassium pumps in skeletal muscle of patients receiving diuretic treatment. *J Intern Med* 1993; 233(2):117–23.

193. Khedun SM et al. Zinc, hydrochlorothiazide and sexual dysfunction. *Cent Afr J Med* 1995; 41(10):312–15.

194. Chen L et al. Electron spin resonance determination and superoxide dismutase activity in polymorphonuclear leukocytes in congestive heart failure. *Can J Cardiol* 1992; 8(7):756–60.

195. Kalra J et al. Oxygen free radicals and cardiac depression. *Clin Biochem* 1994; 27(3):163–8.

196. Mortensen SA. Perspectives on therapy of cardiovascular diseases with coenzyme Q10 (ubiquinone). *Clin Investig* 1993; 71(8 Suppl):S116–23.

197. Sturman JA. Taurine in development. *Physiol Rev.* 1993; 73(1): 119–47.

198. Kobayashi A et al. L-carnitine treatment for congestive heart failure—experimental and clinical study. *Jpn Circ J* 1992; 55(1):85–94.

199. Regitz V et al. Defective myocardial carnitine metabolism in congestive heart failure secondary to dilated cardiomyopathy and to coronary, hypertensive and valvular heart diseases. *Am J Cardiol* 1990; 55(11):755–60.

200. Santos AD et al. Echocardiographic characterization of the reversible cardiomyopathy of hypothyroidism. *Am J Med* 1980; 68(5):675–82.

201. Morris RD et al. Carbon monoxide and hospital admissions for congestive heart failure: evidence of an increased effect at low temperatures. *Environ Health Perspect* 1998; 106(10): 649–53.

202. Davies DF et al. Food antibodies and myocardial infarction. *Lancet* 1974; 1(7865):1012–14.

203. Ironson G et al. Effects of anger on left ventricular ejection fraction in coronary artery disease. *Am J Cardiol* 1992; 70(3):281–5.
204. Middlekauff HR et al. Impact of acute mental stress on sympathetic nerve activity and regional blood flow in advanced heart failure: implications for 'triggering' adverse cardiac events. *Circulation* 1997; 96(6):1835–42.
205. Denollet J et al. Personality, disease severity, and the risk of long-term cardiac events in patients with a decreased ejection fraction after myocardial infarction. *Circulation* 1998; 97(2):167–73.
206. Mills RM et al. Sustained hemodynamic effects of an infusion of nesirtide (human b-type natiuretic peptide) in heart failure. *J Am Coll Cardiol* 1999; 34(8):155–62.
207. Kolata G. Heart study produces a surprise result. *Science* 1982; 218(4567):31–2.
208. Adler Y et al. Colchicine treatment for recurrent pericarditis. A decade of experience. *Circulation* 1998; 97(21):2183–5.
209. Ghatak A et al. Oxy free radical system in heart failure and therapeutic role of oral vitamin E. *Int J Cardiol* 1996; 57(2):119–27.
210. Rasmussen HS et al. Hemodynamic effects of intravenously administered magnesium on patients with ischemic heart disease. *Clin Cardiol* 1988; 11(12):824–8.
211. Shimon I et al. Improved left ventricular function after thiamine supplementation in patients with congestive heart failure receiving long-term furosemide therapy. *Am J Med* 1995; 98(5):485–90.
212. McCarty MF. Fish oil and other nutritional adjuvants for treatment of congestive heart failure. *Med Hypotheses* 1996; 46(4):400–6.
213. Azuma J, Hasegawa H, Sawamura A et al. Therapy of congestive heart failure with orally administered taurine. *Clin Ther* 1983; 5(4):398–408.
214. Corbucci GG et al. L-carnitine in cardiogenic shock therapy: pharmacodynamic aspects and clinical data. *Int J Clin Pharmacol Res* 1993; 13(2):87–91.
215. Cacciatore L et al. The therapeutic effect of L-carnitine in patients with exercise-induced stable angina: a controlled study. *Drugs Exptl Clin Res* 1991; 17(4):225–35.
216. Anand I et al. Acute and chronic effects of propionyl-L-carnitine on the hemodynamics, exercise capacity and hormones in

patients with congestive heart failure. *Cardiovasc Drugs Ther* 1998; 12(3):291–9.

217. Langsjoen PH et al. Long-term efficacy and safety of coenzyme Q10 therapy for idiopathic dilated cardiomyopathy. *Am J Cardiol* 1990; 65(7):521–3.

218. Munkholm H et al. Coenzyme Q10 treatment in serious heart failure. *Biofactors* 1999; 9(2-4):285–9.

219. Langsjoen PH et al. Pronounced increase of survival of patients with cardiomyopathy when treated with coenzyme Q10 and conventional therapy. *Int J Tissue React* 1990; 12(3):163–8.

220. Baggio E et al. Italian multicenter study on the safety and efficacy of coenzyme Q10 as adjunctive therapy in heart failure (interim analysis). The CoQ10 Drug Surveillance Investigators. *Clin Investig* 1993; 71(8 Suppl):S145–9.

221. Watson PS, Scalia GM, Galbraith A et al. Lack of effect of coenzyme Q on left ventricular function in patients with congestive heart failure. *J Am Coll Cardiol* 1999; 33(6):1549–52.

222. Biondi B et al. Impaired cardiac reserve and exercise capacity in patients receiving long-term thyrotropin suppressive therapy with levothyroxine. *J Clin Endocrinol Metab.* 1996; 81(12): 4224–8.

223. Tei C et al. Acute hemodynamic improvement by thermal vasodilation in congestive heart failure. *Circulation* 1995; 91(10): 2582–90.

224. Chen LX et al. Effects of Astragalus membranaceus on left ventricular function and oxygen free radicals in acute myocardial infarction patients and mechanism of its cardiotonic action. *Chung Kuo Chung His I Chieh Ho Tsa Chih* 1995; 15(3):141–3.

225. Leuchtgens H. *Crataegus* special extract WS 1442 in NYHA II heart failure. A placebo controlled, randomized, double-blind study. *Fortschr Med* 1993; 111(20–1):352–4.

226. Weihmayr T et al. Therapeutic effectiveness of *Crataegus*. *Fortschr Med* 1996; 114(1–2):27–9.

227. Chen HC et al. Hemodynamic effects of orally administered Sunitang in humans. *Clin Pharmacol Ther* 1987; 41(5):496–501.

228. Bharani A et al. Salutary effect of *Terminalia arjuna* in patients with severe refractory heart failure. *Int J Cardiol* 1995; 49(3):191–9.

229. Wielenga RP et al. Effect of exercise training on quality of life in patients with chronic failure. *J Psychosom Res* 1998; 45(5): 459–64.
230. Moser DK et al. Voluntary control of vascular tone by using skin-temperature biofeedback-relaxation in patients with advanced heart failure. *Altern Ther Health Med* 1997; 3(1):51–9.
231. Lynch JJ. Decoding the language of the heart: developing a physiology of inclusion. *Integr Physiol Behav Sci* 1998; 33(2):130–6.

3
Chapter Three

Cancer

■ DESCRIPTION

The term cancer encompasses the variety of malignancies affecting humans of all ages. Cancer is a distorted, wild, uncontrolled growth of specific cells which multiply rapidly without restraint, producing a family of descendents which invade and destroy the structure and function of adjacent normal tissues in the organ from which the growth originated. Cancerous cells can migrate through the blood stream or lymph channels to metastasize and compromise the function of organs to which it has spread. The initiatory phase of cancerous growth is triggered by a distortion in the DNA command apparatus of cell nuclei. Many authorities believe that human beings in a single lifetime experience cancer repeatedly, and that on most occasions the immune cellular and chemical defenses defeat the microscopic cancer so quickly that symptoms never make themselves known. Many think that more attention should be directed to the state of the immune system, which, for a variety of reasons, occasionally fails to recognize and target these early growths for destruction before they can become a threat. Damage to DNA in cell nuclei from free oxygen radical proliferation appears to play a key role in initiatory and promotional phases of cancer.

The classical warning symptoms of cancer are:

- Appearance of a new, palpable, growing dermal, subcutaneous, breast, or genital, lump.

- Sudden appearance of lymphadenopathy, most easily palpated in the inguinal, axillary, and neck areas.
- Appearance of unexplained bleeding from the mouth, throat, lungs, bladder, vagina, rectum, or skin lesion.
- Noticeable change in size, pigmentation or shape of a birthmark, mole, or skin blemish.
- Noticeable change in function of a major organ; e.g. unusually persistent diarrhea, constipation, dysphagia, or cough.
- Fatigue of new onset or unexplained weight loss.

■ PREVALENCE

Cancer is a very common in industrialized nations, and is currently responsible for nearly a million deaths each year in the United States. This represents 20 percent of all deaths. Some 1 million new cases are diagnosed yearly. The incidence of cancer has risen 60-fold since 1800, and the risk of cancer for men born in the 1950s is 3-fold higher than it was for men born in the 1880s. Since 1958 alone, the incidence of cancer in men has increased 55 percent. The curve of cancer incidence rises steeply after the age of 60. Prostate cancer is responsible for over 40,000 deaths annually and breast cancer for about the same number. Nearly 1 of every 5 American men will develop prostate cancer in his lifetime and breast cancer will strike 1 out of 9 women. About 20 percent of enlarged prostates are the result of cancer.

However, the SEER (Surveillance, Epidemiology and End Results) report of the 1990–1995 5-year cycle found a 2.6 percent *decline* in cancer mortality, and the National Cancer Institute found similar changes, and a drop of 8.7 percent in those under 65.[1] Mortality in white women with breast cancer increased 0.5 percent annually between 1980 and 1988, and declined 1.6 percent annually from 1989 through 1992, with further declines since. Mortality in black women with breast cancer increased 2 percent per year from 1980 to 1988; the increases slowed to 0.5 percent per year from 1989 to 1992. It may be cautiously assumed that the long increase in cancer incidence has passed its peak.

■ ETIOLOGY AND RISK FACTORS

The incidence of some cancers has a clear hereditary influence, among them are lung and breast cancer.

Dietary and nutritional influences are thought to cause 60 percent of all cancers in women and 40 percent in men. Both carcinogenic substances in the diet, as well as lack of cancer anti-carcinogenic chemicals in foods play important roles. High fat intake including ingestion of large amounts of oxidized fats (those in the process of becoming rancid) are a source of increased free radicals which promote DNA damage. The fat of animal meats also contains hyperconcentrated lipophilic pesticides that also contribute to the incidence of cancer. Studies show total cancer incidence to be positively related to total fat intake. A significant inverse relationship between high polyunsaturated fat intake and the incidence of malignant melanoma is apparent.[2] In a Swiss study, the calculated odds ratio for colon cancer increased 30 percent for each daily serving of refined grains, and 50 percent for each daily serving of red meat.[3]

The highest intakes of sugar are associated with a 4-fold excess risk for cancer of the gall bladder,[4] and high intake of sugar has been linked in epidemiological studies to a markedly increased risk of breast cancer.[5] Cancer of the colon is linked to high sugar intake and deficiency of folic acid. Many studies have found deficiency of fiber is directly related to increased risk of colon and rectal cancers, although one recent study found no relationship. Excess iron has been linked to the development of malignancies, including liver cancer. The odds for prostate cancer in men in the highest quintile of plasma lycopene was 60 percent below that of men in the lowest quintile, with an even stronger inverse association for aggressive prostate cancers.[6] A 1988 study showed that men with low levels of vitamin A were 3 times more likely to develop prostate cancer compared to men with high levels.[7]

Coenzyme Q10 tissue levels are significantly lower in malignant breast biopsy specimens compared to benign ones. Hormones clearly influence breast, endometrial, and prostate cancer. In premenopausal women, DHEA levels are about 10 percent lower in women who subsequently develop breast cancer. High levels of the phytoestrogens equol and enterolactone are associated with a lower risk for breast cancer. They are high in soy-containing foods.

Not all cancerogenic substances are man-made. Carcinogenic psoralen compounds naturally occur in celery, parsnips, figs, and parsley. If mold growth has been encountered, aflatoxins accumulate in seeds, nuts and grains (associated with liver cancer), and cottonseed products contain a carcinogen.

Air pollution elements including particulates, ozone, pesticides, herbicides, fungicides, petrochemicals, and heavy metals all harbor carcinogenic potential. Exposure to petrochemicals, burned diesel fuel exhaust and cyclic and halogenated hydrocarbons result in free radical damage to DNA and lead to cancer formation. Industrial chemicals, including heavy metals (lead, mercury, cadmium, arsenic), solvents (e.g. benzene), chrome and nickel ores, vinyl chloride, asbestos, chlorophenols, and bischloromethylether are cancerogenic. Other carcinogenic chemical sources are defoliants (Agent Orange in Vietnam), coal-tar derivatives in paints, food additives, and nitrosamines from nitrates in cosmetics and in food as preservatives. Chronic use of hair dyes also contributes to the incidence of cancer. Chlorinated hydrocarbons in polluted sources of drinking water raise the all-cancer risk mainly because of the 21 percent increased risk for bladder cancer and 38 percent for rectal cancer.[8] Nations and indigenous tribes with low toxic chemical use and whole food diets have an astonishingly low incidence of cancers.

Cancer risk is increased by exposure to gamma radiation, including nuclear plant workers, those living down-wind from nuclear test sites, and those exposed to diagnostic and therapeutic X-rays. Adults who as children were exposed to X-ray for shrinking adenoids and thymus glands and for treatment of ringworm of the scalp in the era of 1930–1960 have a higher incidence of later leukemia and 4-fold higher risk of thyroid cancer and women have a 2-fold higher risk of breast cancer.[9]

Electromagnetic field exposure appears in some studies to increase risks of some cancers including breast,[10] and there is some evidence for higher incidences of cancer of the head and neck with long-term use of electric shavers. The risk of childhood leukemia in a large Swedish study was very modestly but definitely increased in families living near cross-country high-voltage power transmission lines; other studies have not confirmed this risk. Years of exposure to indoor fluorescent lighting appear to significantly increase the risk of melanoma.[11]

Skin cancer incidence is greatly increased in Caucasians and Asians with histories of long-term ultraviolet exposure, particularly with a history of deep tans and severe sunburns.

Certain drugs appear to enhance the risk for initiation and promotion of cancers. In laboratory rats, Prozac and amitriptyline, given at doses equivalent to therapeutic doses in humans, accelerate the growth of deliberately injected melanomas. When a cancerogenic chemical was administered to laboratory rodents, 20 of 21 given concomitant Prozac and/or amitriptyline developed breast cancers at 15 weeks compared to 4 of 7 animals given placebos.[12]

Antihistamines promote growth of cancers in laboratory animals. In mice, after injection of cancerogenic agents, clear acceleration of sarcoma growth occurred in animals injected with Claritin and Hismanal, and acceleration of melanomas in animals injected with Atarax or Vistaril. These drugs appear to accelerate growth of existing cancers. Among hypolipidemic drugs, the fibrates (e.g., clofibrate) and the statins cause cancer in rodents at levels of exposure close to comparable treatment levels in humans. There are no conclusive human data because of inconsistent and conflicting conclusions and insufficient duration of follow-up. Caution, therefore, is advised in prescribing cholesterol-lowering drugs. Medical editorials have pointed out the significant increased risk of dying with cancer in patients treated by drugs to lower cholesterol (see Chapter 2). Strong positive relationships have been found as well between use of antihypertensive and sedative-hypnotic drugs and the incidence of colon cancer.[13] Chemicals used in chemotherapy for cancer carry a recognizable risk for creating secondary cancers, often years or decades later.

Deleterious personal habits play enormous roles in cancer. Smoking and tobacco significantly increase risks of cancer of the larynx, lung, breast, oral cavity, stomach, esophagus, pancreas, bladder, kidney, cervix, penis, and lymphoma and leukemia by 20 to 2,500 percent. Smoking causes 35 percent of all cancers and 85 percent of lung cancer. In 1997, 175,000 deaths were attributable to smoking and tobacco use. Passive smoking increases the risk of many of the same cancers. Consistent drinking of alcohol increases several-fold the risk of cancers of the mouth, tongue, throat, esophagus, larynx, stomach, liver, colon, rectum, pancreas, breast, and malignant melanoma. 19,000 deaths annually are related to alcohol use. Overweight and frank obesity increase cancer risk; the risk of colon cancer in men with a 43 in. waist is $2\frac{1}{2}$ times the risk in men with a waist measure of 35 in.

Physical deconditioning and lack of exercise play very significant promotional roles in cancer. Authorities estimate that the most active group of men compared to the most sedentary have a reduced all-cancer risk 75 percent lower, with the estimation for women at 45 percent.[14] Cancers best studied for the preventive importance of exercise are carcinoma of the breast, uterus, ovaries, colon, and possibly prostate.

Prospective studies show increases in cancer in persons under chronic, excessive, unmanaged stress, and in persons after acutely stressful events, such as the death of a spouse. In several studies, the manner in which patients cope with stress has been correlated with cancer mortality and cancer progression. Stress decreases antibody formation, interferon synthesis, mitogen-stimulated lymphocyte proliferation, and natural killer (NK) cell cytotoxicity. NK cells are essential in controlling cancers. In animals, stress accelerates tumor initiation, growth, and spread. In one study, NK cell cytotoxicity was suppressed 45 percent in stressed animals compared to controls.[15] Stressed animals have twice as many metastases as controls.

In animals stressed 1 hour before tumor cell injection, a 5-fold increase in metastases was found, compared to unstressed controls.

Two stress studies in humans are illustrative. In women undergoing breast biopsy for suspicious lesions, the level of stress was assessed before the results of the biopsy were known. The chance that a biopsy would be reported back malignant was *15-fold greater* in women who were under severely threatening life events compared to those facing mild to moderate stress.[16] A second study found the risk for recurrence of breast cancer in treated cases was *9-fold greater* in those facing severe rather than mild to moderate stress.[17] Although a recent report discounts the importance of depression, a large number of previous studies have noticed the consistent significant relationship of depression, helplessness, and hopelessness to the onset of various cancers. Depressed patients have a much lower incidence of successful bone marrow transplant survival than non-depressed patients.[18] Patients who express their emotions in socially acceptable ways rather than repressing them and who believe that a lesser amount of adjustment will be necessary to cope with their disease consistently do better.

A widely criticized European study of 2,000 persons spanning over 20 years concluded that suppression of emotion and inability to cope with interpersonal stress lead to hopelessness and helplessness, predisposing to cancer.[19] Behavioral stress management can reduce these risks for development of cancer.

Perceptive observations by those doing interpersonal work with cancer patients sense that cancer is a disease linked to negative emotions of fear, guilt, self-hate, or self-denial; unfinished business with others with whom the patient has had a significant relationship; and resistance to change. These issues cause major resistances to the evolution of emotional, psychological, and spiritual development.[20]

A 30-year study of 1,500 medical students at Johns Hopkins University revealed that the strongest predictor of cancer over the next 25 years was the perception of lack of closeness with parents in childhood.[21]

■ CONVENTIONAL TREATMENT

Following preliminary diagnosis by taking of a history, performing a physical examination and obtaining certain laboratory tests and X-rays, the definitive diagnosis of a cancer rests on obtaining a biopsy. Following the histological diagnosis, surgical excision of the entire tumor mass, or at least most of it, is undertaken. Beside the very small operative mortality with major surgery, long-term postoperative complications include such phenomena as lymphedema of the upper extremity after axillary lymph node dissection for breast cancer, incontinence and impotence after prostate surgery, and vocal cord paralysis after thyroid surgery.

Many patients at this juncture are then advised to undertake further therapy to destroy the remainder of the tumor or prevent recurrence from tiny amounts of tumor unknowingly left behind at surgery. Chemotherapy with various combinations of cytotoxic agents is used to attempt to destroy cancerous tissues manifesting uncontrolled growth. Chemotherapy is highly successful in Hodgkins lymphoma, certain testicular and kidney cancers and childhood leukemias. On the other hand, 70 percent of women with breast cancer whose lymph nodes are negative at the time of surgery are cured without chemotherapy. The record of success for prolongation of life and improvement in quality of life is heterogeneous. Generally, the record for survival in many chemotherapy regimens is not a lot better than survival in persons who reject conventional treatment. John Cairns of the Harvard School of Public Health concluded in 1985 that only about 2–3 percent of those dying with cancer had derived any benefit from chemotherapy.[22] Chemotherapy, of course, is toxic to all rapidly replicating cells, including those of the immune system. This limits the effectiveness and potential for chemicals to destroy all cancer cells. Many combinations of chemotherapeutic drugs cause side effects including nausea, loss of appetite, diarrhea, weight loss, hair loss, and fatigue. An additional hazard is the appearance of secondary cancers later in life, arising from the free-radical damage from the original chemotherapeutic and radiation.

Radiation, in the form of X-ray and radioactive isotope exposure, is used to destroy localized areas of remaining cancer.

Radiation, too, has side effects of inflammation in surrounding normal tissues, diarrhea when the bowel is exposed, and degrees of nausea, loss of appetite, and fatigue. In some types of cancer including leukemia, and breast cancer, radiation is used to destroy the bone marrow, after which the patient is given a bone marrow transplant. Immune suppressants are then necessary to avoid rejection of the transplanted bone marrow.

Newer techniques used in certain cancers involve the use of vaccines and tagged antibodies made from tumor tissue itself. Conventional treatment also now encompasses chemoprevention (e.g., Tamoxifen or raloxifene for women with and at high risk for breast cancer). Four year disease-free survival in advanced melanoma patients, treated with a vaccine from irradiated, cultured melanoma cells harvested from lymph node biopsies, has been reported to more than double survival compared to routine treatment. Similar work is proceeding with vaccines in lymphomas.

In 1992, both the National Cancer Institute and the American Cancer Society held press conferences announcing a change in policy which shifted interest and research funding in the direction of prevention, with emphasis on nutrition. There has been a profuse outpouring of published data relating nutrition to cancer since that time. This is highlighted in the Holistic Treatment of Cancer in following sections. At the same time that this change of emphasis in cancer research was announced, these groups declared that the highly touted and extremely expensive "war on cancer" had been lost. The emphasis on that research and clinical application was on surgery, chemotherapy and radiation, which continue to be the mainstays of conventional cancer management.

■ HOLISTIC TREATMENT

Preventive Measures

Negative nutritional practices to be discouraged in order to affect a decrease in cancer incidence include reduction of fats, particularly oxidized and hydrogenated fats, sugars, and low-fiber dietary content.

Authorities, including the National Cancer Institute and the American Society, are increasingly supportive of the potential for decreasing the risk of malignancy through positive changes, including consumption of increased amounts of fruits, vegetables, fiber and antioxidants, discussed below. Besides the evidence for decreased risk with these foods, hundreds of phytochemicals are being found to have cancer-protective properties as well, including limonene in citrus fruits; allyl sulfides in garlic, onion, leeks and chives; dithiolthiones in broccoli; isothiocyanates from cabbage, cauliflower, kale, Brussels sprouts, broccoli sprouts, collard and other cruciferous vegetables; ellagic acid in grapes; protease inhibitors, phytosterols, isoflavones and saponins in soybeans; caffeic acid found in coffee; ferulic acid (gamma oryzanol) in various grains; phytic acid in grains; glycosinolates in broccoli sprouts; and indulges in a variety of vegetables.

In China and Japan, where low-fat diets high in vegetables and fish are the norm, the incidence of prostate cancer is extremely low. Prostate-cancer rates for first- and second-generation Japanese Americans, on the other hand, are considerably higher than in Japan, probably related to their adoption of an "American" diet. Mounting evidence supports the relationship of high antioxidant intake in food and supplements with a decreased risk of malignancy. In men, for instance, a diet high in vitamin C and dark green vegetables leads to 60 percent reduction in the risk of cancer of the bladder.[23] Protective effects against the risk of brain tumors has been found in children whose mothers' diet in pregnancy had been highest in fruits and fruit juice, vegetables, and vitamins A and C.[24] Incidence of skin cancers was significantly lower in persons with greater intake of foods high in: fish; vegetables in general; beans, lentils, peas, carrots, Swiss chard, pumpkin, and cruciferous vegetables.

The Mediterranean diet is thought to reduce the risk of cancer as well as heart disease. In 600 patients in the Lyon study, the risks of total mortality and cancer deaths were reduced 56 and 61 percent, respectively, compared to controls. The intake of fruits, vegetables, cereals, saturated fat, polyunsaturated fat, and cholesterol were significantly lower and oleic acid and omega-3 fatty acids significantly higher in Mediterranean subjects. Plasma levels of vitamins C and E and omega-3 fatty acids were significantly higher and omega-6 fatty acids significantly lower.[25]

High intake of fruits and vegetables reduced risk of breast cancer 25 percent in premenopausal women; in women who had a positive family history the reduction was 70 percent.[26] The risk for cancers of the mouth/pharynx, esophagus, stomach, colon, and rectum was reduced 30–60% in those with high tomato intake. Tomatoes are high in content of the carotenoid lycopene and low in β-carotene.[27] In a study of 2,500 people, intake of foods with the highest intakes of vitamin C, beta carotene and vitamin A, the risk of lung cancer was reduced 35, 16 and 36 percent, respectively.[28]

Evidence is strong for a 50 percent reduction in the incidence of esophageal cancer in green tea drinkers; it is modest for reduction of gastric, lung, pancreatic, colon, and prostatic cancer.[29] In men with the highest intake of onions, the risk for stomach cancer was 50 percent lower than the risk for those with the lowest onion intake.[30] Inositol hexaphosphate (phytic acid) found in cereals and legumes has anti-carcinogenic properties. This may explain the benefits of high-fiber diets in certain cancers. Soy intake reduces risk and iron intake appears to increase risk for primary liver cancer.

Quercitin, ellagic acid, chlorogenic acid, and genistein, potent antioxidant flavones found in a variety of fruits and vegetables, reduce the bioavailability of cancer-causing substances in laboratory rats and appear helpful in humans as well.

Examples of the benefits of taking micronutrients in the form of supplements follow. In 29,600 Chinese, taking supplements of beta carotene, vitamin E, and selenium significantly reduced the incidence of esophageal and stomach cancer compared to those not on supplements.[31] Taking multivitamin/mineral supplements any time in pregnancy confers a reduced risk for cancer in the offspring; iron, calcium, and vitamin C seem to be most important. The relative risk for dying of stomach cancer appears to be reduced by 25 percent in those with a high intake of vitamin C compared with low intake.[32]

29,000 heavy smoking Finnish males receiving β-carotene 20 mg/day had a death rate 15 percent *higher* than those not taking β-carotene.[33] While the disparity between this result and those of epidemiological trials is not wholly clear, it may be that, since β-carotene and other carotenoids compete for assimilation, the others (lycopene and lutein) are more important than β-carotene in cancer prevention.[34] β-carotene supplements should always be combined with adequate food intake of other carotenoids or a supplement of mixed carotenoids. Subjects with the highest β-carotene levels have a lower risk of mouth cancer than those with the lowest intakes. Mean vitamin A levels are significantly lower in cancer patients compared to healthy subjects.

Men with the highest vitamin E levels had a two-thirds lower risk for melanoma compared to those with lowest intakes, and those with the highest zinc intake had a 50 percent lower risk.

Long-term use of folic acid supplements at 0.4–5.0 mg/day reduced colon cancer 75 percent in a large Harvard women's study compared to those taking no supplements.[35] In a placebo-controlled trial, daily intake of 200 µg of selenium for 7 years reduced total cancer mortality 51 percent compared to placebo; the selenium group experienced a 41 percent reduction in new global cancer incidence, 63 percent reduction in colon cancer, and 70 percent reduction in prostate cancer.[36] A strong association between decreased selenium and oxidative stress was found in patients with breast cancer. Adequate selenium is crucial for synthesis of glutathione peroxidase, an essential endogenous antioxidant enzyme.[37] High selenium intake reduces risk for precancerous colon polyps 75 percent, and selenium blood levels in healthy people are much higher than in melanoma patients.

The use of filtering devices for drinking and cooking water removes the previously mentioned carcinogenic halogenated hydrocarbons.

Within the framework of practicality, working with patients to reduce environmental hazards is obviously wise. Possible initiatives include: challenging smokers to abate their habit; advising the modification of alcohol intake to one drink or less daily; consuming nuts that have been roasted (destroys carcinogenic aflatoxins); reducing air pollution in the home with electronic air filters, HEPA filters, and a negative air ion generator; reducing carcinogenic, halogenated hydrocarbons and heavy metals in drinking and cooking water with a good water filter; avoiding excessive sun exposure, utilizing sunscreens, hats, caps, and long sleeves; avoiding the personal use of pesticides and herbicides as much as possible, and washing carefully when handling petrochemicals and solvents; stopping the use of hair dyes, if used; using full-spectrum fluorescent tubes in light fixtures at work and home; avoiding agricultural areas during pesticide spraying times; moving at the earliest convenient opportunity from a residence within one-half block of high-tension power lines; reducing close exposure to electromagnetic fields—electric clocks, microwaves, television, and video screens; and turning on electric blankets before bedtime, and off at bedtime. Health professionals can limit diagnostic X-rays to those in which the result will make a difference in treatment, and review the carcinogenicity of pharmaceuticals, switching or reducing those that are not absolutely necessary.

Patients can be advised to buy and consume organic produce if possible (see Table 3-1 for the accompanying list of the foods with highest pesticide content and best substitutes).[38]

Walking an hour daily reduces risk of colon and rectal cancer 50 percent compared to sedentary people.[39] As previously mentioned, consistent high-intensity physical activity reduces cancer risk 75 percent in men and 45 percent in women! Intense activity in these studies meant running more than 4 hours or walking more than 12 hours each week.

Herbal research has contributed additional options. A very recent Korean study showed significant reduction in all-cancer incidence in regular Panax ginseng users; the greatest differences were for stomach and lung cancer.[40] Phytoestrogens in soy and other foods occupy the same estrogen receptor sites as the powerful estrogens used in hormone replacement therapy for

TABLE 3-1. FOODS WITH THE HIGHEST PESTICIDE CONTENT AND THE BEST ALTERNATIVE FOODS

High contamination	Best alternatives
Strawberries	Blackberries, blueberries, cantaloupe (US), kiwi, grapefruit, kiwi, oranges, raspberries, watermelon
Bell peppers, green/red	Broccoli, romaine lettuce, peas, asparagus, broccoli, Brussels sprouts, carrots, rtomatoes
Spinach	Asparagus, broccoli, Brussels sprouts, romaine lettuce
Cherries (US)	Blackberries, blueberries, cantaloupe (US), grapefruit, kiwi, oranges, raspberries
Peaches	Cantaloupe (US), red/pink grapefruit, nectarines, oranges, tangerines, watermelon
Cantaloupe (Mexican)	Cantaloupe (US), watermelon
Celery	Broccoli, carrots, romaine lettuce, radishes
Apples	Bananas, cantaloupe (US), grapefruit, kiwi, nectarines, oranges, pears, tangerines, watermelon
Apricots	Cantaloupe (US), red/pink grapefruit, nectarines, oranges, tangerines, watermelon
Green beans	Asparagus, broccoli, Brussels sprouts, cauliflower, peas, potatoes
Grapes (Chile)	Grapes (US, May to December in season)
Cucumbers	Carrots, broccoli, romaine lettuce, radishes

Reproduced, with permission, from Environmental Working Group, Washington, DC.

menopausal women. This appears to block the carcinogenic potential for the powerful estrogens and reduce the incidence of potential cancer.

Mental and emotional factors appear to contribute to risk, and addressing and dealing with depression is important. The studies of Sandra Levy found that women with recurrent breast cancer did remarkably better if they had expressed more joy at baseline testing.[41] Behavioral and cognitive therapy can be of enormous help.

Treatment Options

Nutritional antioxidants exert anti-carcinogenic, immunostimulant, and antimetastatic effects, and act to inhibit cancer at each stage of its development. Since platelet aggregation, a free-radical mediated function, encourages implantation of bloodstream-borne cancer metastases, increasing antioxidant intake becomes important.[42] Reasonable daily doses of antioxidants in treating cancer are 500 µg selenium, 800 IU vitamin E and 4 g vitamin C. In 12 years of follow-up in the Basel study, mortality in cancer patients was significantly associated with low levels of vitamin C and carotenoids. β-Carotene 25 mg daily[43] and 1 g daily of *Spirulina fusiformis*, a blue–green mircoalgae,[44] both significantly regress the lesions and prevent full-blown cancerous changes. Vitamin A has been shown to reduce the incidence of new primary tumors and increase the tumor-free interval in heavy-smoking patients "cured" of lung cancer,[45] and lycopene substantially inhibits the in vitro replication of lung cancer cells. Twenty-one smokers with metaplasia of the bronchial lining given oral doses of folic acid 10–20 mg daily and vitamin B_{12} 750 µg daily for a year significantly decreased incidence of malignancy compared to the controls.[46] Recurring precancerous colon polyps are up to 85 percent diminished in those taking vitamin A 30,000 IU, vitamin C 1 g and D,L-α-tocopherol 70 mg daily. Adequate calcium also significantly reduces risk. Risks are worsened with intake of red meat, total fat, and saturated fat.

In the 1970s, Pauling and Cameron reported benefits of intravenous vitamin C in terminal cancer patients.[47] The pro-oxidant action of ultra-large doses of ascorbic acid is preferentially toxic to tumor cells in vitro and in vivo. The cytotoxicity of ascorbic acid is related to pro-oxidant generation of hydrogen peroxide. Healthy cells have a 10–100-fold greater content of catalase compared to tumor cells, enabling vitamin C to induce cytotoxicity in tumor cells with negligible effects on healthy cells. Many tumor cell types are completely destroyed in laboratory tests by concentrations of 5–40 mg/dl of ascorbic acid, a level which can be achieved by an intravenous infusion of 60–100 g of vitamin C over 10 hours. Documentation of a number of cases of arrest of advanced tumor growth using these doses has been published.[48] Cytotoxicity to tumor cells by high concentrations of vitamin C involves a totally different concept in ascorbic acid pharmacology.

In laboratory rats exposed to radiation, those given vitamin E had significant increased protection against radiation damage to normal cells, including precancerous cell changes. Patients under treatment for cancer of the bladder were randomized to therapy with either an RDA-level multivitamin–mineral daily or an RDA-level multivitamin–mineral plus A 40,000 IU, B_6 100 mg, C 2 g, E 400 IU and Zn 90 mg. Five-year cancer recurrence rates were 91 percent for the RDA vitamin group and 41 percent for the megadose group. And in a study of lung cancer patients on standard chemotherapy and radiation therapy, mega-dose supplements enhanced survival 40–60 percent. Side effects of radiation and chemotherapy were also considerably reduced compared to normal experience.[49] Selenium facilitates immune activity and has anti-cancer activity in animals and in cancer cells in vitro. Incubation of prostate carcinoma cells with physiological levels of zinc in vitro resulted in marked inhibition of cell growth.[50]

Twenty-one end-stage cancer patients who had undergone maximal conventional treatment and classed as untreatable were given 9–18 g daily of evening primrose oil, high in gamma linolenic acid. Most experienced marked subjective improvement.

Analysis of case studies indicates that a strict macrobiotic diet, an extension of a vegetarian diet, is likely to be more effective in long-term cancer management than diets offering a variety of other foods.

An eclectic approach by Nicholas Gonzales, involving an essentially uncooked foods vegetarian diet (regular yogurt, with eggs and fish 3 times a week were allowed); nutritional supplements; up to 80 USP units of proteolytic and up to 40 USP units of lipolytic digestive enzymes daily; and detoxification procedures, has recently demonstrated startlingly long survival in pancreatic cancer, tripling usual 1-year survival and quadrupling usual 2-year survival.[51]

Forty-three patients undergoing a bone marrow transplant receiving standard nutrition, to which the amino acid glutamine 1–2 g daily was added, had significantly less infection and recovered more quickly than those on standard nutrition alone.[52] Glutamine added to chemotherapy regimens in laboratory animals with cancer eliminates the toxic effects of drugs such as methotrexate and inhibits cancer growth.

In studies of animals with cancer, increased physical activity leads to a 25–100 percent retardation in growth rate of experimental sarcomas, adenocarcinomas, hepatomas, and mammary carcinomas. Physical activity appears to be helpful in the treatment of cancer as well as prevention. Increased physical activity in the cancer patient increases appetite, conserves lean tissue, improves functional capacity, slows the clinical course of cancer, pushes back the time of death and improves the quality of life.

Genistein, luteolin, and daidzein, herbal isoflavones from fruits and vegetables, especially soy, inhibit the growth of gastric cancer cells in vitro. Recent in vitro research underscores the benefit of soy, demonstrating that genistein, in a dose-dependent manner involving modest concentrations, induces death of non-small-cell lung cancer cells through apoptosis.[53] Human squamous skin cancer cells in vitro were significantly inhibited by various concentrations of quercitin. Reasonable clinical doses are 400 mg b.i.d. Tangeretin, a naturally occurring flavone in citrus fruit, causes apoptosis in promyelocytic leukemia cells in vitro. So, large amounts of citrus fruits are encouraged. Maitake mushroom extracts appear to have immune-enhancing and anti-cancer properties and may soon be available in the United States.

Biomolecular options stem from a number of isolated observations. The first is a report of a significantly lower incidence of metastases in anticoagulated cancer patients.[54] This report has not led to widespread utilization of this observation. Anti-platelet nutrients also reduce the ability of platelets to participate in the metastatic process. Among these nutrients are essential fatty acids, found as omega-3 oils in cold water fish (salmon, sardines, mackerel), flaxseed oil, soybeans, and in especially concentrated amounts in pumpkin seeds. Another observation is the awareness of the steadily declining levels of dehydroepiandrosterone (DHEA) after the third decade of life. The levels of DHEA in patients with a wide variety of cancers are found to be generally low. Postmenopausal breast cancer appears to be an exception. DHEA has been used with benefit as treatment in some types of cancer, but patients should not embark on this as an adjunctive treatment without professional guidance.

In a 22-year follow-up of 175 breast cancer patients, 6 percent of those who were taking digitoxin for other reasons died of their disease, compared to 34 percent of those not on digitalis dying of their disease. In vitro studies have shown digitalis to possess anti-neoplastic properties. The breast cancers in the digitalis patients were also less aggressive.[55]

Isolated cases of far-advanced metastatic lung cancer have been reported to go into remission when given cimetidine (Tagamet); and far-advanced melanoma has been reported to undergo dramatic regression in 2 of 3 patients with administration of cimetidine. Glutathione, an endogenously synthesized antioxidant enzyme added intravenously to chemotherapeutic cisplatin regimens for advanced ovarian cancer, decreased toxicity and significantly improved prognosis.[56] Significantly better survival and lower recurrence rate in transitional cell carcinoma of the bladder has been accomplished with the addition of *Lactobacillus casei* 1 g t.i.d.[57]

There is preliminary evidence that melatonin is helpful in the treatment of cancer. Patients with brain metastases from solid cancers who received melatonin 20 mg daily in addition to supportive care tripled their survival time at 1 year. Clear improvement in quality of life and performance status was present in 30 percent of the melatonin patients compared to none of the controls. Melatonin 10 mg daily prevented metastases in 40 percent of patients with far-advanced cancers.

Coenzyme Q_{10} 100 mg daily prevents the cardiac toxicity usually seen with adriamycin chemotherapy. In women with breast cancer, advanced liver and metastatic disease has successfully been treated with 400 mg/day.

Relaxation training requiring only 9 hours of training has been shown to significantly reduce cancer pain and use of narcotics and tranquilizers. Hypnotic suggestion also greatly enhances the management of pain in cancer. Patients with malignant melanoma who were enrolled in an intervention group did better than those in a "routine care" group. The intervention group met 1.5 hours weekly for 6 weeks. Group processes and interventions included health and cancer education, enhancement of illness-related problem-solving skills, instruction and practice in relaxation skills, psychological support and the learning of skills promoting positive interactions between patients and health-care professionals. Psychological and immunological testing at 6 months compared to baseline showed significant improvement in immunity, anxiety, and depression compared to "routine care" controls who showed no changes. Imagery enhanced the effects of relaxation on immunity. Over 6 years, the risk of dying was 33 percent less and the risk of recurrence 50 percent less in the intervention group.[58]

In a landmark study of late-stage female breast cancer patients, a 1-year weekly support group including relaxation training greatly enhanced quality of life and more than doubled the survival compared to women treated "routinely."[59] No similar studies in men have been published. Patients with a substantial support system of relatives, spouses and significant others also have a better prognosis, as do married men and men with a confidant.

In well-controlled animal studies, cancer progression has been shown to be inhibited with energy treatments by healers.

■ HOLISTIC CURE OF CANCER

In many of the occasionally published reports of persons recovering from cancer, especially advanced disease, patients have used imagery of their immune systems overcoming or defeating cancer cells and imagery of themselves returning to health. Authoritative research confirms that the efficacy of imagery is highly related to the features of biological imagery (vividness, effectiveness). Guided imagery therapy with skilled professionals can be very helpful and meaningful.

Several thousand case histories of documented "spontaneous" recovery from cancer have been summarized by Brendan O'Regan of the Institute of Noetic Sciences. In many case histories, the "fighting spirit," will to live, and belief in recovery appear to be very important prognostic factors.[60] Most patients who recover from life-threatening cancer have often made a radical change in some aspect of their lives in diet, exercise, attitude, relationships with family members, or sense of connection with God. Patients who achieve a cure of their malignancy often have been able to fully accept their cancer and have used the occasion of their disease as an opportunity to gain some sense of meaning and purpose in their lives. This introspective journey of self-discovery is often so important to them that many actually feel gratitude for the "gift" of cancer.

Participation in the selection of the treatment approach, confidence and belief in the treatment, and confidence in self and the treating physicians, and the ability to evoke a sense of hope seem to be essential in achieving more successful outcomes.

REFERENCES

1. Cole P et al. Declining cancer mortality in the United States. *Cancer* 1996; 78(10):2045–8.
2. Bain C et al. Diet and melanoma. An exploratory case-control study. *Ann Epidemiol* 1993; 3(3):235–8.
3. Levi F et al. Food groups and colorectal cancer risk. *Br J Cancer* 1999; 79(7–8):1283–7.
4. Moerman CJ et al. Dietary sugar intake in the aetiology of biliary tract cancer. *Int J Epidemiol* 1993; 22(2):207–14.
5. Franceschi S, La Vecchia C, Russo A et al. Low-risk diet for breast cancer in Italy. *Cancer Epidemiol Biomark Prev* 1997; 6(11): 875–9.
6. Gann PH et al. Lower prostate cancer risk in men with elevated plasma lycopene levels: results of a prospective analysis. *Cancer Res* 1999 15; 59(6):1225.
7. Hayes RB et al. Serum retinol and prostate cancer. *Cancer* 1988; 62(9):2021–6.
8. Morris RD et al. Chlorination, chlorination by-products and cancer: a meta-analysis. *Am J Pub Health* 1992; 82(7):955–63.
9. Modan B et al. Increased risk of breast cancer after low-dose radiation. *Lancet* 1989; 1(8629):629–31.
10. Loomis DP et al. Breast cancer mortality among female electrical workers in the United States. *J Natl Cancer Inst* 1994; 86(12): 921–5.

11. Beral V et al. Malignant melanoma and exposure to fluorescent lighting at work. *Lancet* 1982; 2(8293):290–3.
12. Brandes LJ et al. Stimulation of malignant growth in rodents by antidepressant drugs at clinical relevant doses. *Cancer Res* 1992; 52(13):3796–3800.
13. Suadicani P et al. Is the use of antihypertensives and sedatives a major risk factor for colorectal cancer? *Scand J Gastroenterol* 1993; 28(6):475–81.
14. Shephard RJ et al. Exercise in the prevention and treatment of cancer—an update. *Sports Med* 1993; 15(4):258–80.
15. Ben-Eliyahu S et al. Stress increases metastatic spread of a mammary tumor in rats: evidence for mediation by the immune system. *Brain Behav Immun* 1991; 5(2):193–205.
16. Chen CC et al. Adverse life events and breast cancer: case control study. *BMJ* 1995; 311(7019):1527–30.
17. Ramirez AJ et al. Stress and the relapse of breast cancer. *BMJ* 1989; 298(6669):291-3.
18. Colon EA et al. Depressed mood and other variables relate to bone marrow transplantation survival in acute leukemia. *Psychosomatics* 1991; 32(4):420–5.
19. Eysenck HJ et al. The prediction of death from cancer by means of personality/stress questionnaire: too good to be true? *Percept Motor Skills* 1990; 71(1):216–18.
20. Shealy CN, Myss CM. *The Creation of Health*. Walpole, NH: Stillpoint, 1988.
21. Thomas CB et al. Closeness to parents and the family constellation in a prospective study of five disease states: suicide, mental illness, malignant tumor, hypertension, and coronary artery disease. *Johns Hopkins Med J* 1974; 134(5):251–69.
22. Cairns J. The treatment of disease and the war against cancer. *Sci Am* 1985; 253(5):51–9.
23. Nomura AM et al. Dietary factors in cancer of the lower urinary tract. *Int J Cancer* 1991; 48(2):199–205.
24. Bunin GR et al. Relation between maternal diet and subsequent primitive neuroectodermal brain tumors in young children. *N Engl J Med* 1993; 329(8):536–41.
25. de Lorgeril M et al. Mediterranean dietary pattern in a randomized trial: prolonged survival and possible reduced cancer rate. *Arch Intern Med* 1998; 158(11):1181–7.

26. Zhang S et al. Dietary carotenoids and vitamins A, C, and E and risk of breast cancer. *J Natl Cancer Inst* 1999; 91(6):547–56.
27. Franceschi S et al. Tomatoes and risk of digestive tract cancers. *Int J Cancer* 1994; 59(2):181–4.
28. Fontham ET et al. Dietary vitamins A and C and lung cancer risk in Louisiana. *Cancer* 1988; 62(10):2267–73.
29. Gao YT et al. Reduced risk of esophageal cancer associated with green tea consumption. *J Natl Cancer Inst* 1994; 86(11):855–8.
30. Dorant E et al. Consumption of onions and a reduced risk of stomach cancer. *Gastroenterology* 1996; 110(1):12–20.
31. Blot WJ et al. Nutrition trials in Linxian, China: supplements with specific vitamin/mineral combinations, cancer incidence, and disease-specific mortality in the general population. *J Natl Cancer Inst* 1993; 85(18):1483–92.
32. Ocke MC et al. Average intake of anti-oxidant (pro)vitamins and subsequent cancer mortality in the 16 cohorts of the seven countries study. *Int J Cancer* 1995; 61(4):480–4.
33. Anonymous. The effect of vitamin E and beta carotene on the incidence of lung cancer and other cancers in male smokers. The alpha-tocopherol and beta carotene cancer prevention group. *N Engl J Med* 1994; 330(15):1029–35.
34. Levy J et al. Lycopene is a more potent inhibitor of human cancer cell proliferation than either alpha carotene or beta carotene. *Nutr Cancer* 1995; 24(3):257–66.
35. Giovannucci E et al. Multivitamin use, folate, and colon cancer in women in the Nurses' Health Study. *Ann Intern Med* 1998; 129(7):517–24.
36. Clark LC et al. Effects of selenium supplementation for cancer prevention in patients with carcinoma of the skin. A randomized, controlled trial. Nutritional prevention of cancer study group. *JAMA* 1996; 276(24):1957–63.
37. Huang YL et al. Association between oxidative stress and changes of trace elements in patients with breast cancer. *Clin Biochem* 1999; 32(2):131–6.
38. Environmental Working Group. 1718 Connecticut Ave NW # 600, Washington, DC, 20009.
39. Giovannucci E et al. Leisure time physical activity, body-size and colon cancer in women. *J Natl Cancer Inst* 1997; 89(13):948–55.

40. Yun TK et al. Non-organ specific cancer prevention of ginseng; a prospective study in Korea. *Int J Epidemiol* 1998; 27(3):359–64.

41. Levy SM et al. Survival hazards analysis in first recurrent breast cancer patients: seven-year follow-up. *Psychosom Med* 1988; 50(5):520–8.

42. McCarty MF. An antithrombotic role for nutritional antioxidants: implications for tumor metastasis and other pathologies. *Med Hypotheses* 1986; 19(4):345–57.

43. Krishnaswamy K et al. A case study of nutrient intervention of oral precancerous lesions in India. *Eur J Cancer B Oral Oncol* 1995; 31B(1):41–8.

44. Mathew B et al. Evaluation of chemoprevention of oral cancer with *Spirulina fusiformis*. *Nutr Cancer* 1995; 24(2):197–202.

45. Pastorini V et al. Adjuvant treatment of stage I lung cancer with high-dose vitamin A. *J Clin Oncol* 1993; 11(7):1216–22.

46. Saito M et al. Chemoprevention effects on bronchial squamous metaplasia by folate and vitamin B_{12} in heavy smokers. *Chest* 1994; 102(2):496–9.

47. Cameron E et al. Supplemental ascorbate in the supportive treatment of cancer: reevaluation of prolongation of survival times in terminal human cancer. *Proc Natl Acad Sci* 1978; 75(9):4538–42.

48. Riordan NH et al. Intravenous ascorbate as a tumor cytotoxic chemotherapeutic agent. *Med Hypotheses* 1995; 44(4):207–13.

49. Jaakkola K et al. Treatment with antioxidant and other nutrients win combination with chemotherapy and irradiation in patients with small cell lung cancer. *Anticancer Res* 1992; 12(3):599–606.

50. Liang JY et al. Inhibitory effect of zinc on human prostatic carcinoma cell growth. *Prostate* 1999; 40(3):200–7.

51. Gonzales NJ et al. Effect of pancreatic proteolytic enzyme treatment of adenocarcinoma of the pancreas, with nutrition and detoxification support. *Nutr Cancer* 1999; 33(2):117–24.

52. MacBurney M et al. A cost evaluation of glutamine-supplemented parenteral nutrition in adult bone marrow transplant patients. *J Am Diet Assoc* 1994; 94(11):1263–6.

53. Lian F et al. p53-independent apoptosis induced by genistein in lung cancer cells. *Nutr Cancer* 1999; 33(2):125–31.

54. Michaels L et al. Cancer incidence and mortality in patients having anticoagulant therapy. *Lancet* 1964; 2(7364):832–5.

55. Stenkvist B. Is digitalis a therapy for breast carcinoma? *Oncol Rep* 1999; 6(3):493–6.

56. Tedeschi M et al. The role of glutathione in combination with cis-platin in the treatment of ovarian cancer. *Cancer Treat Rev* 1991; 18(3):253–9.

57. Aso Y et al. Preventive effect of a *Lactobacillus casei* preparation on the recurrence of superficial bladder cancer in a double-blind trial. *Eur Urol* 1995; 27(2):104–09.

58. Flach J et al. Mind–body meld may boost immunity. *J Natl Cancer Inst* 1994; 86(4):256–8.

59. Spiegel D et al. Effect of psychosocial treatment on survival of patients with metastatic breast cancer. *Lancet* 1989; 2(8688):888–91.

60. O'Regan B, Hirshberg C. *Spontaneous Remission.* Sausalito, CA: Institute of Noetic Sciences, 1993.

4
Chapter Four

Gastrointestinal Disorders

Diarrhea

■ **DESCRIPTION**

Diarrhea can be defined as increased liquidity, frequency, and volume of unformed bowel movements which interfere with the normal activities of daily living. It is often accompanied by abdominal pain, cramping, and excessive gas. Diarrhea is usually a symptom of a temporary gastrointestinal dysfunction, but may be a sign of serious illness. Indicators of more ominous problems are worsening diarrhea lasting longer than a week, bowel movements initiated by urgency, copious loss of fluids, and stools accompanied by pus or blood. The diarrhea of celiac disease, related to reactivity to gluten, a protein in grains, produces a particularly foul-smelling stool. The normal gastrointestinal (GI) transit time from ingestion to stool passage is 12–18 hours.

The gastrointestinal tract is a complex organ having to deal with the breakdown and selective assimilation of all the nutrients necessary to sustain life and the elimination of the residue of that process. Over 500 species of normal bacteria are resident in the gastrointestinal tract, and the number of bacteria exceeds the number of cells in the body by 9-fold. The system of lymph channels in the walls of the small intestine is the largest reservoir of immune function in the body. The lining of the gastrointestinal tract also houses the body's "second brain," known as the enteric nervous system. It produces an entire array of neurotransmitters identical with those produced by the central nervous system. This nerve complex enables the "G-I brain" to act independently, learn, remember, and generate "gut feelings."

■ PREVALENCE

Acute diarrhea has been experienced by nearly everyone. Ordinarily self-limited to 3–4 days, serious complications are seen in dehydration from continuing loss of water and electrolytes in susceptible people. Up to 50 percent of Americans traveling in emerging nations experience diarrhea.

■ ETIOLOGY AND RISK FACTORS

The following factors play major roles in acute diarrhea.

1. Viral and/or bacterial infections from contaminated drinking water or food.
2. Epidemic infections, with *Salmonella typhimurium, E. coli, Shigella*, and *Vibrio cholera* the principal bacteria.
3. Traveler's diarrhea, with parasites or bacteria the usual agents involved.
4. Intestinal or gastric viral "flu."
5. Food allergy and sensitivity, usually due to cow's milk, wheat, coffee, chocolate, egg, corn, orange, pork, beef, chicken, peanuts, and sugar.
6. Drug use and overuse: antibiotics that destroy the balance of normal gut bacteria (acidophilus and bifidus); laxative over-use; excess ingestion of magnesium supplements or medicines, including antacids; corticosteroids; and large doses of vitamin C.
7. Ingestion of milk and milk products by lactose-intolerant patients or fructose by fructose-intolerant patients.
8. Olestra-containing synthesized foods causes diarrhea in a significant number of users. Prescribed for weight loss, it is a synthetic fat not assimilated from the intestine.
9. Intensely experienced emotions including fear and anxiety.

10. Acute exacerbations of the chronic or intermittent diarrhea of inflammatory bowel disease or irritable bowel syndrome (see the following).

Factors in chronic diarrhea include the following:

1. Parasitic infection, most often with *Entamoeba histolytica* or *Giardia lamblia*.
2. Viral infection, including *rotavirus* and acquired immuno-deficiency syndrome.
3. Helminth infestation (worms).
4. Inflammatory bowel disease—Crohn's disease or ulcerative colitis.
5. Resistant bacterial (e.g., *Clostridium difficile*) or fungal (e.g., *Candida albicans*) overgrowth after antibiotic treatment.
6. Irritable bowel syndrome.
7. Diverticulitis.
8. Cancer of the colon.
9. Emotional stress—usually associated with the following issues: fear, distrust, anger, low self-confidence, and threats to personal honor.
10. Malabsorption syndromes including celiac sprue.
11. Laxative overuse.
12. Lactose intolerance; fructose intolerance.
13. Hyperthyroidism.

■ CONVENTIONAL TREATMENT

Symptomatic treatment for diarrhea not resolving in a week or less usually involves maintaining adequate water and electrolyte intake to prevent dehydration. The risk of severe dehydration from diarrhea water loss is, of course, much greater in children and the very elderly. For children not requiring hospitalization, commercially available rehydration solutions are available in pharmacies, or a rehydration solution can be made up at home: $\frac{1}{2}$ tsp of salt and 4 tsp of sugar in 1 quart of filtered or bottled water, given $\frac{1}{2}$ –1 ounce, q 30–90 minutes. Children can be placed on the BRAT diet (bananas, rice, applesauce, toast) since these foods are more easily and completely digested and assimilated. Alcohol, caffeine, milk and dairy products, and artificially flavored foods and chewing gum should be avoided. If the onset of diarrhea quickly follows the start of any new medication, it should be omitted to see if the diarrhea subsides.

Drugs to slow bowel activity include absorbent medicines like Peptobismol, and antimotility opium-derivative medicines such as Lomotil (Rx) and Imodium (OTC). Medications containing attapulgite and kaolin (Donnagel and Kaopectate) are generally less effective. Frequently, pharmaceuticals are prescribed to depopulate offending bacterial, fungal, or parasitic organisms demonstrated on culture or stool examination. When mild to moderate diarrhea does not respond to these measures after about 2 weeks, more extensive diagnostic investigation is undertaken, including stool samples for infectious organisms, parasites, and the presence of occult blood. Other options include upper or lower endoscopy.

■ HOLISTIC MEDICAL TREATMENT

Prevention of epidemic diarrhea including food poisoning is dependent on good personal hygiene, including frequent hand washing, particularly critical in food handlers. A program which can be recommended for effective prevention of traveler's diarrhea includes: using only bottled water (without ice) for drinking, cooking, or teeth-brushing; avoiding raw food or salad which does not have a thick peel, such as bananas or watermelons; using hydrochloric acid tablets following each meal (digest and inactivate parasites); taking heat-resistant acidophilus capsules daily; taking grapefruit seed extract, one tablet or capsule daily; and using the herbal product, Intestinalis, one tablet daily (kills parasites).

Initially, diarrhea should be treated by avoiding any solid foods and limiting intake to water, fruit and vegetable juices, potassium-rich vegetable broth, or non-carbonated soft drinks. Adults should try to consume about 1 pint per hour. With acute diarrhea this helps to avoid dehydration while allowing the body to efficiently eliminate toxic foods, viruses, or bacteria. With chronic diarrhea, this regimen is a convenient step in identifying food allergens. Cow's milk should be omitted if the history suggests lactose intolerance. In infants and young children, breast feeding should be continued, and commercial rehydration solutions can be used. Sports drinks like Gatorade usually do not contain adequate sodium and potassium.

As the diarrhea subsides, the liquid phase can be followed by plain yogurt, vegetable soups, rice or barley broth, cooked fruits (crab apples), garlic, carrots, string beans, eggplant, yams, olives, white rice, sweet rice, and buckwheat. Fats and oils, fried foods, honey, cow's milk, alcohol, caffeine, apricots, plums, sesame seeds, and synthesized products containing the sweeteners sorbitol, xylitol, and mannitol (found in sugarless gums, vitamins, and diet foods) should be omitted. Pectin, found in apples, bananas, carrots, and potatoes, also helps relieve diarrhea.

The diarrhea, weight loss, and abdominal distress of people with celiac disease requires strict avoidance of grains containing gluten, including wheat, barley, rye, and oats. The avoidance of gluten is doubly important: long-term ingestion of gluten in sensitive people carries a much higher risk of colon cancer.[1]

Lactobacillus acidophilus, normally resident in the intestine, is needed following diarrhea to restore the bowel flora. Powdered forms are best in dosages of $\frac{1}{2}$ –1 tsp twice daily. At 250–1,000 mg daily, *Lactobacillus GG*, a variety of *Lactobacillus casei rhamosum*, has been shown to achieve a high rate of cure in patients with recurrent diarrhea from resistant *Clostridium difficile* organisms. Reduction in gastrointestinal and systemic symptoms of food allergy has also been shown with ingestion of *Lactobacillus GG*. Supplementing with bifidobacteria ($\frac{1}{2}$ tsp b.i.d.) reduces the diarrhea of poorly thriving infants.

In pediatric patients, addition of zinc appears to enhance conventional treatment for diarrhea 30 percent, while reducing complications.[2] The treatment of children with vitamin A 100,000–200,000 IU in single doses added to infant feedings every 4 months reduced the risk for diarrhea during epidemics 20 percent.[3] The addition of folic acid 30 mg daily mitigates the diarrhea of celiac disease and aids in the treatment of Crohn's disease.

Several botanical preparations are helpful for their anti-diarrheal action.

1. Blackberry leaf (*Rubus fruticosus*) and raspberry leaf (*Rubus idaeus*) tea, 1 heaping tsp, per cup, $\frac{1}{2}$ cup at hourly intervals.
2. Slippery elm powder (*Ulmus rubra*), 1 ounce in 1 quart of water, simmered down to 1 pint, one tsp q 30–60 minutes.
3. Carob powder, 1 tbsp in 4 ounces of water or applesauce, $\frac{1}{2}$ to 1 tsp q 30–60 minutes, tapering to t.i.d. can help terminate diarrhea.

Several herbs have antimicrobial attributes.

1. Garlic has antibiotic properties against fungal and bacterial organisms, especially *Candida albicans*.
2. Berberine has merit in treating diarrhea from amebiasis, giardiasis and *E.coli*. It is found in goldenseal, Oregon grape and barberry (*Berberis vulgaris*), all used by indigenous peoples for diarrhea. Berberine has also been shown to neutralize certain bacterial toxins, which is helpful in traveler's diarrhea, frequently due to a toxin-producing *E. coli*. Barberry is prescribed 250–500 mg t.i.d.
3. Goldenseal (*Hydrastis canadensis*) is effective in bacterial diarrhea. The dosage for children is $\frac{1}{4}$–$\frac{1}{2}$ tsp t.i.d. in a 1 : 5 tincture; adults: $\frac{1}{2}$–1 tsp or 250–500 mg t.i.d.
4. Peppermint, 3–15 drops in water, q 2–3 h.

A number of homeopathic remedies are used in acute diarrhea but each one is used for treating different symptoms. Common agents used in 12X to 30C potency include aconite, chamomilla, podophyllum, aloe, *Arsenicum album*, and sulfur. It is best to consult a homeopathic practitioner for treatment of acute or chronic diarrhea. In two studies, homeopathy has been shown to eliminate diarrhea more quickly than conventional treatment in childhood diarrhea.[4]

There are several behavioral therapies that are effective in treating some types of chronic diarrhea. Biofeedback training is highly successful in treating the diarrhea of irritable bowel syndrome.[5] It is also often successful well for diarrhea in which stress plays any significant role. Meditation, yoga, and other approaches to management of the sympathetic nervous system are also successful (progressive relaxation, self-suggestion, and autogenics). Psychological studies of adult diarrhea with discernible cause have frequently found that intense feelings and demands on other people are present. Brief therapeutic interventions which may quickly change bowel function often involve evoking an attitude of forgiveness and letting go of intense demands.

Constipation

■ DESCRIPTION

Constipation is a condition of bowel action in which the passage of feces is difficult or abnormally infrequent. Normal bowel habit frequency varies from several bowel passages a day to once daily. Primary constipation is most often related to prolonged transit time within the colon. Primary symptoms include infrequent or irregular bowel movements; pain or straining with bowel movements; passage of small, hard stools; abdominal distention; and, often, fatigue.

Constipation that lasts longer than a week for no apparent reason, often leads patients to seek medical help. The physical examination will include a digital rectal exam to detect any signs of impaction, tenderness, or blood. Depending on the history and findings, diagnostic tests might include: blood count, chemistry panel, thyroid tests, electrolytes, stool analysis, X-ray studies (upper GI and barium enema), and sigmoidoscopy.

■ PREVALENCE

Constipation is easily the most common gastrointestinal complaint in the United States. Nearly everyone has experienced acute or chronic constipation. It is a chronic problem in 2–3% of Americans, who spend more than $400 million a year on laxatives.

■ ETIOLOGY AND RISK FACTORS

A number of physical and psychological factors are implicated in the etiology of this common condition.

The prominent physical factors include:

1. Ingestion of prepackaged, overly cooked foods low in fiber and high in saturated fat.
2. Intake of high amounts of meat, fried foods, cheese, sugar, and refined flour products.
3. Deficient intake of water and other liquids.
4. Eating quickly, with insufficient mastication.
5. Excess intake of coffee, alcohol, and soft drinks which can dehydrate the stool and irritate the colonic mucosa.
6. Deficiency of magnesium and potassium—common with diuretics.
7. Taking calcium and iron supplements and aluminum-containing antacids.
8. Food sensitivities, with or without accompanying diarrhea.
9. Constipating effects of a majority of prescription drugs.
10. Chronic use and abuse of laxatives.
11. Physical inactivity, either chronic lack of exercise or associated with travel or illness.
12. Hemorrhoids, anal fissures.
13. Inflammatory bowel disease (including Crohn's disease), irritable bowel syndrome, and diverticulitis.
14. Neurological disorders including Parkinson's.
15. Outlet inertia with failure of the external sphincter and pelvic floor muscles to relax during straining at defecation.
16. Hypothyroidism.
17. Habitually postponing the urge to have a BM, with feed-back weakening of the defecation signal.

Significant emotional factors include:

1. Anxiety.
2. Depression.
3. Excessive need for control.
4. Obsessive-compulsive tendencies.

5. Fear of making mistakes and need for perfection.
6. Grim determination to carry on in the face of apparently insoluble problems.

■ CONVENTIONAL MEDICAL TREATMENT

Conventional treatment usually involves the use of at least one of four types of laxatives:

1. Bulk producing agents, containing non-digestible fiber, are often the first choice and most effective for mild constipation. Increased fiber enhances proper colon function by providing more substance on which the peristaltic contractions focus their action. These products, such as Metamucil, usually contain psyllium, which is a natural plant fiber. The usual dosage is 1–2 tsp daily with water. Metamucil has additional advantages, including reduction of plasma lipid levels.[6] Methylcellulose products are also used (Citrucel).
2. Hyperosmotic agents such as lactulose, or saline laxatives (Milk of Magnesia) have low profiles of side effects.
3. Stimulant laxatives increase peristalsis by irritating the walls of the large intestine. Bowel movements are usually improved, but to avoid the tendency for their use to promote dependency, use should be limited to no longer than 2 weeks. Examples are Dulcolax, Ex-Lax, and Senokot.
4. Stool softeners hydrate the stools by hygroscopic action. They are often used in combination with stimulant laxatives. Colace and Surfak are popular stool softeners. These should also only be used for short periods while underlying causes are identified and corrected.

Adequate water intake is also essential for re-establishing normal stool consistency.

■ HOLISTIC MEDICAL TREATMENT

Patients should undertake the following dietary initiatives.

1. Reduce or eliminate sugar, milk and dairy products, coffee, alcohol, meat, fats, spicy foods, and processed, refined flour-based products such as white bread and pastries.
2. Increase fiber intake from more raw, preferably organic, fruits (apricots, figs, dates, plums, prunes) and vegetables (beans, lentils, and ground flax and sesame seeds); and/or 1–2 tablespoons of bran (barley or oats) with water at mealtimes, or add bran to cereal or applesauce, 2–3 tbsp daily.
3. Emphasize whole-grain breads, cereals, and whole-wheat flour pastas, brown rice, beans, lentils, and other whole carbohydrates.
4. Increase water intake to at least the minimum requirement ($\frac{1}{2}$ ounce per pound of body weight each day).
5. Olive oil, unrefined, 2 tbsp daily.
6. Masticate food adequately—20–30 chews per mouthful.

Work with patients complaining of constipation to establish consistent healthy habits.

1. Engage in regular aerobic exercise for 30 minutes, 3–5 times weekly.
2. Always answer nature's call and avoid repressing or postponing the natural urge to evacuate.
3. Sit on the toilet at the same time every day, preferably in the morning even if initially no urge is perceived.
4. Practice abdominal breathing while sitting on the toilet.
5. Follow the dietary recommendations.
6. Taper off and stop using laxatives.
7. To re-establish regularity, an herbal laxative containing either cascara or senna at h.s. for 2 weeks may be necessary. If loose stools occur, the dose of the laxative needs to be immediately reduced until a formed stool is established.

Nutritional supplements can be helpful. In addition to dietary fiber, supplements of fiber mentioned above have benefit. The most balanced supplements are Metamucil, Ultra fiber, or Jarrow Gentle Fiber. Supplementary fiber should be introduced slowly— 1 to 2 g daily until 5–10 g daily amounts are reached. Again, adequate water intake is imperative. Supplementary fiber helps reduce absorption of toxins, restore a healthy bacterial balance in the gut, and strengthens immunity. Although disputed, numerous studies have presented evidence of reduction of colorectal cancer risk with high fiber intake; coronary artery disease risk appears 30–40 percent reduced with a high fiber diet,[7] and hypertension reduced approximately 50 percent.[8]

In re-establishing normal bowel function, it is essential to create the proper bacterial balance using probiotics (acidophilus and bifidus).[9] In constipation there is usually a microfloral imbalance, with normal flora being outnumbered by pathogenic bacteria, yeast organisms, and parasites. A high-potency probiotic formula containing both acidophilus and bifidus in powdered form can be given $\frac{1}{2}$ to 1 tsp in water, b.i.d. Bifidus also appears to encourage peristalsis.

Magnesium is essential to peristalsis. The recommended dosage is 400–500 mg daily in a citrate or aspartate form; an excess can cause diarrhea. Potassium 700 mg daily is also beneficial. Vitamin C can usually soften the stool at higher dosages such as 5,000–10,000 mg daily. It can be taken as ascorbic acid with bioflavonoids in gradually increasing doses until constipation subsides. Pantothenate, a variation of pantothenic acid, is markedly helpful for hastening the return of peristalsis after abdominal surgery.

Herbs for constipation include Cascara, Senna, Licorice, Rhubarb, Dandelion root, Fennel seed, Barberry, Psyllium, and Flax. Mixtures often work better, and teas prepared from mixtures and steeped for 20 minutes are also helpful. Cascara, even in these small amounts in tea should not be consumed indefinitely.

Homeopathic remedies used include nux vomica (especially for laxative habituation), Bryonia, Alumina, Calcarea carbonica, and sulfur.

Behavioral medical initiatives including cognitive psychotherapy and biofeedback are often effective in treating constipation. In childhood studies, improvement is significantly accelerated with biofeedback compared to conventional treatment.[10] Adults, too, show up to 80 percent success when biofeedback is used with the outlet inertia type of constipation.[11] The relaxed state promotes markedly more normal autonomic nervous system control of the bowel. Addressing stress, depression, and emotional "gut" issues is essential.

Miscellaneous options include acupuncture which is also used to address functional bowel problems; castor oil packs (see Chapter 10), and massage therapy.

Encourage patients to use eating as an excuse to relax. Thorough, unhurried mastication promotes digestive secretions and peristalsis. Bowel function improves when the body is given a chance to find a brief space of time to just be in a state of low sympathetic arousal.

Irritable Bowel Syndrome

■ DESCRIPTION

Irritable bowel syndrome is a disordered function of small and large intestines presenting as variable symptoms including constipation and diarrhea (often alternating), pain, abdominal distension, burping, flatulence, cramping, nausea, and anorexia. The diarrhea, which is sometimes urgent and explosive, often quickly follows the eating of a meal or occurs soon after awakening. The stools may contain mucus; there is often a feeling of incomplete emptying after evacuation, and large meals tend to aggravate symptoms. Symptoms in women also tend to increase during premenstrual and menstrual phases of the cycle. Anxiety and depression often accompany the physical symptoms. A careful history often establishes the pre-existence of psychological symptoms which have intensified with onset of the physical symptoms. Making the diagnosis requires exclusion of other causes of diarrhea and constipation.

■ PREVALENCE

Irritable bowel syndrome (IBS), also known as spastic or mucous colitis, appears to afflict over 15 percent of the American population. Women outnumber men 2 to 1.

■ ETIOLOGY AND RISK FACTORS

Most textbooks describe the etiology of irritable bowel syndrome as unknown. Many physicians practicing complementary medicine believe the following to be contributory.

1. Food sensitivity or allergy; food offenders most often found to be related, in order of commonness, are milk and milk derivatives, wheat, corn, citrus fruits, eggs, chocolate, nuts, barley, rye, oats, potatoes, onions, tea, and coffee.
2. Intolerance of sugars—sucrose, fructose, sorbitol, mannitol, and lactose, the latter in milk.
3. Intestinal parasitic infestation; an incidence as high as 30–50 percent in IBS has been estimated by some.
4. Candida overgrowth; patients not responsive to food elimination diets often show great improvement with treatment by antifungal antibiotics.
5. Psychological and social stress; in irritable bowel syndrome patients, intestinal motility is accelerated when they are under stress.

■ CONVENTIONAL TREATMENT

Conventional textbooks state that irritable bowel syndrome is poorly understood and that existing therapies are not known to have lasting success. Treatment involves supplying adequate fiber; antispasmodic drugs such as Bentyl, Donnatol, or Levsin; antimotility drugs (Imodium, Lomotil); and avoidance of caffeine and excess alcohol.

■ HOLISTIC TREATMENT

Successful treatment emphasizes a very thorough inquiry for causes and possible triggering factors. These include a careful laboratory search for bacterial and parasitic organisms, utilizing a laboratory especially equipped for testing of stool specimens, such as Great Smokies Laboratory, Asheville, NC. A systematic search for triggering factors from clues in the waxing and waning pattern of symptoms may require journal keeping for correlation of food intake with exacerbation of symptoms.

Dietary options can include the following:

1. Begin with gradual increasing intake of more fiber from vegetables including beans and lentils, adding 1–2 foods each week, taking careful observation of the tolerance of each.
2. The addition of unprocessed psyllium seed powder gradually increased from 1 rounded tsp to 2 tbsp daily tends to stabilize the bowel habit. The use of psyllium seed as a source of fiber circumvents the possibility of sensitivity reactions to wheat or other cereal brans, should they have been used.
3. Water intake should be increased to 6–8 glasses/day, keeping the urine very pale yellow.
4. Thorough mastication and deliberate eating in a relaxed atmosphere is encouraged.
5. Sugar is discouraged. In healthy young male volunteers, reports of urgent defecation are 3 times as common while they were on a diet high in simple sugars.[12] Disruption of intestinal motility is one of the main problems in IBS. Sugar also exacerbates overgrowth of Candida, which has been implicated as an additional factor in IBS.

A food elimination and rechallenge trial should be undertaken if sensitizing food suspicion is high. The conventional doubt that macromolecules cannot be absorbed through the small intestinal mucosa has been strongly refuted.[13] A thoroughgoing food elimination trial can be abbreviated to elimination of the higher suspect foods on the foregoing list under Etiology. Placed on an "oligoantigenic" diet allowing only a limited few foods, IBS patients commonly feel much improved within a week.[14] Food additives can occasionally be problematic, and organically grown foods are desirable. Seventy-five percent of patients who investigate food sensitivities and follow an exclusion diet experience very rewarding improvement.

If Candida overgrowth is demonstrated or strongly suspected, Candida control measures should be instituted, followed by addition of probiotics (acidophillus and bifidus) to the treatment regimen.

Botanical agents of value in IBS include the following. Peppermint oil, 1–3 enteric-coated capsules b.i.d. between meals was found in a German study to lead to twice the clinical improvement and half the pain compared to placebo.[15] Thirty drops t.i.d.a.c. of a combination tincture containing *Valeriana officinalis*, *Passiflora incarnata*, *Pimpinella anisum*, *Filependula ulmaria*, *Dioscorea villosa*, and *Silibum marianum* relieves spasm and improves digestion. A mixture of 20 Chinese herbs, including *Artemesiae capillaris*, *Codonopsis pilosulae*, *Coicis lachyrma-jobi*, *Attractylodis macrocephalae*, *Schisandrae*, and others was also recently shown to be of substantial help in IBS.[16] Teas with antispasmodic properties include chamomile, peppermint, rosemary, valerian, fennel seed, and ginger root. Slippery elm and Marshmallow root add to attempts to increase fiber content of the diet.

Stress experiences and heightened intensity of demands are frequently associated with exacerbations of IBS; these recurrences can be modified by insight-oriented psychotherapy, whose success is augmented by relaxation training and biofeedback practice with biofeedback. Some studies have documented 75 percent improvement in physical and psychological symptoms after several months of regular biofeedback practice.[17] Hypnosis is very effective in irritable bowel syndrome. After an initial series of treatments, the best results occur in patients who return for a reinforcement session of 2–3 times a year.[18] Self-affirmations are particularly effective, especially when repeated in the relaxed state during relaxation, biofeedback, or meditation. An example: "My intestine is healed and serves me well."

The frequently observed tendency for IBS patients to be highly invested in self-criticism or control needs to be recognized so that attempts can be made to modify the attitudes behind these cognitions and behaviors. Acknowledging and resolving the issues surrounding the origin of these predisposing traits stemming from earlier life is of utmost importance. Working with the IBS patient to improve the quality of sleep also reaps significant benefits in bringing symptoms under control.

Intuitive observers link irritable bowel dysfunction to spiritual and psychological issues of gut-level fear, distrust, low self-confidence, personal honor, and self-care. In the hands of experienced practitioners, other helpful approaches include acupuncture, and energy therapies such as Reiki, Therapeutic Touch, Jin Shin Jyutsu, and Jo Rei. Constitutional homeopathic prescribing addresses individual characteristics and symptoms.

Inflammatory Bowel Disease: Crohn's Disease

■ DESCRIPTION

Crohn's disease is an inflammatory disorder involving the entire lining of the small and large bowel. When confined to lower portion of the small intestine, it is called regional enteritis; granulomatous colitis is an older term describing involvement of the colon. The disease manifests with flatulence, anorexia, weight loss, malaise, right lower quadrant pain and tenderness, and is punctuated with intermittent diarrhea and low-grade fevers. Enterocutaneous fistulas may develop in long-standing cases. Small bowel X-rays usually confirm definitive abnormalities in the terminal ileum.

■ PREVALENCE

About 100,000 people in the United States are estimated to be afflicted with Crohn's disease. Women are slightly in the majority. Age of onset is usually between 15 and 40. Over the last four decades, the yearly incidence of new cases of Crohn's disease has consistently and steadily increased.

■ ETIOLOGY AND RISK FACTORS

The causes of Crohn's disease include: genetic predisposition, with 20–40 percent of patients having a positive family history; possible autoimmunological abnormality; psychosocial stress appears to play a fairly strong role; possible infectious causes; and dietary factors.

The presence of anti-Klebsiella antibodies is found in a high percentage of Crohn's patients and patients who have rheumatoid spondylitis. It is known that men with Crohn's are more prone to develop spondylitis. Some authorities think these observations favor an infectious cause of both diseases. Crohn's is also associated with arthritis of the wrists, knees, and ankles. Inflammatory dermal nodules and aphthous ulcers are statistically more common in Crohn's patients.

Crohn's disease is all but unknown in indigenous societies that do not consume calorie-dense and highly refined foods. This dietary influence is thought to be substantial. The diets of people who subsequently develop Crohn's disease have been documented to contain substantially less fruit, vegetables and fiber, and include far more sugar and refined flour foods compared to those who remain healthy.[19] One study found that the amount of sugar consumed by those who later got Crohn's disease was twice that of healthy matched controls.[20]

Abnormal bacteria and yeast organisms often overgrow the small intestine, creating secondary problems. The levels of prostaglandin E2 and leukotrienes, promoters of inflammation, are greatly elevated in the wall of the affected bowel segments. This leads to a distorted pattern of assimilation of nutrients from the affected segments of small bowel. Protein is not properly absorbed, leading to weight loss in many cases. Due to losses in diarrhea or poor assimilation, it is common to have low levels of vitamins A, D, E, C, K, B-complex, magnesium, potassium, calcium, zinc, and iron, the latter from mucosal bleeding. Forty percent of Crohn's patients have depleted zinc levels. Vitamin B_{12} is low 50 percent of the time and folic acid 25–65 percent of the time; repletion may require injections.[21]

■ CONVENTIONAL TREATMENT

Drug treatment is a mainstay of conventional treatment for Crohn's. The most common drugs prescribed are sulfasalazine and cortisone. Sulfasalazine helps control abnormal bacteria and cortisone has a marked anti-inflammatory effect. Both these drugs have undesirable side effects with steady and continuous use. The anemia of Crohn's is addressed by increasing iron intake, and extra dietary protein helps mitigate the typical weight loss. Severe progression of the disease sometimes requires surgery to remove the most severely affected segments of small and/or large bowel, and to manage fistulous tracts. It is estimated, however, that 20 percent of untreated patients experience a spontaneous remission in any given year. In one study, 55 percent of patients receiving a placebo achieved remission, of whom 21 percent remained in remission at the end of the second year of the study; in another study, only 4 percent of those who had been given prior treatment with cortisone remained in remission after 2 years.[22]

A new intravenously administered tumor necrosis factor inhibitor, infliximab, is now being used in resistant cases to reduce signs and symptoms in Crohn's. Administered in 5 mg/kg doses, it affected closure of 55 percent of chronic enterocutaneous fistulas in a recent study.[23]

■ HOLISTIC TREATMENT

The diet predisposing to Crohn's disease, with low fiber and highly refined carbohydrates predominating, is thought to be very significant in the total picture. The diet of choice, therefore, removes sugar and refined flour, and adds vegetable, whole grain and fruit sources of fiber. Meat and dairy products should be omitted or greatly reduced to reduce levels of leukotrienes and the inflammation generated by them. Fish meals (e.g., salmon, halibut, or mackerel), which supply anti-inflammatory prostaglandins and prostacyclin should be consumed 2–4 times weekly.

General and specific micronutrient deficiencies should be acknowledged and addressed. Individual micronutrient daily target amounts to be obtained from a high-potency multivitamin–multimineral combination supplement, or as separate products, include: vitamin A 50,000 IU during acute exacerbations; vitamin C 1–2 g; mixed bioflavonoids, 500 mg; vitamin E 400–800 IU; folic acid 1–20 mg; vitamin B_{12} 200 μg; zinc picolinate 50 mg; and magnesium 600 mg (divided doses). Fish oil 2–3 g b.i.d. or flaxseed oil (one tbsp daily) supply prostacyclin substrates and reduce the frequency of relapses 50–60 percent.[24] Amino acids (not derived from foods likely to be offending—milk and wheat) supply adequate protein and require no digestion before assimilation.

Recognition of possible food sensitivities is addressed with the institution of low-antigenic diets (elemental diets) composed of a small number of foods unlikely to be offending. This dietary approach has generally met with great success. Studies show that elemental diets lead to remission more quickly than the usual response to corticosteroids used in acute exacerbations; remissions with elemental diets are longer than those following steroid treatment.[25] Identified offending foods often need to be omitted indefinitely.

Commonly used herbs include *Echinacea augustifolia*, *Althea officinalis*, *Baptisia tinctora*, *Germanium maculatum*, *Ulmus fulva*, and *Hydrastis canadensis*. These are often combined in a traditional naturopathic formulation, Robert's formula, and its modification, Bastyr's formula.

Stress plays a significant role in Crohn's disease. The consistent practice of relaxation skills, biofeedback and meditation alleviate all inflammatory conditions and improve immune responses with the down-regulation of baseline sympathetic nervous system activity. It cannot be overemphasized: the mind is infinitely more powerful than most can imagine.

The liver, skin, joint, and spine complications of Crohn's disease need to be recognized and treated.

Inflammatory Bowel Disease: Ulcerative Colitis ....

■ DESCRIPTION

Ulcerative colitis is a chronic inflammatory disease of the mucosa and submucosa of the colon, occasionally involving the terminal ileum. The inflammation may be so fulminant that mucosal segments quickly become eroded, creating ulcerated lesions that bleed extremely easily. The disease most commonly announces its presence with bloody diarrhea, cramping, tenesmus, anorexia, malaise, weight loss, and sometimes fever and diaphoresis. Physical examination reveals abdominal tenderness and, in long-standing cases, anal abnormalities including hemorrhoids, fissures, fistulas, and sometimes abscesses. Colon X-rays demonstrate a typical moth-eaten, ulcerative mucosal pattern and sigmoidoscopy usually reveals grossly inflamed patches with ulcerations. A relapsing-remitting pattern commonly ensues, in which phases of partial healing are punctuated by acute exacerbations.

■ PREVALENCE

In the United States, 200,000–400,000 people are thought to have ulcerative colitis. The incidence rate is 100–150 cases per 100,000 people. Typical onset is between the ages of 15 and 35, affecting more women than men, Caucasians more often than Blacks, and those of Jewish descent more often than others. Like Crohn's, it is rarely seen in indigenous cultures.

■ ETIOLOGY AND RISK FACTORS

Textbooks state the cause as unknown. The following are possible contributors:

1. Genetic factors. Positive family histories and Jewish ethnicity increase the odds for occurrence.

2. Nutritional factors. The inflammatory bowel diseases are seen scarcely, if at all, in indigenous peoples on whole food diets.
3. Food allergies. Sensitivity to foods and food additives is not usually mentioned in conventional texts as a possible contributing cause. However, the consistent, substantial improvement during elimination and exclusion diets, and during parenteral feedings, lends great credulity to this probability.
4. Infectious agents. Numerous theories implicate viruses or bacteria.
5. Immunity. The immune theory classifies ulcerative colitis as an autoimmune disease similar to rheumatoid arthritis and lupus erythematosus. Anti-colon antibodies have been demonstrated in some studies.
6. Stress and psychological mechanisms appear to play contributory roles.

Carrageenan, a common stabilizer in synthesized foods, induces ulcerative colitis in guinea pigs. It may exert its damage when combined with the presence of *Bacteroides vulgatus*. The latter is found 6-fold more commonly in ulcerative colitis patients compared to healthy controls.[26] Carrageenan should be avoided in ulcerative colitis patients until further research clarifies the question.

■ CONVENTIONAL TREATMENT

Medications are used to slow the diarrhea, suppress the inflammation, and replace nutritional and blood losses:

1. Azulfidine (sulfasalazine) is the treatment of choice for exacerbations, and chronic prophylaxis to reduce the frequency of recurrences. It often works well, especially in mild to moderate stages of the disease. It should not be prescribed for anyone allergic to sulfas.
2. Olsalazine (Dipentum) is a salicylate derivative that can help maintain improvement once healing is underway.
3. Instillation of retention enemas of short-chain fatty acids (sodium-acetate, sodium-propionate and sodium-butyrate) on a daily basis or b.i.d. is helpful.

4. Aspirin (Rowasa) and cortisone enemas (Cortenema) or rectal foams (Proctofoam) are beneficial, especially when the disease is limited to the rectum.
5. Nicotine skin patches have also been used (ulcerative colitis, for as yet unexplained reasons, is less common in smokers).
6. In acute exacerbations nutrition may need to be maintained by parenteral hyperalimentation.
7. Immunosuppressants such as Imuran and Cyclosporine are used in resistant disease failing other treatments.
8. Low-dose injected heparin led to remission in 12 of 16 acutely ill patients unresponsive to corticosteroids in a 1997 study.[27]
9. Corticosteroids, such as prednisone, given in very large doses, may be necessary to suppress the inflammation in more severe disease. Parenteral steroids are occasionally necessary. The dosages of prednisone or other potent synthetic cortisone derivatives are then slowly tapered to avoid the long-term side effects.

The serious consequences of long-term and high-dose use of steroids include: suppression of the immune system; overgrowth of Candida in the intestine; osteoporosis; weight gain which spares the limbs; moon-faced appearance; development of prominent blood vessels and striae in the dermis; wasting of muscle protein; promotion of diabetes; and loss of neuronal dendrites in areas of the brain.

Rarely, all medical measures fail, and partial or total colectomy become necessary life-saving measures. Patients who have relapsing ulcerative colitis for 15–20 years are at a higher risk for the development of cancer of the bowel and rectum, and need frequent regular reassessment.

■ HOLISTIC TREATMENT

Bowel rest in the acute phase of the disease is usually instituted. With severe symptoms, nutrition needs to be supplied by products that yield essentially no fiber residual, reducing the stimulation and work required by the diseased bowel. Examples are Ultra

Clear or Ultra Clear Sustain from Metagenics, Eugene, OR, or Medipro from Thorne, Sandpoint, ID. In more severe cases of acute onset, as mentioned above, parenteral hyperalimentation with nothing by mouth for several days is necessary to achieve sufficient rest for the bowel. Caloric malnutrition often occurs because of anorexia and poor assimilation of nutrients. Partially predigested proteins, easily assimilable amino acid supplements, and low-fiber elements are necessary dietary constituents in the acute phase of the disease.

Optimum treatment for maintenance utilizes a higher-fiber diet without utilizing wheat bran. Refined carbohydrates and saturated fats should not be included. Two food groups to be avoided because they may trigger exacerbations: the cruciferous vegetables (cabbage, broccoli, cauliflower, kale, Brussels sprouts, turnip, mustard), and, in gluten-sensitive persons, gluten-containing grains (wheat, barley, triticale, rye, and to some extent oats).

Extra-normal amounts of micronutrients are necessary in the acute and chronic phases of ulcerative colitis. A potent, daily, megadose multivitamin/mineral preparation needs to include high amounts of vitamins, minerals, and other supplements listed below. Because sulfasalazine and olsalazine used long-term promote loss of folic acid, extra intake is required. Mineral deficiencies are common. Anemia and iron deficiency occur secondary to persistent bleeding, and extra losses of calcium, magnesium, potassium, and zinc occur with diarrhea. PABA (para-aminobenzoic acid), a B-complex vitamin possessing anti-inflammatory and anti-fibrotic effects, is effective in doses of 2–3 g q.i.d. PABA is helpful in a number of autoimmune diseases, and is known for prolonging survival and improving respiratory exchange in scleroderma.[28]

Daily target intake amounts of micronutrients include: vitamins C 1–2 g; E 800 IU; D 400 IU; K 3 mg; B_{12} 500 µg; folic acid 3–5 mg; B-complex 50 mg each; biotin 300 µg; 50–100 mg of elemental iron (taken with 500 mg of vitamin C and $\geq$ 100 IU of E for better absorption); zinc 100 mg; calcium 500–800 mg; magnesium 300–500 mg; potassium 500–700 mg; selenium 200 µg; mixed bioflavonoids 500–1,000 mg; quercitin 0.5–1.0 g t.i.d.;

omega-3 fatty acids 4–8 g; L-glutamine 3–5 g t.i.d.; and gamma oryzanol 100 mg t.i.d. Gamma oryzanol is derived from rice bran. Omega-3 fatty acids are found in fish and flaxseed oils; they appear to delay, but not prevent, exacerbations of the disease.[29–31]

Food elimination protocols have been mentioned in several gastrointestinal problems. Food sensitivity is the central issue in some ulcerative colitis patients and appropriate exclusion of offending foods from the diet brings significant,' prolonged improvement. Occasionally, elimination of offending foods is *permanently curative*. Cow's milk derivatives, wheat, and sugar are statistically the most likely offenders. Other common offenders are eggs, corn, cocoa, peanuts, oranges, pork, beef, chicken, fish, soy, and tomatoes. Coffee belongs on the list as well. Time spent investigating food sensitivities is often time well spent.

Herbal remedies long in common use include: marshmallow root or licorice root (*Glycyrrhiza glabra*) teas (the latter contraindicated in hypertension); a tincture combining equal parts of *Echinacea*, goldenseal, and geranium, gtts 30 q.i.d.; enteric-coated peppermint oil, two capsules t.i.d.a.c., a combination tincture of equal parts cramp bark, meadowsweet, wild yam, valerian and lemon balm, gtts 20–30 t.i.d.; and Robert's formula or its modification, Bastyr's formula, from Eclectic Institute, Sandy, OR, or NF formulas, Wilsonville, OR (see Crohn's disease).

If dehydroepiandrosterone levels are found to be low, modest replacement doses are helpful, usually 10–20 mg daily for women and 15–25 mg daily for men. When corticosteroids are being used, lower doses can usually be used in enema form, prescribed for preparation by a compounding pharmacist. Injections of liposomal superoxide dismutase, one of the body's potent antioxidant enzymes, have been reported in a small series to be helpful in both ulcerative colitis and Crohn's.[32]

Physicians who have seen many ulcerative colitis patients see a pattern linking acute exacerbations with some acutely stressful life event. Curiously, large studies have linked recurrences to stopping smoking. Why would smoking deter recurrences of this illness? Some believe that denial of smoking, as an outlet for the expression of tension and anxiety, leads to the expression of stress-generated responses in the physical body, including the colon.

Early research in ulcerative colitis revealed that patient conversations, especially at times of recurrences, were often peppered with statements expressing a desire to get rid of their stressful difficulties. Ulcerative colitis and diarrhea have been found in numerous studies and clinical experience to be related to high levels of anger, particularly when the patient possesses no socially acceptable skill for expression of the hostility. The attitude most often underlying anger is hostility; indeed, ulcerative colitis patients are found to have greater hostility, conformity and rigidity compared to controls without ulcerative colitis.[33] The doctor–patient setting may afford patients the opportunity to talk about their hostility and anger without acting them out. Initial precipitating episodes of the disease are also observed to be often related to the loss of an important relationship. Appropriate counseling and personal work to help alter the psychological dynamics, attitudes, and worldview under which the patient is functioning offer potentially striking benefits with attenuation of symptoms and normalization of bowel function. The dysfunction of ulcerative colitis is a local manifestation of a systemic problem, with interaction of psychological, spiritual (beliefs), nutritional, hereditary, allergic, immunological, neurological, and endocrinological issues. An approach to anything resembling a cure requires addressing all issues.

One of the successful initiatives employed in this and other stress-modulated illnesses lies in the incorporation of techniques that teach the acquisition of the relaxed state, achieved through biofeedback, meditation, imagery, quiet contemplation, autogenics or progressive relaxation. Hypnotherapy, too, particularly as part of a multidimensional approach, can be of enormous assistance.

The spasms and cramping of ulcerative colitis may respond to acupuncture. Acute-disease homeopathic remedies in 12X to 30C potency used in ulcerative colitis include *Arsenicum album* for burning and intense cramping, phosphorus for painless diarrhea, prostration and thirst, and sulfur for urgent early morning diarrhea. Constitutional prescribing is the province of the thoroughly experienced practitioner.

Peptic Ulcer

■ DESCRIPTION

Peptic ulcers are the ulcerations, or canker-sore-like erosions, usually less than 0.8 cm in diameter, penetrating the gastric and duodenal mucosa and muscularis mucosa. The defect in the surface lining is the result of excessive erosive action of stomach acid and pepsin, a major digestive enzyme secreted by lining cells of the stomach. The mucosal surfaces are ordinarily naturally protected against ulcerative erosions. Gastric ulcers can occur in any portion of the stomach. They are occasionally the earliest sign of malignancy, in contrast to duodenal ulcers, which are almost never cancerous.

Ulcers may be present in early stages without causing symptoms. When symptomatic, ulcer is heralded by the onset of gnawing or burning upper abdominal pain about an hour after meals, usually later in the day or evening, rather than in the morning. Associated gastroesophageal reflux disease (GERD) may also give prominent symptoms of heartburn. Patients usually experience prompt relief from ulcer symptoms with eating or ingestion of antacids.

The diagnosis is made on the basis of the typical history and physical examination with mild epigastric tenderness in the midline or slightly to the right of midline. The diagnosis is confirmed by an upper GI X-ray study or by endoscopy. Endoscopy or a positive ELISA serum antibody test can confirm the presence or absence of *Helicobacter pylori*. The rapid urease test confirms the presence of *H. pylori* in antral biopsies with 90 percent sensitivity and 100 percent specificity. The urea breath test identifies the presence of *H. pylori* with nearly 100 percent sensitivity and specificity. In the last 10 years, *H. pylori* has been discovered to be present in 90 percent of those with duodenal, and 75 percent of those with gastric ulcers. It is clear, however, that other co-morbidity factors must also be present, since only about 15–20 percent of those infected with *H. pylori* will actually develop ulcers. *H. pylori* is implicated in the etiology of ulcers, but appears to not be the sole causative agent.

■ PREVALENCE

Lifetime ulcer incidence affects about 10 percent of the population. The ratio of men to women is about 4 : 1. One hundred years ago the ratio was reversed. Duodenal ulcers are four times as common as gastric ulcers. Eighty to 90 percent of duodenal ulcers recur within 2 years; this is reduced to below 25 percent with eradication of *H. pylori* infection. The incidence of malignancy in gastric ulcers appears to be about 2–5 percent.

■ ETIOLOGY AND RISK FACTORS

The major causes of ulcers are:

1. Excess acidity and pepsin from the stomach, overwhelming the normal slightly alkaline condition of the small intestine. Gastric secretions, with a pH of about 2, are potentially extremely corrosive to duodenal mucosa.
2. Reduced efficacy in the normal protective mechanisms defending the gastric and duodenal mucosa against erosion. These include (a) production of large quantities of mucin which constantly coats the gastric surface, in addition to (b) the ability of the stomach to regenerate its mucosal lining within a few hours.

Among the factors that promote ulceration or compromise the natural protection of the lining of the stomach and duodenum are:

1. Ingestion of aspirin and non-steroidal anti-inflammatory drugs (Motrin, Advil, ibuprofen, Indocin, Clinoril, Feldene,

Relafen, Tolectin, Voltaren). NSAIDs and aspirin are gastric and intestinal mucosal irritants, and frequently cause damage and variable amounts of bleeding.

2. Cortisone derivatives (prednisone, prednisolone, Medrol) reduce the resistance of the gastric mucosa.

3. Caffeine in coffee, and soft drinks and alcohol also contribute to this loss of protection.

4. Fried and highly spiced foods and chili powder are contributory. Smoking accelerates the discharge of gastric contents into the duodenum and reduces the capacity to neutralize their acidity by inhibiting the pancreatic secretion of bicarbonate. Smoking is highly associated with the incidence of ulcers, less favorable response to treatment and doubled mortality from complications.

5. Deficiencies of nutrients (see holistic treatment, following).

6. Stress is strongly related to the risk of ulcer development. A particularly aggressive and ominous type of "stress ulcer" is a feared complication, which may develop in patients experiencing life-threatening medical or surgical emergencies. This latter phenomenon is common enough that intensive-care unit physicians caring for such patients usually anticipate such an event and take steps to prevent it. The opinion of many authorities notwithstanding, the tension induced by significant and unmanaged stress is almost a universal factor in the etiology of ulcers. The history of patients with ulcers is often one of many exacerbations and remissions. Added stress often heralds recurrences.

7. The Zollinger–Ellison syndrome (pancreatic islet-cell gastric-stimulating tumors) exhibits a pattern of recalcitrant symptoms.

8. Blood type O patients are more susceptible for unknown reasons.

Complications of ulcers include: sudden searing pain from perforation; mild bleeding manifested by dark or black, tarry-looking stools; and massive bleeding manifested by "coffee-grounds" emesis. Any of these complications constitutes an emergency and must be handled as such.

■ CONVENTIONAL TREATMENT

The conventional management of ulcers involves the prescribing of pharmaceuticals, while occasionally resorting to surgery for complications.

Antacids which are commonly prescribed or self-selected by patients include Maalox, Mylanta, Amphojel, Digel and Aludrox; disadvantages of these aluminum-containing medications include the displacing of calcium in the body, and possible aluminum toxicity including accumulation of aluminum in the brain, thought by some to contribute to Alzheimer's dementia. Other antacids include Tums and calcium carbonate (may cause acid rebound), and Rolaids, Alka-Seltzer, and Bromo-Seltzer (these contain sodium that may affect blood pressure and cardiac function).

H2 antagonists block acid secretion (e.g., Zantac, Tagamet, Pepcid, Axid). These drugs, formerly available by prescription only, but now over-the-counter are widely advertised and used. With an active ulcer, relief of symptoms is prompt and healing usually occurs within 1–2 months. Disadvantages include suppression of acid secretion to the point of hindering digestion, side effects of nausea and diarrhea, and the suppression of vital nutrient absorption including vitamin B_{12} and zinc.[34] Unusual side effects include headaches, depression, liver toxicity, impotence, and breast enlargement in men. Cimetidine (Tagamet) may also reduce immune defenses.[35]

Proton-pump (acid-pump) inhibitors include Omeprazole (Prilosec), and Prevacid. These drugs are potent inhibitors of gastric secretion and recommended for treatment not exceeding a month in duration. Carafate (sucralfate) is a prescription agent which promotes ulcer healing by adhering to the ulcer surface and promoting healing through this protective action. Cytotec is a prostaglandin E1 analogue which offers mucosal protection against the gastric erosions caused by NSAIDs. It is prescribed to prevent gastric ulcers during NSAID therapy.

Antibiotics for *H. pylori* treatment reduce the incidence of relapse and lengthen intervals between episodes. Current standards suggest better results with triple-therapy antibiotics. A higher eradication rate is achieved when antibiotics are combined with bismuth subsalicylate, found in Pepto-Bismol. Patient compliance appears to be compromised with use of three agents at once.

Several decades ago, surgery was commonly done for recurrent and persistent ulcers and recurrences were common. The problem with surgery in this disease is similar to that in many situations: *partial gastrectomy or anastomosis of the stomach to the fourth segment of duodenum did not alter the underlying causative mechanisms.* The advent of H2 antagonists greatly reduced the need for surgery. Ulcer disease today becomes a surgical emergency only with uncontrollable bleeding, perforation, or gastric outlet obstruction. Mortality rates for these surgical emergencies approach 20 percent.

■ HOLISTIC TREATMENT

Intake of NSAIDs needs to be carefully monitored to reduce dosages and find alternatives with fewer gastrointestinal side effects. NSAID use multiples the risk for upper GI bleeding 5-fold compared to non-NSAID users.[36] Less toxic alternatives are often available for the management of musculoskeletal pain and arthritis (see Chapter 10). Smoking abatement is equally important, using a multifaceted approach including biofeedback, cognitive therapy, exercise, and acupuncture. Overuse of alcohol, often a problem in ulcer disease, is addressed with similar approaches. Part of that approach is to emphasize control and reduction of intake as a way of honoring the needs of the body and treating it in a caring way.

There is strong evidence that oxidative stress plays an important role in *H. pylori*-infected ulcer patients; increased antioxidant intake is a logical step in treatment. Daily intake of nutrients which are helpful are: vitamin A 50,000 IU for treatment of an active ulcer and 10,000–25,000 for maintenance; zinc 30 mg balanced with copper 2 mg;[37] vitamin C 1–3 g (inhibits *H. Pylori* growth in vitro);[38] *Lactobacillus acidophillus* (inhibits *H. pylori* growth);[39] vitamin E 400–800 IU; vitamin B-complex (50 mg of each element); high fiber (reduces risks of recurrence about 50 percent compared to recurrences during previous low-fiber diet);[40] omega-3 oils (prevent NSAID-induced ulcers in animals); bananas or banana plantain (fed to animals prevents and heals ulcers). In humans, low intake of potassium has predicted a higher ulcer incidence; this may explain why bananas, containing potassium, yield positive benefits); bioflavonoids exhibit anti-ulcer activity (5 g of catechin reduces histamine levels and inhibits *H. pylori*); cabbage juice (prepared from a blender, 1–2 pints q.i.d., established in older research as helpful in healing ulcers);[41] and glutamine, in doses of 1.5–3 g in divided doses.

The tradition of utilizing milk and milk products in ulcer treatment was terminated by evidence that increasing milk intake is associated with increasing the risk of ulcers. Research from mid-century established milk and other foods—chicken, wheat, corn, eggs, beef, tomato, coffee, tea, oranges, avocados, peaches, potatoes, barley, chocolate, grapes, peanuts, and spices—as potential sensitizing agents in gastric and duodenal irritation. In 30 patients in whom milk sensitivity had been identified in food trials, application of a few drops of milk to the gastric lining introduced through an endoscope resulted in immediate swelling, erosions, and bleeding in all 30.[42] Persons with recurrent ulcerations deserve a food elimination trial and elimination of any identified offenders. A nutritional plan omitting sensitizing foods is highly successful. *Failing to eliminate food offenders almost always results in a continuing cycle of recurrence.*

Beneficial herbal agents in the armamentarium include:

1. Deglycyrrhizinated licorice is quite successful and has been shown to have effects comparable to H2 antagonists in both duodenal and gastric ulcers. Anti-*H. pylori* activity has been shown as well, possibly explaining the lower recurrence rate with DGL compared to H2 antagonists. Dosage: two 380 mg tablets t.i.d. on an empty stomach, 20 minutes a.c. Lower doses may be used for maintenance and prophylaxis. The ten-

dency for licorice to raise blood pressure is circumvented by
removal of the glycyrrhizin.[43]

2. Ginger root strengthens the mucosa of the upper gastrointestinal tract. Nutrition stores carry 250 mg capsules to be taken
q.i.d., and it can be prepared as a strong tea prepared from
the blended fresh root.

3. Bastyr's formula (modified Robert's formula), relatively unre-
searched, has a long tradition of use in Naturopathic settings
and a long history as a home-remedy.

4. Ayurvedic botanical remedies and other botanicals are used,
including a mixture of slippery elm and goldenseal powder
mixed in a 2 : 1 ratio, two capsules q.i.d.

5. Aloe vera juice, 1–2 tbsp q.i.d. also has a long folk-medicine
history.

Regular practice of the elements of a sound stress management program is essential in attempting to realize a cure. Utilizing
relaxation through biofeedback or meditation, imagery to modify
the competitive striving often found to be present, regular aerobic
physical exercise, and establishing a pattern of sound sleep are
important components of such a program. The perfectionism pattern frequently found in association with duodenal ulcer can be
modified with insight, practice, and cognitive psychotherapy.

Since studies show the incidence and severity of ulcers to be
highly correlated with a lack of positive life-events,[44] strategizing
ways of enhancing loving self-treatment, improving relationships,
and finding social support is important. The quality of the relationship with the patient also bears on the outcome. One study in
patients with bleeding ulcers found that positive results were 3
times as common when a medication was given with confidence
and positive enthusiasm by a caring physician compared to the
offering of medication by a nurse without authority or enthusiasm;
in reality, both "medications" were placebos.[45] Belief in the success of treatment greatly enhances the potential for better healing.

Insightful observers of human behavior relate ulcer disease to
issues of self-responsibility, self-esteem, oversensitivity to criticism, and fear of rejection. These observations correlate exceed-

ingly well with conventional psychosomatic research mentioned earlier.[46]

Acupuncture, too, has success in achieving relief from nausea and reducing gastric acidity, utilizing acupoints including the left calf zusanli acupoint.[47]

Homeopathic remedies include Nux vomica for the type-A person who gets heartburn following overindulgent eating; Ignatia for a tendency to eat foods that cause symptoms; Bryonia for after-meal tenderness worsened by movement; and Chamomilla for indigestion following anger and irritability.

Gallbladder Disease

■ DESCRIPTION

The principal disruptions of healthy function of the gallbladder are cholecystitis and cholelithiasis. They commonly present together. Gallstones are mixtures of cholesterol, calcium and bile pigments. A combination of decreased bile salts or increased cholesterol leads to the formation of free cholesterol (insoluble in water), which can precipitate as solid particles which develop into stones of variable size. When stones become larger than the caliber of the gallbladder duct, the obstruction of the release of bile from the gallbladder announces itself with pain, inflammation, indigestion, and nausea. The pain is typically in the right upper quadrant of the abdomen, directly over the liver and gallbladder, and usually starts after consumption of fatty foods. Pain may also be referred to the right upper aspect of the back and right shoulder. A vast majority of gallbladder disease is associated with stones. Very rarely, rupture occurs secondary to the intense pressure generated when the gallbladder duct is completely obstructed, rapidly becoming a surgical emergency. Confirmation of the suspected diagnosis of gallstones is made by ultrasound examination. X-rays may reveal the presence of stones containing calcium; contrast medium studies are necessary to demonstrate non-calcified stones.

Stone formation requires cholesterol saturation of the bile, biliary stasis, and a nucleating agent (bacteria, calcium salts, proteins, pigments) triggering particle formation.

■ PREVALENCE

Gallstones and cholecystitis are common in Western cultures. In the United States, autopsy surveys confirm gallstones in 8 percent of men and 20 percent of women over the age of 40. About 65 percent of people who develop gallstones are asymptomatic. Estimates of the number of cholecystectomies done each year in the United States range from 300,000 to slightly under 1 million.

■ ETIOLOGY AND RISK FACTORS

Risk factors for gallstones include:

1. Being female.
2. Being of northern European or Native American descent.
3. Being over the age of 30.
4. Consuming a high fat, high sugar, low fiber, low calcium diet.
5. Having coexisting alcoholic cirrhosis.
6. Being infected with the liver fluke (in the Orient).
7. Being significantly overweight.
8. Participating in weight loss programs increases risk. During weight loss on a very low-calorie diet, bile acid formation decreases, allowing cholesterol in the bile to become less soluble, increasing crystal and stone formation.
9. Excessive sunbathing for Caucasians. Compared to sun-avoiders, the risk for gallstones in Caucasian sunbathers is doubled, with risk increasing to *26-fold greater for those who always sunburned.*[48]
10. Taking problematic drugs; oral contraceptive agents increase risk 2–3-fold; hypolipidemic agents clofibrate and gemfibrozil carry a moderate to high risk for gallstone formation due to higher excretion of cholesterol in the bile; and postmenopausal estrogen replacement increases risk.

11. Increased hepatic secretion of cholesterol (obesity, advanced age, estrogen therapy), and decreased hepatic secretion of bile salts and phospholipids.
12. Having other diseases (diabetes, Crohn's disease, cystic fibrosis, cirrhosis).

■ CONVENTIONAL TREATMENT

After confirmation of the diagnosis, three choices face the conventional physician: surgery, medical treatment—"watchful waiting," or dissolution of stones with drugs.

When gallbladder attacks recur, cholecystectomy is still the predominant recommendation. With the advent of laparoscopic surgery, convalescence has been accelerated and hospitalization time shortened. Endoscopic sphincterotomy has also met with success in allowing stones to pass. The disadvantages of surgery are:

1. A very small risk of operative complications, including unrecognized damage to the common bile duct.
2. The 5 percent chance of incomplete removal of all stones at surgery including those in the common bile duct.
3. The 7–27 percent risk of recurrence of newly formed stones in the common bile duct within 5 years of surgery . Symptoms of common duct stones (post-cholecystectomy syndrome) are very similar to the original symptoms. This complication again shows that *surgery does not alter the underlying process creating the presence of stones.*
4. Five percent chance that a planned laparoscopic procedure will be converted to an open one, due to unforeseen problems.

Variants of laser lithotripsy performed endoscopically for common duct stones are also in use. Again, the recurrence rate for new stone formation would be expected to be substantial.

There has been a shift in the philosophy of gall bladder disease management over the last decade with the realization that most patients with gallstones can be managed non-surgically. "Watchful waiting" is becoming more acceptable; the occurrence of an obstructed gallbladder with imminent danger of rupture is quite rare. Conventional medical measures emphasize:

1. medications for pain relief in the acute attack, and no food by mouth for 24–48 hours;
2. a low fat diet;
3. weight reduction;
4. initiatives to lower cholesterol;
5. maintenance of adequate hydration.

Treatment with the stone-dissolving drug Actigall (ursodeoxycholic acid) has achieved only about 30 percent success. Its use is limited to non-calcified stones, requires months of treatment, and has a 50 percent recurrence rate within 5 years.

■ HOLISTIC TREATMENT

Prevention is more easily accomplished than curative treatment. Regular aerobic physical exercise has recently been reported to reduce the incidence of gallstones 20 percent below levels seen in sedentary persons.[49]

Persons on a low-fat, high vegetable and fruit diet have a significantly lower incidence of gallstones.[50] By increasing the bile acid production to keep cholesterol more soluble, fiber reduces the absorption of deoxycholic acid which also reduces the solubility of cholesterol. Some studies demonstrate significant benefits,[51] but other reviews have concluded fiber offers little benefit. High intake of sugar more than doubles risk for gallstones, and highest intakes of calcium reduce risk 70 percent.[50]

Supplements of benefit in managing gallstones are:

1. Vitamin C 1–3 g daily improves bile composition and reduces stone formation risk; women ingesting higher amounts of vitamin C have been shown to reduce the risk of stones and the need for cholecystectomy 25 percent.[52]
2. Vitamin E is also part of a complete program, since studies have found that low levels of vitamin E cause gallstones in animals.

3. B-complex vitamins (choline, folic acid, and B_{12}) have lipo-tropic activity, decreasing fat deposition in the liver. When used with substances that increase bile secretion (see botanicals, below), these lipotropic agents increase bile solubility and prompt dissolution rather than formation of stones.
4. Phosphatidylcholine (lecithin) 0.5 g b.i.d. and choline 1 g daily can both be used to increase solubility of cholesterol in the bile.
5. Methionine, an essential amino acid, exhibits lipotropic activity.
6. Taurine—a non-essential amino acid—increases bile acid production in doses of 40 µmol/kg daily, and may be helpful in doses of 500 mg t.i.d. if there is a positive family history, or if gallstones are present.[53]
7. Adequate water is essential to prevent even mild dehydration from decreasing the solubility of bile salts and increasing the likelihood of stone formation. The classical 6–8 glasses daily is a requisite.

Any individual foods that are found to cause symptoms need to be avoided. Dr. J. C. Breneman found in the 1960s that a series of gallbladder patients were totally free of recurrences while on an elimination diet permitting only beef, rye, rice, soybeans, spinach, beets, cherries, peaches, and apricots. On challenge testing, the foods provoking gallbladder symptoms (with the percentage affected) were eggs (93), pork (64), onion (52), fowl (35), milk (25), coffee (22), oranges (19), corn, beans, and nuts (15), apples and tomatoes (6). Treatment with antihistamines accelerated recovery, giving further impetus to the belief that gallbladder disease has a significant allergic factor.[54] Physicians practicing complementary medicine have found this approach very rewarding.

Herbs which increase bile production by the liver (with dried extract dosages t.i.d.) include:

1. dandelion (*Taraxacum officinalis*) dried root 4 g,
2. silymarin (*Silybum marianum*) 100–200 mg,
3. celandine (*Chelidonium majus*) 1 : 5 tincture gtts 15–20 t.i.d.,
4. artichoke (*Cynara scolymus*) leaf extract 500 mg,

5. tumeric (*Curcuma longa*) 300 mg,
6. boldo (*Peumus boldo*) dried leaves 250–500 mg.

Betaine, a plant derivative, has been shown to have lipotropic activity, decreasing fat deposition in the liver. Peppermint oil, 5 drops t.i.d., is helpful in treatment of acute phases of the disease, and may even help in dissolution of stones. Gallstones may also be dissolved by a combination of natural plant terpenes (menthol, menthone, pinene, borneol, cineole, citral, and camphene). One such combination preparation, Rowachol, used alone, achieved dissolution of stones 42 percent of the time, and when combined with the drug Actigall, succeeded 73 percent of the time.[55]

Use of castor oil packs, also mentioned elsewhere, placed over the right upper quadrant of the abdomen and right flank is used to modify pain and promote healing.

Classical individualized *homeopathy* and *acupuncture*, especially for pain, may both be helpful. For acute homeopathic prescribing in 12X to 30C potencies, Colocynthis is used for colicky pain, Chelidonium for pain radiated to the right scapula, and Lycopodium for pain aggravated with deep inhalations.

REFERENCES

1. Holmes GK et al. Malignancy in coeliac disease—effect of a gluten free diet. *Gut* 1989; 30(3):333–8.
2. Sazawal S et al. Zinc supplementation in young children with acute diarrhea in India. *N Engl J Med* 1995; 333(13):839–44.
3. Baretto ML et al. Effect of vitamin A supplementation on diarrhea and acute lower-respiratory-tract infections in young children in Brazil. *Lancet* 1994; 344(8917):228–31.
4. Jacobs J et al. Treatment of acute childhood diarrhea with homeopathic medicine: a randomized clinical trial in *Nicaragua*. *Pediatrics* 1994; 93(5):719–25.
5. Blanchard EB et al. Adaptation of a multicomponent treatment for irritable bowel syndrome to a small-group format. *Biofeedback Self Regul* 1987; 12(1):63–9.
6. Anderson J. Amer Academy of Family Physicians 1996 annual meeting Nov 1996. *Fam Pract News* 1996; 26(21):13.

7. Rimm EB et al. Vegetable, fruit and cereal fiber intake and risk of coronary heart disease among men. *JAMA* 1996; 275(6):447–51.
8. Ascherio A et al. A prospective study of nutritional factors and hypertension among US men. *Circulation* 1992; 86(5):1475–84.
9. Saliminen S et al. Lactulose, lactic acid bacteria, intestinal micro-ecology and mucosal protection. *Scand J Gastroenterol Suppl* 1997; 222:45–8.
10. Benninga MA et al. Biofeedback training in chronic constipation. *Arch Dis Child* 1993; 68(1):526–35.
11. Papachrysostomou M et al. Effects of biofeedback on obstructive defecation: reconditioning of the defecation reflex? *Gut* 1994; 35(2):252–6.
12. Yodrick MM et al. Comparison of the effects of a diet high in simple sugars on bowel function in healthy, lactose-tolerant men. *J Am Diet Assoc* 1992; 92(9):1121–3.
13. Walker WA et al. Uptake and transport of macromolecules by the intestine. Possible role in clinical disorders. *Gastroenterology* 1974; 67(3):531–50.
14. Nanda R et al. Food intolerance and the irritable bowel syndrome. *Gut* 1989; 30(8):1099–1104.
15. May B et al. Efficacy of a fixed peppermint oil/caraway oil combination in non-ulcer dyspepsia. *Arzneimittelforschung* 1996; 46(12):1149–53.
16. Bensoussan A et al. Treatment of irritable bowel syndrome with Chinese herbal medicine. *JAMA* 1998; 280(18):1585–9.
17. Guthrie E et al. A controlled trial of psychological treatment for the irritable bowel syndrome. *Gastroenterology* 1991; 100(2):450–7.
18. Whorwell PJ et al. Physiological effects of emotion: assessment via hypnosis. *Lancet* 1992; 340(8811):69–72.
19. Thornton JR et al. Diet and Crohn's disease: characteristics of the pre-illness diet. *Br Med J* 1979; 2(6193):762–4.
20. Mayberry JF et al. Increased sugar consumption in Crohn's disease. *Digestion* 1980; 20(5):323–6.
21. Steger GG et al. Folate absorption in Crohn's disease. *Digestion* 1994; 55(4):234–8.
22. Meyers S et al. Natural history of Crohn's disease: an analytical review of the placebo lesson. *Gasteroenterology* 1984; 87(5):1189–92.

23. Present DH et al. Infliximab for the treatment of fistulas in patients with Crohn's Disease. *N Engl J Med* 1999; 340(18):1398–1405.

24. Belluzzi A et al. Effect of an enteric-coated fish-oil preparation on relapses in Crohn's disease. *N Engl J Med* 1996; 334(24):1557–60.

25. Hiwatashi N. Enteral nutrition for Crohn's disease in Japan. *Dis Colon Rectum* 1997; 40(10 suppl):S48–S53.

26. Hentges DJ. *Human Intestinal Microflora in Health and Disease.* New York: Academic Press, 1983.

27. Evans RC et al. Treatment of corticosteroid-resistant ulcerative colitis with heparin—a report of 16 cases. *Aliment Pharmacol Ther* 1997; 11(6):1037–40.

28. Zarafonetis CJ et al. Retrospective studies in scleroderma: effect of potassium para-aminobenzoate on survival. *J Clin Epidemiol* 1988; 41(2):193–204.

29. Stenson WF et al. Dietary supplementation with fish oil in ulcerative colitis. *Ann Intern Med* 1992; 116(8):609–14.

30. Bennet JD et al. Use of alpha-tocopherylquinone in the treatment of ulcerative colitis. *Gut* 1986; 27(6):695–7.

31. Dronfield MW et al. Zinc in ulcerative colitis: therapeutic trial and report on plasma levels. *Gut* 1977; 18(1):33–6.

32. Niwa Y et al. Effects of liposomal-encapsulated superoxide dismutase on active oxygen-related human disorders. *Free Radic Res Commun* 1985; 1(2):137–53.

33. Engel G. Studies of ulcerative colitis, III—the nature of the psychologic process. *Am J Med* 1955; 19:231–56.

34. Sturniolo GC et al. Inhibition of gastric secretion reduces zinc absorption in man. *J Am Coll Nutr* 1991; 10(4):372–5.

35. Hast R et al. Decrease in helper (T4+) lymphocytes following cimetidine treatment for duodenal ulcer. *Clin Exp Immunol* 1986; 64(11):114–18.

36. Garcia Rodriguez LA et al. Risk of upper gastrointestinal bleeding and perforation associated with individual non-steroidal anti-inflammatory drugs. *Lancet* 1994; 343(8900):769–72.

37. Frommer DJ et al. The healing of gastric ulcers by zinc sulphate. *Med J Austr* 1975; 2(21):793–6.

38. Banerjee S et al. Effect of gut *Helicobacter pylori* and its eradication on gastric juice ascorbic acid. *Gut* 1994; 35(3):317–22.

39. Bhatia SJ et al. *Lactobacillus acidophilus* inhibits growth of *Campylobacter pylori* in vitro. *J Clin Microbiol* 1989; 27(10): 2328–30.
40. Aldoori WH et al. Prospective study of diet and the risk of duodenal ulcer in men. *Am J Epidemiol* 1997; 145(1):42–50.
41. Vargha G et al. Standardized cabbage factor complex for peptic ulcers. Report of animal experiments and 162 ambulatory cases. *J Am Women's Assoc* 1963; 18(6):460–3.
42. Reimann HJ et al. Gastric mucosal reactions in patients with food allergy. *Am J Gastroenterol* 1988; 83(11):1212–18.
43. Turpie AG et al. Clinical trial of deglycyrrhizinized liquorice in gastric ulcer. *Gut* 1969; 10(4):299–302.
44. Hui WM et al. Life events and daily stress in duodenal ulcer disease: a prospective study of patients with active disease and in remission. *Digestion* 1992; 52(3–4):165–72.
45. Gliedman LH et al. Reduction of symptoms by pharmacologically inert substances and by short-term psychotherapy. *Arch Neurol Psychiatr (Chicago)* 1958; 79(3):819–25.
46. Shealy N, Myss C. *The Creation of Health*. Walpole, NH: Stillpoint. 1988.
47. Tougas G et al. Effect of acupuncture on gastric acid secretion in healthy male volunteers. *Digestive Dis Sci* 1992; 37(10):1576–82.
48. Pavel S. Sunbathing and gallstones. *Lancet* 1992; 339(8787) 241–2.
49. Leitzmann MF et al. The relation of physical activity to risk for symptomatic gallstone disease in men. *Ann Intern Med* 1998; 128(6):417–25.
50. Moerman CJ et al. Dietary risk factors for clinically diagnosed gallstones in middle-aged men. A 25-year follow-up study (the Zutphen study). *Ann Epidemiol* 1994; 4(3):248–54.
51. Moran S et al. Effects of fiber administration in the prevention of gallstones in obese patients on a reducing diet. A clinical trial. *Rev Gastroenterol Mex* 1997; 62(4):266–72.
52. Simon JA et al. Ascorbic acid supplement use and the prevalence of gall bladder disease. *J Clin Epidemiology* 1998; 51(3):257–65.
53. Wang WY et al. Effect of a taurine-supplemented diet on conjugated bile acids in biliary surgical patients. *JPEN J Parenter Enteral Nutr* 1991; 15(3):294–7.

54. Breneman JC. Allergy elimination diet as the most effective gall-bladder diet. *Ann Allergy* 1968; 26(2):83–7.

55. Ellis WR et al. Pilot study of combination treatment for gall stones with medium dose chenodeoxycholic acid and a terpene preparation. *Br J Med (Clin Res Edition)* 1984; 289(6438):153–6.

5

Chapter Five

Neurological Disease

Tension Headache

■ DESCRIPTION

Tension headache is the descriptor for the steady, constant, dull ache and pressure sensation, bilaterally involving the entire head from the temples to the cervical muscles. The pain is thought to result from entrapment of substance P in contracted, tense muscles. The trapezius, cervical, and temporal muscles may be quite tender, even when the intensity of the headache is mild. Tension headache is occasionally severe enough to interfere with sleep. Women are more prone to headaches during the premenstrual and menstrual days of the cycle; symptoms are more common in patients who are fatigued or depressed, and in those who are sleep deprived. Other structures which can contribute to headache pain include the temporomandibular joint, teeth, and inner ears. Most tension headaches do not signal serious disease and will resolve spontaneously.

■ PREVALENCE

Headaches are among the most common of human afflictions. For most patients, a headache is an occasional inconvenience which resolves spontaneously, but for an estimated 45 million Americans, it is a recurring affliction, and, at worst, a debilitating experience, seriously interfering with activities of daily living. The incidence in men and women is equivalent, and there is an even distribution across all age groups from teenagers to the elderly.

■ ETIOLOGY AND RISK FACTORS

Tension headaches are thought to be caused by sustained contraction of the occipito-frontalis, cervical, and trapezius muscles, the result of exaggerated poor postural head positioning, or by excessive tension triggered by stress. They can be initiated by the facial muscular tension of eyestrain, holding constant postures for long periods of time, reading with the head in a constant position, tensing the jaw in anger, bruxing the teeth at night, or even chewing gum for a long time. A listing of more common causes and triggers includes:

- stress
- poor posture
- muscle tension
- fatigue, lack of sleep, and overwork syndrome
- deficient exercise pattern
- eyestrain
- sinus problems
- recent root canal treatments
- temporomandibular joint dysfunction
- cervical spine mechanical problems
- hypothyroidism and low adrenal function
- premenstrual syndrome
- artificial sweeteners (up to 14 percent of those ingesting aspartame experience headache[1])
- alcohol has been ingested in a disproportionately high portion of patients prior to onset of headache[2]
- carbon monoxide exposures
- trichloroethylene, an industrial solvent, consistently causes headache and other toxic symptoms. The main exposure is to workers in industry.[3] Contamination of water supplies has also been associated with a 50 percent incidence of headache following exposure.
- anxiety and depression.

■ CONVENTIONAL TREATMENT

The most commonly used medications are NSAIDs (e.g., ibuprofen), aspirin or acetominophen (Tylenol). All three can have harmful gastrointestinal, hepatic, and renal side effects. When recurring headaches are accompanied by depression, antidepressants are frequently prescribed (see Chapter 8). Physical therapy is sometimes also utilized.

■ HOLISTIC TREATMENT

Nutrition

Because tension headache is so often related to increased stress, replacement of micronutrients which are depleted in times of stress is essential. The most critical are antioxidant vitamins C, E, and β-carotene, B-complex and minerals calcium, magnesium, potassium, zinc, manganese, and selenium. A mega-dose multi-vitamin-mineral product can easily meet all these needs.

Physical Activity

A well-conceived regular exercise program lessens the incidence of tension headache, presumably through the dissipation of tension during vigorous activity.

Biofeedback and Relaxation

Learning and regularly practicing biofeedback or any of the systematic relaxation approaches achieves a 50–90 percent reduction or elimination in both severity and frequency of tension and migraine headache.[4,5]

Meditation

Similar results are achieved with learning and practicing meditation.[6] Hypnosis and autogenic training have significant success with headache.[7] Self-hypnosis has been particularly helpful in children and teenagers.[8] These approaches to the process of change are enhanced by other stress management initiatives including imagery and repetitions of affirmations.

Acupuncture in skilled hands is often very effective in acute and chronic-recurrent tension headache and has also been used intermittently for prevention.[9] Acupressure applied to the thumb-index finger web of the hands works often enough to be worth suggesting.

Therapeutic touch has been shown to provide a substantial, sustained improvement in headache patterns. Other energy therapies have success as well.[10]

Botanical Options

Aromatherapy. Patients using an aromatic combination of peppermint oil, eucalyptus oil and alcohol applied to the temples and forehead relaxed their scalp muscles, experienced greater general relaxation, manifested better cognitive performance, and experienced noticeably less intensity to the headache. Prescribe 5–10 drops of each b.i.d. to t.i.d.[11,12] Rosemary oil (1 part oil to 10 of vegetable oil) massaged into the temples and forehead has also been used with success.

A liquid preparation of capsaicin used intranasally has significant research-backed success.[13]

Other herbs commonly used as teas or tinctures include white willow bark (*Salix alba*, associated with aspirin development); Jamaican dogwood; valerian and Kava kava, especially when headache is accompanied by marked anxiety and tension; and meadowsweet (*Filipendula ulmaria*, contains salicylic acid).

Manual Therapies

The literature regarding chiropractic manipulation for headache is mixed, but a number of studies conclude it is helpful, especially when compared to treatment with antidepressant drugs.[14] Craniosacral osteopathic treatment has substantial benefits in helping patients cope with tension symptoms.

Massage therapy also has its advocates, research showing beneficial effects of massage in patients with chronic tension headache.[15]

Reflexology research has also demonstrated effectiveness for headache.[16]

Homeopathy

Constitutional prescribing can be sought from experienced practitioners. For symptomatic treatment, the following remedies in 12X to 30C dilution, taken as 3–5 pellets q 1–4 h until relief appears can be prescribed: Aconitum, Belladonna, Bryonia, Gelsemium, Arnica, and Nux vomica.

Migraine

■ DESCRIPTION

Migraines are the most common presentation of vascular headache, which also includes cluster headaches. Most authorities think that distorted blood flow to the brain triggers migraine episodes, but the mechanism involved is disputed. Blood flow during a migraine episode can be so severely compromised that stroke-like effects are occasionally seen as a residual.

Serotonin levels in those predisposed to migraine appear to be low in most cases.[17] The low serotonin levels are thought to lower pain threshold, a fact utilized in serotonin agonist drugs in treatment. Serotonin, a neurotransmitter with multiple functions, including the entrainment of arteriolar dilation, is stored in thrombocytes; in migraine subjects, platelets exhibit accelerated agglutination, releasing significantly more serotonin, but accompanied by inflammation-inducing compounds including histamine, leading directly to the pain of migraine.[18] An unusually high percentage of migraineurs also have mitral valve prolapse, a condition which theoretically could damage platelets as they traverse the mitral valve, possibly contributing to the pathological cascade of events in migraine.

The classical migraine headache is unilateral, and is frequently preceded by an "aura" of visual disturbances consisting of bright spots, zigzagy lines, blind spots, or temporary loss of part of the ipsilateral visual field. The ensuing throbbing, pounding pain is often severe and incapacitating. Untreated, the pain can last for hours or days and is often severe enough to also induce nausea and emesis. It is often accompanied by excruciating sensitivity to light, forcing the patient to seek relief in a darkened room. Typical age of onset is before age 35. The symptoms in children tend to be more systemic, with nausea, malaise, vertigo, and abdominal pain more prominent than the headache itself. Migraine episodes recede with age; the incidence in post-menopausal women diminishes greatly.

Cluster headaches are also unilateral, presenting as a steady retro- or peri-orbital piercing pain. Cluster headaches also strike people in their 20s and 30s, with typical onset at night or early morning.

■ PREVALENCE

About 15 percent of men and 25 percent of women have experienced at least one migraine headache at one time or another.[19] Cluster headaches, though much less frequent, are 6-fold more common in men than women. Migraine occurs in children as well, although more difficult to diagnose because the presenting symptoms are less classical.

■ CAUSES AND RISK FACTORS

Migraines can be caused or triggered by:

- Genetic predisposition, with one-half of migraine patients giving a positive family history. This predilection may explain why migraine-prone patients have low baseline levels of serotonin.
- Oxygen-free-radical activity markers are elevated, explaining the aberrant activity of platelets in migraineurs.[20]
- Smoking.
- Excessive and deficient sleep.
- Fatigue and exhaustion.
- Food sensitivities (see holistic treatment).

- Tyramine containing foods[21] (see conventional treatment).
- Withdrawal from caffeine reverses the arterial constriction effect of caffeine.
- Food additives and drugs (nitrates, monosodium glutamate, nitroglycerin).
- Rebound from withdrawal of analgesic or vasorelaxant drugs.
- Deficiency of magnesium; serum and red blood cell levels are notably below those in healthy people, increasing susceptibility to arterial constriction.[22]
- Weather changes, barometric shifts, sun exposure.[23]
- Eyestrain and excessive sunglare from snow or water.
- Stress often triggers episodes. The classical history is the onset of the headache in easing of tension immediately after an acutely stressful episode has ended. Studies have described the precipitation of headache in migraineurs by submission to a stressful interview in which the patient has little control.[24]
- Migraines are more common before and during premenstrual and peri-menstrual times and in women taking oral contraceptive agents. They are less common in pregnancy and postmenopausally. In migraine-prone pregnant women, headaches are much more common if pre-eclampsia is present; both conditions are related to lower levels of magnesium.
- Intense emotional experience and reactivity. Anxiety and depression are strongly related to vascular headaches of both cluster and migraine varieties. Perceptive observers of migraine think there is a strong association with intense organized activity to attempt to manage feelings of anxiety.
- Studies have shown that migraine patients include a disproportionate number of people with chronic candidiasis (see Chapter 13). In those with high positive candida antibody titers, a great majority experience marked improvement or cessation of migraines when the yeast infection is treated.[9]

■ CONVENTIONAL TREATMENT

Prescriptions written for migraine include drugs from a number of classes including narcotics, antidepressants, vasoconstrictors, beta-blockers, muscle relaxants and 5-hydroxytryptophan agonists. Zomig (zolmitriptan) and Imitrex (sumatriptan) are 5-hydroxy-tryptophan agonists. These drugs require long-term treatment of at least 60 days for potential benefits to appear. Ergotamines (Ergomar, Wigraine) are the most commonly used class of pharmaceuticals in acute migraine; ergotamine is vaso-constrictive, preventing the vasodilatory phase thought to trigger pain. Midrin is also a commonly used vasoconstrictor. Beta blockers (Inderal) also have a place in drug treatment. Suddenly stopping vasoconstrictors (ergotamine) or analgesics can trigger a rebound headache and a perceived need for more medication. *Drugs have no impact on reducing the frequency of migraine episodes unless continually taken.*

Because high tyramine content in certain foods can trigger excess elaboration of norepinephrine and encourage vaso-constriction, avoiding the following foods is often suggested: cheeses, pickled herring, fermented sausages (pepperoni, salami, bologna), overripe avocados and fruits, red wine, sherry, and red wine vinegar.

■ HOLISTIC TREATMENT

Nutrition

Nutritional initiatives in prevention include decreasing fats from land-animals and increasing foods that inhibit platelet aggregation including vegetable oils, onion, garlic and fish oils.[26] Emphasis should also be given to whole foods with high antioxidant vitamin and mineral content, given the apparent free-radical participation in the migraine process.

Supplements

Supplements of antioxidants beta-carotene and vitamins E and C give beneficial results.[26] Vitamin B_2 (riboflavin) 400 mg daily for

3 months has been shown to reduce migraine frequency by two-thirds.[27] IV injection of folic acid 15 mg in one study achieved total subsidence of acute headache within 1 hour in 60 percent, with great improvement in another 30 percent.[28]

Since magnesium-deficient patients are more subject to vascular headache, adequate intake (400–600 mg/day) from food or supplements is essential.[29] Intravenous injection of 1 g of magnesium over 10 minutes terminates an acute migraine within minutes in many and substantially helps in over 50 percent of patients.[30] IV use of folic acid in the acute attack is also strikingly successful.

Omega-3 oils (EPA and DHA, 14 g daily in divided doses) greatly reduce intensity and frequency of migraines.[31] Gamma-linolenic acid (GLA) is also therapeutic.[26] Melatonin 10 mg each evening for 2 weeks can terminate episodes of cluster headaches in 3–5 days.

5-Hydroxytryptophan 300 mg b.i.d. works well for prevention of migraine[32] when used long term.

Food Eliminations

In several studies of foods and migraine, a majority of migraineurs improves on elimination diets, and food rechallenge confirms specific food offenders.[33] The commonest offenders, in order of frequency, appear to be cow's milk, wheat, rye, corn, orange, eggs, tomato, beef, pork, yeast, shellfish, coffee, tea, and chocolate. A food elimination trial, begun with elimination of these most common offender foods from the diet, or using the more systematic approach described in Chapter 1, may bring great relief.

Herbal Treatment

Feverfew (*Tenacetum parthenium*) 0.25 to 0.5 parthenolide content daily has markedly helpful effects in migraine.[34] Dried ginger 500 mg q.i.d.[35] and Pueraria root also provide substantial benefit with reduced frequency and intensity of migraine episodes.[36] Intranasal instillation of capsaicin has been shown to induce remissions in cluster headache. Skullcap and Meadowsweet have also been used.

Homeopathy

Systematic constitutional prescribing is the province of the trained homeopathic physician. In 12X to 30 C concentration, symptomatic remedies include *Iris versicolor* for those headaches in which blurred vision is prominent; *Singuinaria* for right-sided migraine originating in the neck; *Lac defloratum* for frontal migraine preceded by an aura; and *Natrum muriaticum* for headache of hammer-like quality.

Other Options

Transcutaneous electrical nerve stimulation (TENS) treatment achieves considerable success.[37]

Massage therapy is effective as adjunctive treatment.

Physical Exercise

Appropriate regular aerobic exercise—brisk walking, jogging, sports activities, gardening, low-impact aerobics, and water aerobics are among the options that release tension from the system and diminish the frequency and intensity of migraine episodes.[38]

Mental and Emotional Treatment

Cognitive therapy. An understanding of the interrelationships of attitudes, conditioned responses, emotional state and disease as well as the dynamics of the change process can be enormously helpful. Many patients with headache and migraine feel trapped by their circumstances and distressed by the wide disparity between the way life is and the way it should be. Releasing the demands (the "shoulds") with a strong dose of forgiveness can lead to dramatic changes, which can often be quickly accomplished in the clinical setting.

Biofeedback and relaxation. Learning and regularly practicing biofeedback or any of the relaxation approaches achieves a *45–80 percent reduction or elimination* in both migraine headache severity and frequency.[39] Practicing regular meditation also results in impressive progress, potentially eliminating or reducing the need for medication. Hypnosis also has significant success with headache.[40] Self-hypnosis can be particularly helpful in children and teenagers.

Manual Methods

Chiropractic treatment in one study gave comparable results to medical and physical therapy management.[41]

Acupuncture in skilled hands can be very effective in migraine treatment. Forty percent of patients in one study achieved a 50–100 percent reduction in severity and frequency of migraine episodes.[42] Among acupoints which can be used also for acupressure are ho-ku in the index finger-thumb web of the hand, B2 below the inner aspect of the eyebrow, and GB20 and GV16 bilaterally and over the C1 vertebra just below the cranium.

Therapeutic touch has been shown to provide substantial, sustained improvement in headache patterns. Other energy therapies have success as well.

Multiple Sclerosis

■ DESCRIPTION

Multiple sclerosis (MS) is a disease manifesting in progressive loss of neurological sensory and motor functions. Anatomically, the process involves the degeneration of lipoprotein content of the myelin sheath of motor and sensory nerves. Neurons then lose their ability to propagate electrical impulses. The disease has a tendency to be progressive, and in severe cases, walking often becomes difficult, weakness of arm and hand movement ensues, speech may become slurred, and urinary incontinence sometimes develops. Fatigue is a frequent accompanying symptom. The disease may progress slowly and steadily or assume a relapsing/remitting pattern with long periods of stability between episodes of deterioration. Treatment measures can stabilize the condition for many years.

Early diagnosis of this disease is difficult. The early symptoms in order of frequency are:

1. motor—muscular weakness, clumsiness, dropping of objects, leg-dragging,
2. sensory—numbness, tingling, paresthesias, heaviness, tightness,
3. balance—lightheadedness, vertigo, ataxia,
4. visual—blurring, blindness, double vision, haziness,
5. pain—occasionally experienced.

Diagnostic tests, though non-specific, are used to confirm the suspected diagnosis. The most helpful are delayed nerve conduction and abnormalities on MRI of the brain.

■ PREVALENCE

The incidence of multiple sclerosis varies from 50 to100 affected persons per 100,000 population in higher latitudes in both northern and southern hemispheres to 5–10 persons per 100,000 near the equator. 350,000 Americans are thought to have the disease. In Switzerland and Norway, the incidence is significantly lower in mountainous regions and higher at lower altitudes and along the seacoast. In most areas, women with MS outnumber men 3 to 2. Onset is commonly between the ages of 20 and 40. The incidence has significantly increased since early descriptions about 1850. MS is uncommon in emerging nations.[43]

■ ETIOLOGY AND RISK FACTORS

The cause of multiple sclerosis is unknown. The leading theories are:

- Genetic—first-degree relatives of MS patients have an increased risk of the disease.
- Autoimmune reactions.[44]

- Viral infections, with theories of different agents postulated from time to time.
- Abnormal intestinal permeability has been found in over a quarter of multiple sclerosis patients.[45] Malabsorption has also been suggested as a contributing cause.[41]
- Nutritional factors, including high dairy and animal food sources, high saturated animal fat content, and deficiency of omega-3 fatty acids.
- Free-radical damage. Low levels of glutathione peroxidase, an antioxidant enzyme, appears to be present in greater numbers of MS patients than healthy controls.[47]
- High levels of proinflammatory prostaglandins of the arachidonic acid cascade and leukotrienes.[48,49]
- Environmental toxins—petrochemicals and solvents may trigger free-radical reactivity.[50]
- Heavy metal toxicity. A 1998 case-control study found an odds ratio of 2.6 for multiple sclerosis in those who had 15 silver–mercury fillings compared to those who had none, although the difference was not statistically significant.[51] A 1999 study found no differences in body mercury, but a 20 percent higher incidence of multiple sclerosis in those with decayed, missing, and filled teeth.[52] Visual evoked potential latencies in MS patients were significantly reduced 6 months after removal of silver–mercury amalgam fillings.[53]
- Vitamin D deficiency. The incidence of MS is greater at higher altitudes and higher latitudes. The evidence for the importance of vitamin D in protection against multiple sclerosis is circumstantial, but compelling.[54]
- Threatening stressful experience is more than twice as common in the 6 months preceding the initial bout of MS symptoms.[55,56]

■ CONVENTIONAL TREATMENT

Most conventional practitioners believe that the disease is inevitably progressive. Besides supportive care for complications, measures often utilized include concentrated courses of cortico-steroids with exacerbations. Based on the autoimmune theory, immune suppressant drugs are also used, including Cytoxan and methotrexate. These drugs appear to have short-term benefit, but demonstration of long-lasting results is lacking. Intravenous gamma globulin 20–30 g daily for 5 days with boosters every 2 months reduces relapses 70 percent in the first year of treatment. Beta-interferon is a drug that has been prescribed in recent years with varying degrees of success in up to 30 percent of patients.

■ HOLISTIC TREATMENT

Physical Treatment

Nutrition. The extremely low-fat diet pioneered by Dr. Roy Swank in Portland, OR, has shown remarkable stabilizing effects in mild to moderate MS. Even including patients with advanced disease, insti-tution of a low-fat diet supplying less than 20 g of fat daily resulted in a 35-year mortality rate of 31 percent compared to 81 percent for those ingesting more than 20 g daily. He and others emphasize the extreme importance of treatment as early as possible.

His regimen calls for:

1. saturated fat intake of ≤ 10 g daily with 40–50 g of polyun-saturated oils daily,
2. complete prohibition of margarines, shortening, and hydro-genated oils,
3. > one teaspoonful of cod liver oil daily (high in omega-3 oils),
4. normal amounts of protein, with emphasis on fish (at least 3 servings per week).

To limit fat intake to 10 g daily, the diet greatly restricts animal pro-tein which has a higher fat content. In restricting animal protein and animal fat, the diet greatly reduces the intake of lipophilic pes-ticides, herbicides, and fungicides which are hyperconcentrated in the fat of animals. This may be one reason why the diet works well. The diet also reduces platelet adhesion, reduces autoimmune responses, and increases essential fatty acid levels in the bloodstream and spinal fluid. These effects probably globally reduce the entry of toxins into the central nervous system.

Supplements

- Omega-3 oils from fish sources are essential (3–6 1-g capsules b.i.d.) and can be obtained from flaxseed oil as well (1 tsp daily).[58]
- Daily antioxidants, especially vitamin E 400–1,200 IU are important. A high-dose multivitamin–mineral preparation will supply most needs.
- Vitamin B_{12} by injection in massive doses has been shown to improve nerve electrical conduction time. A reasonable dose is 1–10 mg from daily to weekly.[59] Patients can easily be instructed to self-administer injections at home.

Food sensitivities. A small study in the 1950s demonstrated positive food reactions in about 40 percent of MS patients and found that elimination of offenders led to complete or substantial remission in 10 percent, and clinically significant improvement in 20 percent.[60] Attempts to replicate this finding have not met with success.

Mercury toxicity. Improvement in function with removal of mercury amalgam dental fillings has been reported but no large-scale studies have been published. Removal of amalgam fillings is expensive and the potential benefits need to be individually assessed. Significant improvement in hearing loss associated with multiple sclerosis was reported in 1997 in a small series of patients whose amalgam fillings were removed.[61]

Exercise. Although exercise is the last thing that fatigued MS patients think they can do, studies document improvement in upper- and lower-body strength and significant gains in scores on anxiety and depression tests. Holistic physicians, physical therapists, and sports medicine trainers can be helpful. If deterioration of function after exercise beyond the expected 12–24 hours of muscle tiredness is reported, the exercise should be reduced; the correct balance of challenge is critical.[62]

Biomolecular Options

Autoimmune diseases are thought by many to be related to distorted intestinal assimilation with failure to appropriately absorb all the needed nutrients and prevent absorption of toxins, incompletely digested food substances, and potentially toxic organisms and chemicals which can cause abnormal responses by the immune system. Those who take seriously the assimilation research suggest that patients undertake extensive evaluation of stool specimens sent to laboratories who specialize in this work. Vigorous treatment of abnormalities is undertaken to normalize the balance of organisms in the intestine and repair the function of the intestinal mucosa with probiotics and a balance of nutrients.

Preliminary experimental research with natural alpha-interferon derived from leucocytes has shown encouraging results with a high percentage of remission in initial 2-year treatment periods. Treatment in the United States will not be generally available until further research is completed.[63]

Bee venom therapy, enthusiastically embraced by a small number of holistic physicians in the United States, has been researched and shown to be beneficial in reported cases. Large-scale controlled trials have not been done.

Botanical Options

Forty-four percent of MS patients noted benefit in symptoms and strength during treatment with Padma 28 (a combination herbal product), 2 tablets t.i.d. for a year.[64]

Mental, Emotional, Attitudinal, and Belief

Cases of complete recovery from MS with permanent remission of all symptoms and resumption of all functions have been reported, just as cases of recovery from far advanced cancer, intractable coma and amyotrophic lateral sclerosis (Lou Gehrig's disease) have been reported. These possibilities are enhanced in a climate of positive attitudes and beliefs. Communication with patients should tell this story, letting the patient accept what he or she chooses from the doctrine of hope. Patients should be encouraged to find positive supportive people with whom to associate; to read the stories, and listen to the cases of recovery. Their quality of life will be enhanced.[65]

Attention Deficit Hyperactivity Disorder

■ DESCRIPTION

Attention deficit disorder (ADD) encompasses a group of conditions including those previously called "minimal brain dysfunction," "hyperkinetic disorder," and "minimal brain damage." Attention deficit disorder is seen with and without a component of hyperactivity. The identifying diagnostic features of ADD patients are:

- distractibility, inattention, short attention span, lack of perseverance, failure to finish, not listening, poor concentration,
- dysfunctional memory and thinking, forgetful,
- poor listening,
- poor organizational skills, loses things,
- emotional instability,
- often bored, spacey,
- specific learning disabilities.

Hyperactivity features are:

- impulsivity, acting before thinking, abruptly shifting in activity, unable to stay seated quietly, settled only while participating in, or watching rapid-fire activity,
- hyperactive squirming and fidgeting, talking excessively,
- interrupting, difficulty taking turns,
- perceptual motor impairment,
- general coordination deficit,
- disorders of speech and hearing.

Electrocardiographic (EEG) abnormalities may be abnormal and soft neurological signs present. Positive emission tomography

(PET) scans of the brain have demonstrated that the prefrontal lobes, which function to organize and sequence thinking and behavior and maintain a mental focus, are hypoactively energized in ADHD children and adults. This phenomenon is significantly more demonstrable when scans are done following a stressful experience. Laboratory tests to screen for food allergens, subnormal thyroid functioning, abnormal glucose tolerance, and heavy metal toxicity may be done.

Children with ADHD often have converse reactions to medications, becoming "hyper" with sedatives (including antihistamines) and sedated with stimulants.

■ PREVALENCE

About 2–3 percent of the population is said to have a predisposition to hyperactivity and/or attention deficit disorder. Boys outnumber girls at least 5 to 1. However, distressing disparities exist: ADD and ADHD are diagnosed in about 6 percent of children in the United States, but in only about 1 percent in the United Kingdom. The most common age at which the diagnosis is made is 6 or 7.

■ ETIOLOGY AND RISK FACTORS

Risk factors, based on published studies and broad experience, include:

- Genetic influences. Some authorities believe that predisposing hereditary influences are present in 4 of 5 children with a diagnosable condition.
- Associative environmental factors often mentioned include poor prenatal maternal health, maternal exposure to alcohol, illicit drugs, nicotine and heavy metals, birth hypoxia, and low birth weight.
- Brain EEG with high theta activity.[66]
- Low levels of norepinephrine metabolites.[67]

- Predisposition to hypoglycemia. Hyperkinetic children have very flat glucose tolerance curves.[68]
- Standard fluorescent lighting has been associated as a contributing cause.
- Recurrent otitis media is associated with increased risk.[69]
- Heavy metal toxicity—higher amounts of lead and aluminum have been found in ADHD children.[70]
- Thyroid resistance. In 18 families with patterns of ADHD, 50 percent of adults and 75 percent of children had resistance to thyroid hormone. The odds for ADD were 3-fold higher in thyroid-resistant patients.
- Specific nutrient deficits. Iron deficiency is associated with decreased attentiveness and attention span, decreased persistence and decreased voluntary activity.[71] Deficiencies of vitamins C, B_1, B_3, B_5, B_6, and bioflavonoids have all been implicated. Fatty acid deficiency, as well, has been found.[72] The beginnings of this deficit may date from infancy; breast-fed children have higher levels of essential fatty acids compared to bottle-fed children. Bottle-fed children also have higher levels of manganese which is associated with an increased incidence of learning problems.
- Sensitivity to foods and food additives.[73] The most common food offenders to be cow's milk, wheat, corn, tomato, yeast, soy, citrus, grapes, eggs, peanuts, cane sugar, and chocolate. The most common additives found to be problematic are the red, yellow, and blue FD&C dyes. Double-blind studies show some children to be unequivocally sensitive to tartrazine food colorings. Over 5,000 food additives are in use in the US today: anti-caking agents, synthetic antioxidants (BHA, BHT), bleaches, colorings, flavorings, emulsifiers, fillers, preservatives, thickeners, mineral salts, and vegetable gums. About 10 pounds of additives are consumed by each person in the US each year.
- Social and family isolation are often aggravating factors; the isolation stems from inability of family members and

friends to accommodate to the fact that the ADHD child is different, often disruptive, and the central focus of the family.

■ CONVENTIONAL TREATMENT

The emphasis of conventional treatment is placed on pharmaceutical intervention. Over 2 million U.S. school children are currently taking the stimulant Ritalin. Other drugs which are used include Dexedrine, Adderall, Cylert, SSRI antidepressants (Prozac, Zoloft), tricyclic antidepressants (desipramine), anti-seizure drugs (Tegretol, Depakote), and clonidine (an antihypertensive drug with sedative properties which helps impulsiveness and aids in sleep). Associated bouts of recurring otitis media in children should be given high priority for treatment to break the cycle and eradicate underlying predisposing factors (see following).

Side effects of medications include up to $1-1\frac{1}{2}$ in. of cumulative growth retardation with the stimulants; vacation and summer drug holidays may help to attenuate this effect. Drug abuse is a hazard among teenagers and young adults using the stimulant medications.

■ HOLISTIC TREATMENT

Physical Treatment

Vitamin, mineral supplements. A potent megavitamin trial in ADHD children which includes part of the suggested amounts listed above can easily be undertaken with no fear of side effects.[74] Target dosages of nutrients which have been shown to alter hyperactive and ADD behavior in upper half of hyperactive children and teenagers (the most severely affected) are:[75]

- iron—20–100 mg daily depending on deficits,
- vitamin C—1 g daily,
- pyridoxine (B_6)—100 mg t.i.d.,
- thiamin (B_1)—100 mg t.i.d.,
- niacinamide—500 mg b.i.d.,

- pantothenic acid as calcium pantothenate, 400 mg b.i.d.,
- bioflavonoids—500–1,000 mg daily of mixed bioflavo-noids.

Helpful amino acid supplements

- L-tryptophan, prescription-available through compound-ing pharmacists (1–3 g at h.s. without food for sleep); or 5-hydroxytryptophan, available from health food stores and holistic practitioners (50–250 mg at h.s.), both gentle options to help the sleep of ADHD patients whose rest is often disrupted.
- DL-phenylalanine (500–1,500 mg mid-morning and mid-afternoon on empty stomach) helps maintain mental focus.
- L-tyrosine, precursor for dopamine, a stimulant neuro-transmitter (500–1,500 mg b.i.d. on an empty stomach).

Food elimination. Elimination diets for 1–2 weeks followed by rechallenge with eliminated foods, one at a time, often brings to light offending foods; an appropriate elimination diet often results in substantial improvement (see Chapter 1). Most studies with positive results report 50–60 percent improvement. In one of these, forty-two percent of hyperactive children showed nearly 60 percent significant improvement with less hyperactivity on a diet eliminating artificial flavors, colorings, preservatives, caffeine, monosodium glutamate, chocolate, and individually parent-sus-pected foods.[76] Physicians affiliated with the American Academy of Environmental Medicine also use hyposensitization procedures, administering desensitizing intradermal injections of antigens of foods to which the patient was sensitive, greatly reducing reactiv-ity and all associated symptoms.[77]

Environment

Standard fluorescent lighting is related to ADHD in some studies; for patients not responding to other measures, replacement of standard fluorescent tubes by full-spectrum tubes should be tried. New standard size full-spectrum light bulbs should shortly be available. And, for children and young adults who are not responding to dietary and food elimination protocols, lead levels should be checked. One of the least expensive tests is a hair mineral analysis which accurately identifies heavy metal toxicities.

Biomolecular Options

Persistent antibiotic treatment for recurrent otitis media in children frequently alters the gastrointestinal flora, permitting overgrowth of candida. Patients may need to be checked and treated for candidiasis, which, when present, often alters gut mucosal integrity, leading to distorted immune interactions with food antigens, and to generalized inflammatory reactions with increased free-radical activity. This may explain why antioxidants such as grape seed extract are sometimes found to be helpful.

If thyroid resistance is suspected, it needs to be confirmed and treatment instituted.

Chelation has been shown to markedly improve hyperactivity in children in whom lead levels were elevated.[78]

Botanical Treatments

- Hypericum (St. John's wort) 300 mg t.i.d. for the depression commonly associated with ADHD.
- *Ginkgo biloba* 80 mg b.i.d. improves circulation and may enhance frontal lobe activity although positive studies are not all in agreement.
- Kava kava has helpful anti-anxiety effects (see Chapter 8).
- Valerian for evening and night sedative effects, tincture 1 : 5, 1–1$\frac{1}{2}$ tsp or fluid extract 1 : 1, $\frac{1}{2}$–1 tsp at bedtime.
- Mentalin, an Ayurvedic herb containing Gotu kola (*Centella asiatica*) for improving memory and relieving depression (4–6 tablets daily).

Homeopathic treatment needs to be highly individualized and managed by skilled practitioners.[79] Symptomatic treatment involves 3–5 pellets of 12X to 30 C concentrations q 1–4 h of the following remedies: *Chamomille* for irritability; *Argentum nitricum* for anxiety in children; and *Arsenicum album* for sleep.[80]

Craniosacral manipulation. This gentle specialized manner of working with the craniosacral rhythm of the body has been reported to have considerable success.[81]

Mental and Emotional Treatment Options

Hyperactive children would seem to be unlikely candidates for relaxation training. They often, however, seem to look upon the challenge much like the challenge of computer games to which they are often attracted. Children learn biofeedback and relaxation skills quickly. EEG biofeedback training teaches the skills to affect a basic change in predominant brainwave function, and when persistently practiced can be of substantial help.[82] Studies have shown the benefits of biofeedback to outscore those of Ritalin.[83]

Alzheimer's Disease

■ DESCRIPTION

Alzheimer's disease is the most common of the dementia disorders of aging. The earliest manifestation is memory loss for recent and contemporary events. Forgetfulness, disorientation, confusion, and mood changes, language deterioration, including depression, are also common symptoms. Later symptoms include motor disabilities, tremors, disinhibited behavior, incontinence, and hallucinations. The Alzheimer's process is usually progressive, often leading to paranoia, inability to manage activities of daily living, and eventual need for institutionalization where 24-hour care is available. The typical autopsy brain lesions found in Alzheimer's dementia are formations of plaque and neurofibrillary tangles, and abnormal depositions of beta-amyloid protein, particularly concentrated in the hippocampus, the center of memory and intellectual functioning. With disease progression, there is increasing atrophy and cellular death in many parts of the brain.

Alzheimer's disease (AD) can easily be confused with other causes of dementia. Among them are multi-infarct dementia, cerebral arterial insufficiency, pernicious anemia, Parkinson's disease, Huntington's chorea, drug side effects, environmental toxins, nutritional deficiencies, alcoholism, and depression. Since some of these causes are more treatable, it is important to be as precise as possible in making a diagnosis.

An extensive investigation must include a carefully taken history (often with a relative present), physical examination, psychological tests (the Mini-Mental Status Examination and/or the Alzheimer's Disease Assessment Scale), and often a neurological consultation; laboratory tests, a CT scan, and EEG are usually necessary to rule out other conditions and confirm the diagnosis.

Fingerprint patterns with increased numbers of ulnar loops (loops deviating medially toward the fifth finger) predominating over radial loops, whorls and arches, are 3 times as common in Alzheimer's dementia patients compared to patients without dementia, making this phenomenon a significant marker for predisposition to AD.[84] The reason for the association is unclear.

PREVALENCE

More than 4 million patients living today in the US have been diagnosed with Alzheimer's disease or dementia. Alzheimer's is the commonest cause of senile dementia, affecting 10 percent of those over 65 and an alarming 50 percent of those over 85. Several million additional elderly have early dementia changes not yet formally diagnosed.

ETIOLOGY AND RISK FACTORS

Physical

Genetic. The risk for AD is markedly higher if first-degree relatives have manifested Alzheimer's changes.

Nutritional. Research shows that the free radical markers in brain tissue of Alzheimer's patients are twice as high compared to healthy patients of the same age who have no dementia.[85,86]

This oxidative stress is now thought to be the primary cause. Alzheimer's patients also have lower levels of antioxidant nutrients compared to healthy elderly controls, due to depletion of the antioxidant reserves by increased free-radical activity. Alzheimer's patients are deficient in vitamins B_1, B_6, B_{12}, folic acid, magnesium, zinc, and selenium.[87,88] Niacin (B_3) deficiency can simulate Alzheimer's disease. Functional elderly subjects with no diagnosed problems who have had lower blood levels of vitamins E, C and β-carotene in the past, as well as the present, score higher on dementia tests.[89] Deficient serum levels of docosahexaenoic acid (an essential fatty acid) are also associated with diminished cognitive function.[90] High levels of glutamate have neurotoxic brain effects; levels are higher in Alzheimer's patients.[91]

Toxicity

The role of aluminum and mercury in contributing to Alzheimer's disease is disputed. The concentration of these minerals in brain tissue at autopsy is significantly higher in those who had Alzheimer's versus those who did not. Alzheimer's is more common in patients who have used more axillary antiperspirants containing aluminum,[92] those who lived in districts with higher aluminum content in the water supply,[93] and those whose aluminum blood levels were higher. Aluminum is known to be absorbed from many sources (see below). Mercury in animals accumulates to a modest extent in brain tissue and induces a histological appearance in the brain indistinguishable from the neurofibrillary tangles found in the brain tissue of Alzheimer's patients. Some but not all studies have found higher mercury levels in Alzheimer's patients.[94] Other studies show that mercury absorbed from silver–mercury amalgam dental fillings is the major source of the body burden of mercury in most people. Both minerals are described as animal toxins by the Environmental Protection Agency.

Prescription medications can cause side effects simulating Alzheimer's; the commonest classes of drugs to manifest side effects of mental confusion are: tranquilizers (valium-type medications); antidepressants; anti-seizure drugs; anti-Parkinson drugs; antihypertensives; cancer chemotherapy agents; interferon; antiarrhythmic drugs; and muscle relaxants.

In persons who do not have genetic markers for Alzheimer's, smoking is a risk factor.

Disease Associations

A recent prospective report showed that men who had elevated systolic blood pressures in the 1960s had detectably lower mental abilities 25–30 years later in 1990. Chronically hypertensive individuals are at risk for atherosclerosis, a major contributor to "multi-infarct dementia," a deterioration of cognitive functions frequently indistinguishable from Alzheimer's. AD is also significantly increased in those with a history of chronic uncompensated hypothyroidism.

Biochemistry

Immune and inflammatory chemicals moieties have been identified in brain tissue of AD patients, suggesting that a strong inflammatory component is involved in the degenerative process.

Physical Inactivity

Groups of elderly persons who lack physical activity have poorer cognitive function and slower reaction times than more active groups.[95]

Mental and Emotional Factors

Low "idea density" in childhood and early adulthood appears to be related to increased risk of Alzheimer's. This implies that children and young people need adequate challenge and stimulation to think broadly and develop a wide spectrum of mental images and ideas.[96]

Social Health

Medical intuitive Caroline Myss discusses the recent cultural shift in the social position of many elderly from being "wisdomkeepers" in society to being elderly dependents as a major contributor to Alzheimer's dementia. She senses the withdrawal of contact with surrounding family and friends in AD as a metaphor for the withdrawal and separation of the elderly into isolation and institutionalization in society.

■ CONVENTIONAL TREATMENT

Conventional approaches have little to offer Alzheimer's patients. Among the drugs used, seligiline, and cholinesterase inhibitors tacrine and donepezil may have some benefit in retarding deterioration. Seligiline also has antioxidant properties. Diarrhea may be a side effect of cholinesterase inhibitors. Amantadine, a drug used to prevent influenza, is reported helpful in some cases and is worth trying at 300 mg b.i.d. Reports have also recently emerged that highlight benefit with anti-inflammatory medications such as aspirin and non-steroidal anti-inflammatory drugs (e.g., ibuprofen).

■ HOLISTIC TREATMENT

Nutritional Supplements

High antioxidant intake is important in preventing and offsetting the free-radical damage associated with AD. A potent multivitamin–multimineral can supply most of the needed elements including folic acid (see Chapter 1). Research shows that the elderly who have higher levels of vitamins C (1–2 g daily), E (400–1,200 IU daily), β-carotene (10,000–25,000 IU daily), and B_6 (50–100 mg daily) do best on tests of memory, recognition and vocabulary.[97,98] Supplements of B_1 (300–2,000 mg/day) and B_{12} (1 mg weekly by injection or 1 mg b.i.d. p.o.) help stabilize or improve mood and cognitive functions.[99,100]

Patients with early Alzheimer's who increase zinc intake in food or supplements (zinc 45 mg daily)[101] do better.

Added intake of monosaturated fatty acids improves cognitive function tests.[102] Omega-3 fatty acids from fish, flaxseed oil, or algae sources are also a feasible option (100–300 mg daily of docosahexaenoic acid content).

Acetyl L-carnitine 2–3 g daily retard deterioration and achieves moderate reversal of some of the memory, attention, and mood alterations in Alzheimer's patients.[103]

NADH (nucleotide adenine dehydrogenase) 10 mg once daily before breakfast improves functioning in AD patients.[104] Phosphatidylserine, another endogenous substance, 100 mg t.i.d., also evokes noticeable improvement.[105] Coenzyme Q_{10}, 100 mg daily, has been used widely in Japan. If benefit is achieved with this endogenous, biosynthetic supplement, treatment needs to be continued indefinitely.[106]

The suggestion has been made that women taking estrogen for hormone replacement post-menopausally may have a lower incidence of AD. Several well-done studies now dispute this conclusion. If estrogen is prescribed, natural hormones have less possibility for problematic side effects (see Chapter 7). DHEA, if blood levels prove deficient, can be taken as a supplement (usual doses 10–25 mg daily). Melatonin has quite recently been reported to be useful in Alzheimer's.[107] Appropriate doses are 3–10 mg daily.

Environmental Options

Although the importance of aluminum and mercury in Alzheimer's dementia is still debated, since they are both identified to be toxic to the human body, excessive contact should be avoided. To reduce aluminum exposure, recommend that patients:

- Utilize deodorants without aluminum antiperspirants.
- Use stainless steel instead of aluminum cookware.
- Use glass bottles rather than aluminum cans if colas and beer are consumed.
- Avoid aluminum-containing antacids.
- Avoid storage of highly acidic or alkaline foods in aluminum foil.
- Avoid salt, baking powder, and pastry mixes with aluminum.

- Use a water filter to remove heavy metals from drinking and cooking water; certified city water supplies can contain excessive amounts of aluminum.
- Ingest extra supplements of magnesium to oppose aluminum absorption.
- Take citric acid and citrate forms of mineral supplements cautiously because they increase aluminum absorption.

To reduce mercury exposure:

- If patients are having dental caries filled or replaced, they can choose plastic or porcelain options rather than silver–mercury amalgam material. The extra cost may well be worth it.
- Avoiding high intake of coastal fish with high mercury contamination is wise.

In a 2-year research project, intramuscular injections of the chelating agent desferrioxamine significantly slowed the rate of decline in patients with early Alzheimer's disease.[108] Desferrioxamine removes heavy metals from the body.

If the onset of Alzheimer's-like symptoms in a patient seems to be associated with the starting of a new prescribed medication, toxic side effects should be suspected.

Herbal Options

Given research evidence, *Ginkgo biloba* extract, 80 mg b.i.d. is worth trying; it has a 60 percent chance of slowing the progression and even partially reversing symptoms.[109] One study also noted improvement in the electroencephalograms. A long-term trial of several months is necessary. The subtle benefits of many supplements may only become apparent when notable deterioration follows cessation of the substances.

Homeopathy

Comprehensive constitutional prescribing must be individualized by experienced homeopathic practitioners. Three to four pellets q 1–4 h of the following symptomatic remedies are used at 12X to

30 C concentrations: Helleborus for patients who stare vacantly and answer questions slowly; silica for mental deterioration with high anxiety; *Argentum nitricum* for impulsive behavior with high irritability; and alumina for slow responsiveness and generalized demented vagueness.[110]

Exercise

For maintenance of mental function, challenging physical activities are essential. Forty-five to 60 minute workouts of brisk walking or other aerobic activity several times each week are important. Alzheimer's patients in nursing homes who participate in bouncing a beach ball across a circle of a dozen seated patients were shown to be more functional and lived twice as long as a comparable group which only reminisced about old times. Physical activity is an indispensable element of every health maintenance program.

Mental and Emotional Options

Continued intellectual challenge is clearly beneficial in retarding the progression of Alzheimer's. New challenges including classes, reading and playing games requiring mental skill such as board games (chess for example), card games, crossword, and jigsaw puzzles are all helpful.

Social Health

Accepting social challenges has also been shown to prevent or postpone the dementia-like changes of advancing age. Patients who attempt to remember names, develop new skills, interact socially and conversationally with others maintain their alertness better and longer.

REFERENCES

1. Van den Eeden SK et al. Aspartame ingestion and headaches: a randomized crossover trial. *Neurology* 1994; 44(10):1787–93.
2. Lipton RB et al. Aspartame as a dietary trigger of headache. *Headache* 1989; 29(2):90–2.

3. Waters EM et al. Trichloroethylene. I. An overview. *J Toxicol Environ Health* 1977; 2(3):671–707.
4. Arena JG et al. Electromyographic biofeedback training for tension headache in the elderly: a prospective study. *Biofeedback Self Regul* 1991; 16(4):379–90.
5. Grazzi L et al. A therapeutic alternative for tension headache in children: treatment and 1-year follow-up results. *Biofeedback Self Regul* 1990; 15(1):1–6.
6. Benson H et al. Physiologic correlates of meditation and their clinical effects in headache: an ongoing investigation. *Headache* 1973; 13(1):23–4.
7. Spinhoven P et al. Autogenic training and self-hypnosis in the control of tension headache. *Gen Hosp Psychiatry* 1992; 14(6):408–15.
8. Gysin T et al. Clinical hypnosis therapy/self hypnosis for aspecific and episodic headache or migraine and other defined types of headaches in children and adolescents. *Schweiz Med Wochenschr Suppl* 1994; 62:64–6.
9. Hansen PE et al. Acupuncture treatment of chronic tension headaches—a controlled cross-over trial. *Cephalalgia* 1985; 5(3):137–42.
10. Keller E et al. Effects of therapeutic touch on tension headache pain. *Nurs Res* 1986; 35(2):101–6.
11. Gobel H et al. Effect of peppermint oil preparations on neurophysiological and experimental algesimetric headache parameters. *Cephalalgia* 1994; 14(3):228–34.
12. Gobel H et al. Effectiveness of Oleum Menthae Piperitae and paracetamol in therapy of headache of the tension type. *Nervenarzt* 1996; 67(8):672–81.
13. Marks DR et al. A double-blind placebo-controlled trial of intranasal capsaicin for cluster headache. *Cephalalgia* 1993; 13(2):114–16.
14. Boline PD et al. Spinal manipulation vs. amitriptyline for the treatment of chronic tension-type headaches: a randomized clinical trial. *J Manip Physiol Ther* 1995; 18(3):148–54.
15. Pustjarvi K et al. The effects of massage in patients with chronic tension headache. *Acupunct Electrother Res* 1990; 15(2):159–62.
16. Launso L et al. An exploratory study of reflexological treatment for headache. *Altern Ther Health Med* 1999; 5(3):57–65.

17. Anonymous. Treatment of migraine attacks with sumatriptan. The Subcutaneous Sumatriptan International Study Group. *N Engl J Med* 1991; 325(5):316–21.

18. Kagaya A et al. Serotonin-induced desensitization of serotonin 2 receptors in human platelets via mechanism involving protein kinase C. *J Pharmacol Exp Ther* 1990; 255(1):305–11.

19. Rubenstein E, Federman DD. *Scientific American Medicine*. New York: Scientific American, 1987; 11(XL):1–5.

20. Tozzi-Ciancarelli MG et al. Oxidative stress and platelet responsiveness in migraine. *Cephalalgia* 1997;17(5):580–4.

21. Hannington E et al. Preliminary report on tyramine headache. *Br Med J* 1967; 2(551):550–1.

22. Seelig MS. Interrelationship of magnesium and estrogen in cardiovascular and bone disorders, eclampsia, migraine and premenstrual syndrome. *J Am Coll Nutr* 1993; 12(4):442–58.

23. Arregui A et al. High prevalence of migraine in a high-altitude population. *Neurology* 1991; 41(10):1668–9.

24. Marclussen RM et al. A formulation of the dynamics of the migraine attack. *Psychosom Med* 1949; 11(5):251–6.

25. Heuser G et al. *Candida albicans* and migraine headaches: a possible link. *J Adv Med* 1992; 5(3):177–87.

26. Wagner W et al. Prophylactic treatment of migraine with gamma-linolenic and alpha-linolenic acids. *Cephalalgia* 1997; 17(2):127–30.

27. Schoenen J et al. High-dose riboflavin as a prophylactic treatment of migraine: results of an open pilot study. *Cephalalgia* 1994; 14(5):328–9.

28. Kopjas TL et al. The use of folic acid in vascular headache of the migraine type. *Headache* 1969; 8(4):167–70.

29. Facchinetti F et al. Magnesium prophylaxis of menstrual migraine: effects on intracellular magnesium. *Headache* 1991; 31(5):298–301.

30. Mauskop A et al. Intravenous magnesium sulphate relieves migraine attacks in patients with low serum ionized magnesium levels: a pilot study. *Clin Sci (Colch)* 1995; 89(6):633–6.

31. Glueck CJ et al. Amelioration of severe migraine with omega-3 fatty acids: a double-blind, placebo-controlled clinical trial. *Am J Clin Nutr* 1986; 43(4):710.

32. Titus F et al. 5-Hydroxytryptophan versus methysergide in the prophylaxis of migraine. Randomized clinical trial. *Eur Neurol* 1986; 25(5):327–9.

33. Mansfield LE et al. Food allergy and adult migraine: double-blind and mediator confirmation of an allergic etiology. *Ann Allergy* 1985; 55(2):126–9.

34. Murphy JJ et al. Randomised double-blind placebo-controlled trial of feverfew in migraine prevention. *Lancet* 1988; 2(8604):189–92.

35. Mustafa T et al. Ginger (*Zingiber officinale*) in migraine headache. *J Ethnopharmacol* 1990; 29(3):267–73.

36. Xiuxian G et al. *Radix Puerariae* in migraine. *Chin Med J* 1979; 92(4):260–2.

37. Solomon S et al. Treatment of headache by transcutaneous electrical stimulation. *Headache* 1985; 25(1):12–15.

38. Lockett DM et al. The effects of aerobic exercise on migraine. *Headache*. 1992; 32(1):50–4.

39. Holroyd KA et al. Pharmacological versus non-pharmacological prophylaxis of recurrent migraine headache: a meta-analytic review of clinical trials. *Pain* 1990; 42(1):1–13.

40. Simpson I et al. Hypnotherapy and the GP. *CMAJ* 1991; 144(7):908–9.

41. Parker GB et al. A controlled trial of cervical manipulation of migraine. *Aust N Z J Med* 1978; 8(6):589–93.

42. Lenhard L et al. Acupuncture in the prophylactic treatment of migraine headaches: a pilot study. *NZ Med J* 1983; 96(738):663–6.

43. Cutler RWP. Demyelinating disease. In: Dale CD, Federman DD, eds., *Scientific American Medicine* 1997; 11(IX):1–5.

44. Antonovsky A et al. The life crisis history as a tool in epidemiological research. *J Health Soc Behav* 1967; 8(1):15–21.

45. Yacyshyn B et al. *Digestive Dis Sci* 1996; 41(12):2493–8.

46. Gupta JK et al. Multiple sclerosis and malabsorption. *Am J Gastroenterol* 1977; 68(6):560–5.

47. Szeinberg A et al. Decreased erythrocyte glutathione peroxidase activity in multiple sclerosis. *Acta Neurol Scand* 1979; 60(5):265–71.

48. Neu I et al. Leukotrienes in the cerebrospinal fluid of multiple sclerosis patients. *Acta Neurol Scand* 1992; 86:586–7.

49. Cooper RL et al. Multiple sclerosis: an immune legacy? *Med Hypotheses* 1997; 49(4):307–11.
50. Landtblom A et al. Organic solvents and multiple sclerosis: a synthesis of the current evidence. *Epidemiology* 1996; 7(4): 429–33.
51. Bangsi D et al. Dental amalgam and multiple sclerosis: a case-control study in Montreal, Canada. *Int J Epidemiol* 1998; 27(4):667–71.
52. McGrother CW et al. Multiple sclerosis, dental caries and fillings: a case-control study. *Br Dent J* 1999; 187(5):261–4.
53. Siblerud RL et al. Evidence that mercury from silver dental fillings may be an etiological factor in reduced nerve conduction velocity in multiple sclerosis patients. *J Orthomolec Med* 1997; 12(3):169–72.
54. Hayes CE et al. Vitamin D and multiple sclerosis. *Proc Soc Exp Biol Med* 1997; 216:21–7.
55. Grant I et al. Severely threatening events and marked life difficulties preceding onset or exacerbation of multiple sclerosis. *J Neurol Neurosurg Psychiatry* 1989; 52(1):8–13.
56. Warren S et al. Emotional stress and the development of multiple sclerosis: case-control evidence of a relationship. *J Chronic Dis* 1982; 35(11):821–31.
57. Swank RL et al. Effect of low saturated fat diet in early and late cases of multiple sclerosis. *Lancet* 1990; 336(8706):37–9.
58. Bates D et al. Polyunsaturated fatty acids in treatment of acute remitting multiple sclerosis. *Br Med J* 1978; 2(6149):1390–1.
59. Kira J et al. Vitamin B12 metabolism and massive-dose vitamin B12 therapy in Japanese patients with multiple sclerosis. *Intern Med* 1994; 33(2):82–6.
60. Ehrentheil OF et al. Role of food allergy in multiple sclerosis. *Neurology* 1952; 2(5):126–9.
61. Siblerud RL et al. Evidence that mercury from dental amalgam may cause hearing loss in multiple sclerosis patients. *J Orthomolec Med* 1997; 12(4):240–4.
62. Petajan JH et al. Impact of aerobic training on fitness and quality of life in multiple sclerosis. *Ann Neurol* 1996; 39(4):432–41.
63. Squillacote D et al. Natural alpha interferon in multiple sclerosis: results of three preliminary series. *J Intern Med Res* 1996; 24(3):246–57.

64. Korwin-Piotrowska T et al. Experience of Padma 28 in multiple sclerosis. *Phytother Res* 1992; 5:133–6.
65. Crawford JD et al. Stress management for multiple sclerosis patients. *Psychol Rep* 1987; 61(2):423–9.
66. Mann CA et al. Quantitative analysis of EEG in boys with attention-deficit-hyperactivity disorder: controlled study with clinical implications. *Pediatr Neurol.* 1992; 8(1):30–6.
67. Hanna GL et al. Urinary catecholamine excretion and behavioral differences in ADHD and normal boys. *J Child Adolesc Psychopharmacol* 1996; 6(1):63–73.
68. Langseth L et al. Glucose tolerance and hyperkinesis. *Food Cosmet Toxicol* 1978; 16(2):129–33.
69. Reichman J et al. Learning disabilities and conductive hearing loss involving otitis media. *J Learn Disabil* 1983; 16(5): 272–8.
70. Tuthill RW. Hair lead levels related to children's classroom attention-deficit behavior. *Arch Environ Health* 1996; 51(3):214.
71. Krause M, Mahan L. Nutritional care in disease of the nervous system and behavioral disorders. In LK Mahan (ed.) *Food, Nutrition and Diet Therapy.* Philadelphia: Saunders, 1984: 654–70.
72. Stevens LJ et al. Essential fatty acid metabolism in boys with attention-deficit hyperactivity disorder. *Am J Clin Nutr* 1995; 62(4):761–8.
73. Egger J et al. Controlled trial of oligoantigenic treatment in the hyperkinetic syndrome. *Lancet* 1985;1(8428):540–5.
74. Kershner J et al. Megavitamins and learning disorders: a controlled double-blind experiment. *J Nutr* 1979; 109(5):819–26.
75. Colgan M et al. Do nutrient supplements and dietary changes affect learning and emotional reactions of children with learning disabilities? A controlled series of 16 cases. *Nutr Health* 1984; 3(1–2):69–77.
76. Carter CM et al. Effects of a few food diet in attention deficit disorder. *Arch Dis Child* 1993; 69(5):564–8.
77. Egger J et al. Controlled trial of hyposensitisation in children with food-induced hyperkinetic syndrome. *Lancet* 1992; 339(8802):1150–3.
78. David OJ et al. Lead and hyperactivity. Behavioral response to chelation: a pilot study. *Am J Psychiatry* 1976; 133(10):1155–8.

79. Reichenberg-Ulman J, Ullman R. *Ritalin-Free Kids: Safe and Effective Homeopathic Medicine for ADD and Other Behavioral and Learning Problems.* Rocklin, CA: Prima, 1996.
80. Blumenthal M. (ed.) *The Complete German Commission E Monographs.* Boston: Integrative Medicine Communications, 1998:107, 160.
81. Block MA. *No More Ritalin: Treating ADHD without Drugs.* New York: Kensington Books, 1996.
82. Lubar J et al. Evaluation of the effectiveness of EEG neurofeedback training for ADHD in a clinical setting as measured by changes in T.O.V.A. scores, behavioral ratings, and WISC-R performance. *Biofeedback Self Regul* 1995; 20(1):83–99.
83. Potashkin BD et al. Relative efficacy of Ritalin and biofeedback treatments in the management of hyperactivity. *Biofeedback Self Regul* 1990; 15(4):305–15.
84. Weinreb HJ et al. Fingerprint patterns in Alzheimer's disease. *Arch Neurol* 1985; 42(1):50–4.
85. Butterfield DA et al. Amyloid beta-peptide-associated free radical oxidative stress, neurotoxicity, and Alzheimer's disease. *Methods Enzymol* 1999; 309:746–68.
86. Bermejo P et al. Determination of malondialdehyde in Alzheimer's disease: a comparative study of high-performance liquid chromatography and thiobarbituric acid test. *Gerontology* 1997; 43(4):218–22.
87. Levitt AJ et al. Folate, vitamin B12 and cognitive impairment in patients with Alzheimer's disease. *Acta Psychiatr Scand* 1992; 86(4):301–5.
88. Gibson GE et al. Reduced activities of thiamine-dependent enzymes in the brains and peripheral tissues of patients with Alzheimer's disease. *Arch Neurol* 1988; 45(8):836–40.
89. Schmidt R et al. Plasma antioxidants and cognitive performance in middle-aged and older adults: results of the Austrian Stroke Prevention Study. *J Am Geriatrir Soc* 1998; 46(11):1407–10.
90. Kyle DJ et al. Low serum docosahexaenoic acid is a significant risk factor for Alzheimer's dementia. *Lipids* 1999; 34 Suppl:S245.
91. Miulli DE et al. Plasma concentrations of glutamate and its metabolites in patients with Alzheimer's disease. *J Am Osteopath Assoc* 1993; 93(6):670–6.

92. Graves AB et al. The association between aluminum-containing products and Alzheimer's disease. *J Clin Epidemiol* 1990; 43(1):35–44.
93. Martyn CN et al. Geographical relation between Alzheimer's disease and aluminum in drinking water. *Lancet* 1989; 1(8629): 59–62.
94. Hock C et al. Increased blood mercury levels in patients with Alzheimer's disease. *J Neural Transm* 1998; 105(1):59–68.
95. Satoh T et al. Walking exercise and improved neuropsychological functioning in elderly patients with cardiac disease. *J Intern Med* 1995; 238(5):423–8.
96. Snowdon DA et al. Linguistic ability in early life and cognitive function and Alzheimer's disease in late life. Findings from the Nun Study. *JAMA* 1996; 275(7):528–32.
97. Joseph JA et al. Long-term dietary strawberry, spinach, or vitamin E supplementation retards the onset of age-related neuronal signal-transduction and cognitive behavioral deficits. *J Neurosci* 1998; 18(19):8047–55.
98. Morris MC et al. Vitamin E and vitamin C supplement use and risk of incidence Alzheimer disease. *Alzheimer Dis Assoc Disord* 1998; 12(3):121–6.
99. Blass JP et al. Thiamine and Alzheimer's disease. A pilot study. *Arch Neurol* 1988; 45(8):833–5.
100. van Goor L et al. Review: cobalamin deficiency and mental impairment in elderly people. *Age Ageing* 1995; 24(6): 536–42.
101. Constantinidis J et al. The hypothesis of zinc deficiency in the pathogenesis of neurofibrillary tangles. *Med Hypotheses* 1991; 35(4):319–23.
102. Solfrizzi V et al. High monosaturated fatty acids intake protects against age-related cognitive decline. *Neurology* 1999; 52(8):1563–9.
103. Salvioli G et al. L-acetylcarnitine treatment of mental decline in the elderly. *Drugs Exp Clin Res* 1994; 20(4):169–76.
104. Birkmayer JG et al. Coenzyme nicotinamide adenine dinucleotide: new therapeutic approach for improving dementia of the Alzheimer type. *Ann Clin Lab Sci* 1996; 26(1):1–9.
105. Crook TH et al. Effects of phosphatidylserine in age-associated memory impairment. *Neurology* 1991; 41(5):644–9.

106. Imagawa M et al. Coenzyme Q10, iron, and vitamin B6 in genetically-confirmed Alzheimer's disease. *Lancet* 1992; 340(8820): 671.
107. Pappolla MA et al. Alzheimer beta protein mediated oxidative damage of mitochondrial DNA: prevention by melatonin. *J Pineal Res* 1999; 27(4):226–9.
108. MacLachlan DR et al. Desferrioxamine and Alzheimer's disease: video home behavior assessment of clinical course and measures of brain aluminum. *Ther Drug Monit* 1993; 15(6):602–7.
109. LeBars PL et al. A placebo-controlled, double-blind, randomized trial of an extract of *Ginkgo biloba* for dementia. North American EGB Study Group. *JAMA* 1997; 278(16):1327–52.
110. Blumenthal M. (ed.) *The Complete German Commission E Monographs*. Boston: Integrative Medicine Communications, 1998.

Chapter Six

Endocrine Diseases

Diabetes Mellitus ....

■ DESCRIPTION

Diabetes mellitus is a chronic, disordered regulation of carbohy-drate, protein and fat metabolism, in which the blood glucose is improperly controlled. Type I disease results from a lack of insulin production in the beta-cells in the islets of the pancreas, whereas type II disease results from resistance to utilization of insulin at receptor sites on cell membranes. When insulin is deficient or sub-optimally utilized, body cells become fuel-depleted, while the blood glucose rises to excessively high levels.

The classical signs of diabetes are excessive thirst and appe-tite, frequent urination, and weight loss. The diagnosis of diabetes depends on the finding of a morning fasting blood sugar level of 140 mg/dL or greater on at least two occasions or a blood sugar concentration of 200 mg/dL or more at 2 hours after the ingestion of 75 g of sugar. If the diagnosis is in doubt, a 6-hour glucose–insu-lin tolerance test measuring blood glucose and insulin levels at hourly intervals after ingestion of 75 g of glucose in 10 ounces of water may be undertaken. Over 50 percent of patients whose glu-cose tolerance test was normal have an abnormal glucose–insulin tolerance test.

In juvenile-onset (type I) diabetics, marked deprivation in glu-cose availability in brain cells can lead to diabetic coma, and the excess burning of fat for fuel can lead to diabetic ketoacidosis. In adult-onset type II diabetics, stress combined with dehydration can lead to hyperosmolar non-ketogenic coma. Ketoacidosis and hyperosmolar non-ketogenic coma are life-threatening emergency situations requiring urgent hospitalization.

Long-term complications of diabetes include nephropathy, retinopathy, and peripheral neuropathy. Diabetics tend to have premature onset of atherosclerosis, heart attacks, strokes, and compromised circulation. Loss of circulation to the legs can lead to skin deterioration and pregangrenous changes in the feet. Diabetics with high sugars lack the ability to convert sorbitol to fructose; a majority of the complications mentioned above are associated with the accumulation of high sorbitol in body cells. Thyroid function also becomes impaired in uncontrolled diabetes.[1]

The characteristics of type II diabetes mellitus are:

- onset at any time from early adulthood on,
- may or may not become insulin-dependent.

The characteristics of type I are:

- onset in infancy, childhood, and young adulthood up to about age 35,
- results from total destruction of the beta-cells of the islets of the pancreas, the site of insulin production,
- inevitably insulin-dependent.

■ PREVALENCE

Diabetes in the United States involves about 4 percent of the population. About 600,000 new cases are diagnosed each year, and diabetes is the seventh leading cause of death. Diabetes is all but absent among indigenous peoples, making it a disease of developed nations. Ninety percent of patients have type II disease, so-called "adult onset" diabetes while the remainder have type I diabetes of "juvenile onset." The incidence of diabetes in the American people has been increasing a little over 5 percent each year. Type II disease is more common in African-Americans,

Hispanics, and Native American Indians. One of every 5 persons over 65 is affected.

■ ETIOLOGY AND RISK FACTORS

Type I Disease

- Heredity plays some role.
- Early exposure to bovine milk as a risk factor is attracting mounting evidence (see below).
- Nitrates metabolized to *N*-nitroso compounds have been shown to produce islet beta-cell damage and may be problematic; cured meats including ham, bacon, and smoked meats, and drinking water contain significant amounts of nitrates.[2]
- Diet, exercise, and stress management are very important for optimal disease control.

Type II Disease

- Hereditary factors play a major role.
- Insulin resistance is a major factor.
- Sucrose intake and lack of exercise decrease insulin receptors on cell membranes.
- There is a strong association with obesity.
- Diabetics tend to have lower levels of testosterone and DHEA,[3] especially in states of hyperinsulinism.[4] The clinical application of these findings is uncertain at this time.
- Oxidative stress. Lipid peroxidation products are significantly higher in erythrocytes of diabetics, and even higher in diabetics with complications. Type II diabetics have lower levels of antioxidants (vitamins E, C, glutathione, and superoxide dismutase),[5] so deficiency of antioxidant nutrients plays a role. Leucocyte vitamin C is 33 percent below levels in non-diabetics in spite of equivalent oral intake.[6]

- Insufficiency of vitamins B_6 and biotin [7] increases risk.
- Deficient levels of magnesium, calcium, potassium, zinc, and manganese.[8] Mean serum magnesium levels in diabetics are 16 percent below those of healthy people, and levels in patients with diabetic retinopathy are 23 percent lower.[9] Serum zinc levels are 25 percent lower in juvenile type I patients compared to healthy peers.[10]
- Smoking. The risk of developing type II disease for those smoking more than 25 cigarettes daily is twice as great as the risk in non-smokers.[11] Smoking accelerates progression of diabetic nephropathy five-fold over the rate in non-smokers.[12]
- Sedentary lifestyle doubles the risk for development of type II disease.[13] Sedentary lifestyle increases mortality 4-fold over those in the high exercise category.[14]
- Psychological stress contributes to onset of type II diabetes and deteriorates glucose control in patients who have the disease.[15] In Swedish children, age 5–9, loss or threatened loss of parent relationships increased the risk of developing type I diabetes 80% compared to a group with low loss experiences.[16]
- Taking certain drugs increases risks for induction of diabetes; these include corticosteroids, estrogens, oral contraceptive agents, thyroid preparations, catecholamines, diuretics, antidepressants and other psychotropics, chemotherapeutic agents, and isoniazid.

Astute psychologists and skilled diagnosticians see diabetes as a disorder related to personal maturation and self-responsibility, with resentment or fear on having to take responsibility for another person or for oneself, anger at being neglected or ignored while constantly giving to others, discomfort with codependent excuse-making for irresponsible behavior or attitudes of others, intense efforts to prevent others from maturing into self-responsibility resulting in less need for them, and resentment in children when parents, out of ineptitude or immaturity, demand to be parented by the children.[17]

■ CONVENTIONAL MEDICAL TREATMENT

Management of diabetes begins with proper nutritional control, decreasing simple sugars, decreasing fat and increasing starch consumption to 60–70 percent of caloric intake. In juvenile diabetics, insulin becomes required, sometimes after a "honeymoon" period during which sugar is transiently easier to control. Proper insulin adjustment, based on adequate blood sugar readings, is imperative. In "brittle" diabetics, an insulin pump may be used.

In type II diabetics, a properly constituted diet is equally important. Appropriate exercise is prescribed. Ninety percent of type II diabetics are overweight and weight loss for these obese persons becomes very desirable. Prescription of oral anti-diabetic agents is common. Frequently prescribed agents include first-generation (Diabinese, Tolinase, Orinase) and second-generation (Diabeta, Glucotrol, Micronase) sulfonylureas and newer agents including metformin (Glucophage). Sulfonylurea drugs can cause hypoglycemia; death from heart attack or stroke is also significantly higher compared to patients controlled by diet, weight loss, and exercise alone.

The metformin drugs can lead to acidosis and increased cardiovascular mortality in susceptible patients, and must be used with caution in congestive heart failure. Metformin also raises homocysteine levels; extra supplemental folate is required to neutralize this effect.[18] Thiazolidinediones (Rezulin) reduce insulin resistance. They are not recommended for initial therapy and are to be used in combination with other agents. Hepatic toxicity can be occasionally severe and life threatening. Precose, an alpha-glucosidase inhibitor which prevents absorption of carbohydrate, is contraindicated in ketoacidosis, and chronic intestinal inflammatory disease, and induces moderate flatulence and diarrhea in some patients. When diet and oral drugs do not sufficiently control glucose levels, insulin treatment is undertaken. The addition of Humalog (human recombinant insulin) to the armamentarium has facilitated glucose control for some patients.

Conventional management emphasizes careful attention to the monitoring of patients for diabetic complications, including neuropathy, accelerated atherosclerosis, nephropathy, retinopathy, sexual dysfunction, and neurogenic loss of bladder control.

■ HOLISTIC MEDICAL TREATMENT

Prevention

Dietary initiatives. Vegetarians consuming meat or poultry less than once a week had a 38 percent lower risk of developing diabetes than omnivores in one study, probably because of high fiber intake.[19]

Cow's milk sensitivity. Children fed cow's milk in their first 90 days of life are 50 percent more likely to develop type I diabetes compared to those who are exclusively breast fed.[20] IgA antibodies to a cow's milk protein, beta-lactoglobulin, were found significantly more often in newly diagnosed diabetic children compared to healthy controls. Islet cell antibodies were present in 92 percent of the diabetic children but only 3 percent of nondiabetic children.[21] In sibling-pair studies (one sibling has type I diabetes, the other does not), in which HLA alleles for susceptibility to and protection from diabetes were identical, IgG and IgA antibodies to bovine milk albumin and beta-lactoglobulin were significantly higher in the diabetic sibling.[22] IgG antibodies to bovine insulin are also suspected (bovine insulin differs from human insulin by only 3 amino acids).[23] Studies have also shown an 88 percent correlation between the amount of milk consumed by children and the risk of diabetes.

Beta-cell autoimmunity precedes the development of type I diabetes. Eleven percent of 3 year olds with pancreatic islet beta-cell autoimmunity had been given infant vitamin supplements compared to 32 percent of those with no beta-cell autoimmunity. Vulnerable beta-cells appeared to be protected by antioxidants.[24] Although the cow's milk issue is still very controversial, at this point in our understanding, there is wisdom and nothing lost in recommending exclusive breast feeding for infants for at least 3–

6 months and the sparing use of cow's milk in early childhood until final research conclusions can be reached. If breast feeding is not possible, alternative milk sources (goat, rice bran, soy) should be used.

Supplements. Long-term treatment in prediabetic patients with doses of nicotinamide of 1 g daily (vitamin B_3) appear to significantly extend the "honeymoon" period in type I disease.[25] Glycosylation of serum proteins in healthy volunteers was reduced 47 percent during ingestion of 1 g of vitamin C daily; this finding carries a very clear implication for postponement or prevention of type II disease by increasing antioxidant effects.[26]

Habits

- Obesity is a highly significant predictor of adult-onset diabetes, particularly in those with a genetic family predisposition. In one study, a body mass index of over 26 incurred a future risk for diabetes 330 percent higher than the risk in those with a BMI of less than 24.[27] Obesity is a more specific predictor of diabetes than lack of exercise.[28]
- Smoking. In persons who have abated smoking, the risk of developing type II diabetes drops 20 percent in only two years.[11] Attempts to stop are paramount.
- Exercise. A 35-year study found a 42 percent risk reduction for developing type II diabetes with consistent aerobic exercise at least once a week.[27]

Stress management is unequivocally related to both prevention and control. The stress of marital or personal separation is linked to onset of diabetic symptoms, and to onset of complications.[29] Poorly managed stress increases cortisone, increasing insulin requirements. In experiments with dietary intake and exercise held constant, episodes of elevated blood sugar, diabetic acidosis, and near-coma can be induced by intentional exposure to stress.[30] Learning and applying stress management skills helps prevent diabetic crises.

■ TREATMENT

Diet

The best general overall diet invites omission of simple sugars and processed grains, and emphasizes high complex carbohydrate, fiber, fruit and vegetable intake with modest protein, and low-fat consumption. Snacks of candy bars compared to equicaloric fruit with peanuts require 70 percent more insulin,[31] and sucrose should consequently be discouraged. Starchy foods vary significantly in the degree to which they raise blood sugar levels. Optimal foods in diabetes are those whose glycemic index is low.[32] Among the better low glycemic foods are legumes (beans, peas, peanuts, soybeans); vegetables such as carrots and beets; pasta, especially whole wheat flour; grains including parboiled rice and bulgur (cracked wheat) and bran cereals; whole grain breads such as pumpernickel; fruit (apples, oranges); fructose; dairy milks; and nuts. High fiber foods (whole grains, vegetables, and fruits) lower blood sugar and insulin levels and decrease insulin requirements. Onion and garlic have both been shown to have blood sugar lowering effects and can be used liberally with benefit.

Peoples with high coldwater fish consumption have a significantly lower incidence of diabetes. Vegetarians who consume very little or no sucrose are known to better handle blood sugar. Neuropathic pain of diabetic origin was completely alleviated in 80 percent and partially relieved in 20 percent of diabetics who adhered to a program of exercise and a vegan diet of unrefined foods for 25 days.[33] Renal function in type I patients with clinical nephropathy treated with a diet containing less than 0.6 g of protein/kg of ideal body weight daily and less than 1 g of phosphorus daily deteriorated 67 percent more slowly over 3 years compared to controls on a standard American Diabetic Association diet.[34]

Nutritional supplements. Beneficial supplements are catalogued below.

1. Vitamin C. Diabetics given vitamin C 1 g/day for 3 months had an 18 percent reduction in HbA_1c.[35] Sorbitol, thought to be

related to many adverse findings in diabetes, was reduced about 50 percent in diabetics ingesting 2 g daily of vitamin C for 3 weeks.[36]

2. Vitamin E. Elderly diabetics improved glucose disposal 44 percent after taking vitamin E 900 mg daily for 4 months.[37] In type I diabetics, compromised retinal circulation was restored to normal, and elevated creatinines restored to normal or significantly improved with administration of 1,800 IU of vitamin E daily for 4 months.[38]

3. Vitamin B_1. About half of diabetics given thiamin 10 mg daily for a month improved glucose disposal.[39]

4. Vitamin B_3 (niacin) has markedly beneficial effects on serum lipids, which is important for diabetics. Doses above 3 g daily, however, compromise glucose control.[40]

5. Vitamin B_6 (pyridoxine). Even in diabetics whose erythrocyte vitamin B_6 status is normal, double-blinded studies have shown that 50 mg of pyridoxine daily improves blood sugar control 6 percent. Pyridoxine alpha-glutarate, a form of B_6, given 600 mg t.i.d. for 4 weeks to type I diabetics achieved a drop in fasting blood sugar and improvement in HbA_1c of 30 and 32 percent, respectively, with 24 and 24 percent, respectively, for type II diabetics. After cessation of the treatment, all values returned to previous levels within 3 weeks.[41]

6. Vitamin B_{12}/folate injections in patients with neuropathy have achieved significant benefits.[42]

7. Raising plasma biotin decreases fasting blood sugars; blood sugars of type II diabetics taken off insulin and given 16 mg of biotin daily for 1 week decreased blood glucose from 13 to 7 mmol/L.[43]

8. Inositol, given 500 mg b.i.d. to diabetics with peripheral neuropathy, has been noted to significantly improve nerve sensation.[44] Blood sugar control has not appeared to benefit.

9. Magnesium levels in diabetics with cardiac complications are significantly lower than in those without cardiac problems.[8] Magnesium levels in elderly persons are more deficient than levels in younger persons. And insulin production and utiliza-

tion in type II patients is greatly enhanced with magnesium 400–800 mg daily.[45]

10. Zinc tends to be utilized in higher amounts in diabetics and zinc supplementation is a wise precaution (30 mg daily).[46]

11. Manganese is commonly low in many people, including diabetics; 5–15 mg/day is a reasonable supplemental intake.

12. Chromium aids insulin action, reduces HbA_1c levels, reduces fasting glucose levels,[47] and reduces required doses of oral hypoglycemic agents.[48] The doses in these two studies were 1,000 and 200 μg daily, respectively. Chromium picolinate 200 μg daily also improves blood sugar control when insulin is being used.[49]

13. Iron stores are elevated in 50 percent of poorly controlled type II diabetics. The most accurate index of iron stores is a blood ferritin. In one study, lowering ferritin levels with IV desferrioxamine 10 mg/kg twice weekly for up to 13 weeks improved glycemic control and lowered triglycerides in 90 percent of patients getting the chelation, in spite of stopping oral hypoglycemic drugs.[50] Excess iron stores can also be reduced through blood donations and avoiding iron in supplements.

14. Vanadium 50 mg b.i.d. for 4 weeks in type II patients improved fasting glucose 20 percent.[51]

15. Supplementation with omega-3 fatty acids enhances insulin binding to cell membranes. Eicosapentaenoic acid given to diabetics significantly inhibits platelet aggregation, but because some reports have reported adverse effects in very high dosages, intake should not exceed 2.5 g daily. Red blood cell deformability, which is decreased in diabetics, improves to normal with omega-3 oils from sardine oil, 2–3 g daily, after only 4 weeks. Greater red blood cell membrane rheology (deformability) improves microcirculation in diabetics.[52]

16. Gamma linolenic acid, 480 mg daily, significantly improved neurological deterioration in diabetics with peripheral neuropathy compared to placebo patients.[53] Sources of GLA are evening primrose oil, borage oil, and black currant oil.

Biomolecular options

- DHEA and testosterone are consistently significantly lower in diabetics compared to levels in healthy persons. In animals, DHEA improves diabetic control. Present research will shed light on the possibilities for human use.
- Alpha lipoic acid 600 mg b.i.d. has added a new dimension in treatment, with benefits in diabetic neuropathy as well as glucose disposal.[54]
- L-carnitine experimentally improves insulin sensitivity in insulin-resistant type II diabetics[55] and may be of benefit in neuropathy.
- Taurine 500 mg t.i.d. normalized platelet aggregation found to be accelerated in type I patients.[56]
- Gabapentin, an epilepsy drug, in doses of 900–3,600 mg daily gave relief from the pain of diabetic neuropathy, although a quarter of patients had bothersome side effects.[57]

Exercise. In type I diabetics, the mortality rate of those regularly engaging in moderate or strenuous exercise is *70 percent lower* than the mortality of those exercising minimally or not at all.[14] Some authorities boldly state that those in the top echelon of regular aerobic exercise frequency and intensity *do not get* type II diabetes. In male type II diabetics, mean blood sugar 2 hours post-sugar-load fell from 227 to 170 mg/dL and blood insulin from 172 to 106 μU/mL after exercising on a treadmill at 60 percent of maximal heart rate, 60 minutes daily, for only 1 week. Four out of every 5 had *normal glucose and insulin tolerance tests at the end of the week.*[58] Exercise evokes marked increases in insulin receptor sites and insulin utilization, diminishing insulin resistance. Resistance exercise also improves blood glucose control.

Herbs

1. Two bioflavonoids, catechin (1 g daily) and quercitin (400 mg b.i.d.) appear to stimulate insulin action and have been shown to scavenge free radicals.[59] Quercitin inhibits sorbitol

accumulation, and appears to be helpful in controlling symptoms of diabetic neuropathy.[60]

2. Aloe, 1/2 tsp daily for 4–14 weeks in type II patients, has been shown to reduce fasting blood glucose.[61]

3. Type II patients given 100 or 200 mg/day of ginseng for 8 weeks improved fasting glucose levels and resulted in weight loss. Those receiving 200 mg/day demonstrated improvement in HbA$_1$c. Normalization of fasting blood sugars was achieved in 4 times as many patients treated with ginseng compared to those treated with placebo.[62]

4. Compared to baseline control values, non-insulin-dependent patients given 100 g/day of defatted fenugreek seed powder for 10 days decreased their fasting blood sugars 30–65 percent.[63]

5. *Momordica charantia* (bitter melon), prepared as a juice of the unripe tropical Asian fruit, lowered blood sugar in 3 of 4 type II diabetics tested (25–50 g or 2 ounces t.i.d.).[64]

6. *Gymnema sylvestre* is an Ayurvedic glucose-lowering botanical. Research utilizing doses of 400 mg daily as supplement to conventional treatment has shown significant reductions in glucose disposal, HbA$_1$c, and required doses of other medications.[65]

7. In patients with type II disease due to liver cirrhosis, 600 mg of silymarin daily significantly reduces average fasting blood sugar, HbA$_1$c, daily insulin need, fasting insulin levels, and blood free-radical levels.[66]

Mental and emotional treatment. Diabetics who learn to incorporate stress management techniques have far better diabetic control. Biofeedback, relaxation practices, autogenic training, and meditation can play major roles in managing stress, improving diabetic control, and reducing deleterious effects, mediated in part through reduction in corticosteroid synthesis and release. Two of three diabetic subjects with recalcitrant, non-healing diabetic ulcers of the lower extremity showed significant healing after 20 sessions of thermal biofeedback at the ulcer site, plus hand warming training and home practice.[67] In a recent study, type II diabetic patients learned and practiced yoga b.i.d. After 40 days, mean fasting glucose fell from 135 to 100 mg/dL and dosages of required hypoglycemic drugs fell significantly.[68]

Control of blood sugar is known to deteriorate during periods of depression. In a study of cognitive behavioral therapy in type II diabetics, not only was a significant remission from depression achieved, but HbA₁c levels also showed significant improvement.[69] Psychotherapy approaches for depression have been shown to work better than the use of drugs, many of which actually tend to make blood sugar control worse.[70] Smoking abatement also needs to be a major goal of counseling.

In a case history report of a male diabetic successfully treated for incontinence with hypnosis, concomitant 36 percent decrease in insulin requirements was inadvertently observed.[71]

Diabetics participating in interactive sessions regarding information-seeking and medical decision-making show significantly fewer physical limitations in activities of daily living and significantly better sugar control than those not offered this kind of opportunity. In every disease process, patient involvement in being informed and participating in decisions predicts a better outcome.

■ REVERSAL

Case history reports in juvenile-onset type I diabetics have shown reversal of diabetic retinopathy when excellent blood sugar control is achieved. High doses of niacin in newly diagnosed juvenile diabetics have been reported to reverse the glucose handling problems and prevent the onset of full-fledged disease. The children's doses used in successful trials were 100–200 mg daily. Not all studies have confirmed this phenomenon.

Fifty percent of type I patients were found to have totally reversed their retinopathy after being given subcutaneous daily injections of 100 μg of vitamin B_{12} for 2 years in addition to their insulin.[72]

Type II diabetics who have required oral anti-diabetic drugs and/or less than 20 units of insulin daily, on assuming a lifestyle leading to optimum weight, diet, supplements and exercise, are frequently found on retesting to be non-diabetic and requiring no insulin or medications. At a minimum, improvement in lifestyle factors may eliminate or reduce insulin and drug requirements in type II patients while improving glucose control. The arteriosclerotic complications of diabetes can likewise be controlled and at least modestly reversed with good blood sugar control and adoption of the measures discussed under coronary heart disease in Chapter 2.

Epicatechin, a flavonoid extracted from the bark of *Pterocarpus marsupium*, long used in Ayurvedic medicine, has shown promise in pancreatic beta-cell regeneration in animals.[73] It is not yet available in the US.

Hypothyroidism

■ DESCRIPTION

Hypothyroidism is the condition in which there is compromised synthesis, availability, absorption, or utilization of thyroid hormone, slowing the metabolic activities of the body. The primary active thyroid hormone produced within the thyroid gland is thyroxin (T4). Thyroxin is converted into triiodothyronine (T3) to control the metabolic activity of thousands of cytoplasmic enzymes.

Hypothyroidism causes a myriad of symptoms affecting virtually every organ. Symptoms vary from subtle "sub-clinical" symptoms to abject life-threatening myxedema. The most common symptoms and signs are fatigue, weight gain, constipation, cold intolerance, bradycardia, dry and flaky skin, hair loss, brittle nails, decreased immune function, recurrent infections, constipation, hypermenorrhea, dysmenorrhea, aggravated PMS symptoms, infertility, decreased male libido, increased incidence of miscarriages in pregnancy, subtle edema, loss of the outer third of the eyebrows, depression, slow reflexes, hypertension, and hyperlipidemias.

Currently, the thyroid-stimulating hormone (TSH) is the most reliable blood test used to diagnose hypothyroidism and monitor thyroid function. The TSH is a highly sensitive test, and in some instances where TSH is elevated, indicating low thyroid hormone production, the serum T4 may be normal. With previous reliance on the T4, many cases of clinical hypothyroidism went undetected. The more expensive TRH stimulation test will detect some cases of hypothyroidism not found with the usual thyroid profile including the TSH.

When the cause of hypothyroidism is insufficient conversion of T4 to T3, or insufficient uptake by the cells, "tissue resistance" is said to be present. In this situation, the TSH and T4 blood tests are usually normal, while the patient is exhibiting all the clinical signs of hypothyroidism.

Among the ways to clinically assess hypothyroidism are the slowed return phase on testing for the ankle jerk, and a subnormal basal body temperature. Although rejected by many conventional practitioners, this method has worked well in the hands of many complementary physicians.[74,75] A description for the patient follows:

> Shake down any mercury thermometer before retiring. On awakening, before arising place the thermometer under the arm for 10 minutes to obtain the axillary temperature. Obtain the average for at least 6 days. Menstruating women should begin on the last menstrual day. The normal axillary basal temperature averages 97.6–98.2°F. Especially if the mean temperature is 97.0°F or less, hypothyroidism is suspect, if other clinical signs support the diagnosis.

■ PREVALENCE

About 2 percent of adults in the United States are estimated to have moderate to severe hypothyroidism,[76] with another 10 percent manifesting mild thyroid deficiency.[77] The vast majority of those with hypothyroidism are women. The incidence increases with age.

■ ETIOLOGY AND RISK FACTORS

Hypothyroidism results from: primary failure of the thyroid gland to synthesize sufficient thyroxin; secondary failure due to inappropriate stimulation by TSH from the anterior pituitary; failure of adequate conversion to triiodothyronine; diminished cellular uptake and utilization of T3; or overproduction of reverse T3 (Wilson's syndrome). Over 90 percent of all cases are caused by primary failure of the thyroid gland.

Factors that contribute to the hypothyroid state are:

- heredity—usually a parent or grandparent with hypo-thyroidism,
- advancing age,
- deficiencies of nutrients involved in T4 synthesis—iodine, selenium, copper, tyrosine; and vitamins A, C, E, B_2, B_3, and B_6,
- deficiencies of nutrients involved in the conversion of T4 to T3—zinc, copper, and selenium,
- stress—excessive cortisol levels appear to reduce conversion of T4 to T3,
- Hashimoto's thyroiditis, a major cause of primary gland failure, is an autoimmune disorder in which anti-thyroid antibodies react to slowly destroy the thyroid gland itself,
- intended or unintended consequences of treatment for hyperthyroidism with radioactive iodine,
- heavy metal toxicity from mercury, lead, cadmium, and chemical contamination may be important factors interfering with thyroid hormone effect on the cells of the body.

■ CONVENTIONAL MEDICAL TREATMENT

The standard treatment for hypothyroidism is replacement with synthetic thyroid (Synthroid). However, some patients appear to be unable to convert T4 to T3 normally, and one recent animal study has suggested that a mixture may have better results.[78] And, some practitioners have thought that T3 (Cytomel) actually works better in some patients.

■ HOLISTIC MEDICAL TREATMENT

The primary treatment is thyroid hormone replacement. Because natural thyroid (Armour thyroid) from the glands of slaughter animals contains a mixture of T4 and T3 as well as its precursors, it is the preferred choice by many practitioners of complementary medicine. Because T3 is assimilated erratically from the digestive system, patients taking it can experience fluctuations of their thyroid blood level. Close clinical and blood test monitoring initially help to establish the correct dose for any form of thyroid supplement. Iron and thyroid compete for absorption and their ingestion should be separated by at least 2 hours.[79] High intake of oat bran and soybean fiber appear to do the same thing, causing a marked rise in the TSH.[80]

Nutrition. Certain foods, supplements, and herbs can strengthen thyroid function. The foods which support and enhance thyroid function include:

1. Fish, sea vegetables (kelp, dulse, arame, hijiki, kombu, nori, wakame), root vegetables (potatoes), and sea-salt supply iodine. Iodized salt does also, but some brands still contain aluminum.
2. Beef, oatmeal, chicken, seafood (especially oysters), liver, dried beans, bran, seeds (especially pumpkin seeds), nuts, and tuna supply zinc.
3. Liver and other organ meats, eggs, yeast, legumes, nuts, and raisins supply copper.
4. Soy foods, beef, chicken and fish supply tyrosine, substrate for thyroxin.

Foods that naturally tend to diminish thyroid function include broccoli, spinach, cabbage, Brussels sprouts, mustard greens, turnips, kale, peanuts, pine nuts, millet, peaches, and pears. Antihistamines and sulfa drugs can also have this affect.

Supplements

1. Iodine—200–500 μg daily, present in many multiple supplement products.
2. Vitamin B-complex—25–50 mg daily.

3. Beta-carotene—10–25,000 IU daily.
4. Zinc—15–30 mg daily.
5. Magnesium—400–500 mg daily.
6. Copper—2–3 mg daily.
7. Selenium—200–250 µg daily.[81]
8. Tyrosine—300–1000 mg daily.
9. Omega-3 fatty acids—1–2 g daily.
10. Iron—18 mg daily (especially for menstruating women and if anemia is present).

Herbs. Tinctures of kelp (*Alaria esculenta*), bladderwrack (*Fucus vesiculosis*), and Irish moss (*Chondrus crispus*) gtts 10 daily to b.i.d., or capsules 500–2,000 mg daily to b.i.d. have been used extensively. Teas containing equal parts of Horsetail (*Equisetum arvense*), oatstraw (*Avena sativa*), alfalfa (*Medicago sativa*) and gotu kola (*Centella asiatica*) also supply essential minerals.

Exercise. People with hypothyroidism also often derive significant benefit from aerobic exercise, probably as a result of enhanced circulation, greater cellular uptake of thyroid hormone, and increasing metabolism during and following the exercise time. Exercise should be performed for at least 30 minutes 3 times weekly.

Homeopathy. Homeopathic glandulars have been employed in hypothyroidism, and individualized acupuncture protocols may be helpful in correcting hormonal imbalances.

Mental and emotional treatment. In animal studies, it appears that stress markedly adversely affects thyroid hormone production, mediated through corticoid receptor downregulation and inhibition of TSH release in animal studies.[82] There is also evidence that stress increases levels of rT3 (reverse T3), shown during fasting and post-surgically.[83] Autonomic nervous system fibers have purportedly been described in carefully stained histological sections of thyroid tissue; their significance remains to be shown. Addressing appropriate strategies for hypothyroid patients to manage stress with greater efficacy is effective therapy. Yoga has a tradition of helpfulness for hypothyroidism.

REFERENCES

1. Pittman CS et al. Impaired 3,5,3'-triiodothyronine (T3) production in diabetic patients. *Metabolism* 1979; 28(4):333–8.
2. Kostraba JN et al. Nitrate levels in community drinking waters and risk of IDDM. An ecological analysis. *Diabetes Care* 1992; 15(11):1505–8.
3. Barrett-Conner E et al. Lower endogenous androgen levels and dyslipidemia in men with non-insulin-dependent diabetes mellitus. *Ann Intern Med* 1992; 117(10):807–11.
4. Nestler JE et al. Dehydroepiandrosterone: the "missing link" between hyperinsulinemia and atherosclerosis? *FASEB J* 1992; 6(12):3073–5.
5. Parthiban A et al. Oxidative stress and the development of diabetic complications—antioxidants and lipid peroxidation in erythrocytes and cell membrane. *Cell Biol Int* 1995; 19(12): 987–93.
6. Cunningham JJ et al. Reduced mononuclear leucocyte ascorbic acid content in adults with insulin-dependent diabetes mellitus. *Metabolism* 1991; 40(2):146–9.
7. Coggeshall JC et al. Biotin status and plasma glucose in diabetics. *Ann NY Acad Sci* 1985; 447:389–92.
8. Zhang WG et al. Hypomagnesemia and heart complications in diabetes mellitus. *Chin Med J* 1987; 100(9):719–22.
9. Ceriello A et al. Hypomagnesemia in relation to diabetic retinopathy. *Diabetes Care* 1982; 5(5):558–9.
10. Hepburn DA et al. Hypoglycemic convulsions cause serious musculoskeletal injury in patients with IDDM. *Diabetes Care* 1989; 12(7):932–7.
11. Rimm EB et al. Prospective study of cigarette smoking, alcohol use, and the risk of diabetes in men. *BMJ* 1995; 310(6979): 555–9.
12. Sawicki PT et al. Smoking is associated with progression of diabetic nephropathy. *Diabetes Care* 1994; 17(2):126–31.
13. Manson JE et al. A prospective study of exercise and incidence of diabetes among U S male physicians. *JAMA* 1992; 268(1):63–7.
14. Moy CS et al. Insulin-dependent diabetes mellitus, physical activity, and death. *Am J Epidemiol* 1993; 137(1):74–81.
15. Surwit RS. Role of stress in the etiology and treatment of diabetes mellitus. *Psychosom Med* 1993; 55(4):380–93.

16. Hagglof B et al. The Swedish diabetes study: indications of severe psychological stress as a risk factor for type 1 (insulin-dependent) diabetes mellitus in childhood. *Diabetologia* 1991; 34(8):579–83.

17. Shealy N, Myss C. *The Creation of Health*. Walpole, NH: Stillpoint, 1988.

18. Aarsand AK et al. Folate administration reduces circulating homo-cysteine levels in NIDDM patients on long-term metformin treatment. *J Intern Med* 1998; 244(2):169–74.

19. Snowdon DA et al. Does a vegetarian diet reduce the occurrence of diabetes? *Am J Pub Health* 1985; 75(5):507–12.

20. Verge CF et al. Environmental factors in childhood IDDM. A population-based, case-control study. *Diabetes Care* 1994; 17(12):1381–9.

21. Dahlquist G et al. An increased level of antibodies to beta-lacto-globulin is a risk determinant for early onset type-1 (insulin dependent) diabetes mellitus independent of islet-cell antibodies and early introduction of cow's milk. *Diabetologia* 1992; 35(10): 980–4.

22. Saukkonen T et al. Significance of cow's milk protein antibodies as risk factor for childhood IDDM: interactions with dietary cow's milk intake and HLA-DQB1 genotype. Childhood Diabetes in Finland Study Group. *Diabetologia* 1998; 41(1):72–8.

23. Vaarala O et al. Cow milk feeding induces antibodies to insulin in children—a link between cow milk and insulin-dependent diabetes mellitus? *Scand J Immunol* 1998; 47(2):131–5.

24. Norris J. Univ. Colorado Health Sciences Center, American Diabetes Assoc. Annual Meeting, San Francisco, July 1996. *Fam Pract News* 1996; 26(14):4.

25. Vague P et al. Nicotinamide may extend remission phase in insulin-dependent diabetes. *Lancet* 1987; 1(8533):619–20.

26. Vinson JA et al. Inhibition of protein glycation and advanced glycation end products by ascorbic acid and other vitamins and nutrients. *J Nutr Biochem* 1996; 7(12):659–63.

27. Helmrich SP et al. Physical activity and decreased occurrence of non-insulin-dependent diabetes mellitus. *N Engl J Med* 1991; 325(3):147–52.

28. Serrano RM. Relationship between obesity and the increased risk of major complications in non-insulin-dependent diabetes mellitus. *Eur J Clin Invest* 1998; 28 suppl 2:14–17.

29. Bresater LE et al. Foot pathology and risk factors for diabetic foot disease in elderly men. *Diabetes Res Clin Pract* 1996; 32(1–1):103–9.

30. Hinkle LE et al. Experimental study of life situations, emotions and the occurrence of acidosis in a Jew. *Am J Med Sci* 1949; 217:130.

31. Oettle GJ et al. Glucose and insulin responses to manufactured and whole-food snacks. *Am J Clin Nutr* 1987; 45(1):86–91.

32. Behme MT et al. All bran versus corn flakes: plasma glucose and insulin responses in young females. *Am J Clin Nutr* 1989; 50(6):1240–3.

33. Crane MG et al. Regression of diabetic neuropathy with vegan diet. *Am J Clin Nutr* 1988; 48(3):926.

34. Zeller K et al. Effect of restricting dietary protein on the progression of renal failure in patients with insulin-dependent diabetes mellitus. *N Engl J Med* 1991; 324(2):78–84.

35. Davie S et al. Effect of vitamin C on glycosylation of proteins. *Diabetes* 1992; 41(2):167–73.

36. Vinson JA et al. In vitro and in vivo reduction of erythrocyte sorbitol by ascorbic acid. *Diabetes* 1989; 38(8):1036–41.

37. Paolisso G et al. Pharmacologic doses of vitamin E improve insulin action in healthy subjects and non-insulin-dependent diabetic patients. *Am J Clin Nutrition* 1993; 57(5):650–6.

38. Bursell SE et al. High-dose vitamin E supplementation normalizes retinal blood flow and creatinine clearance in patients with type 1 diabetes. *Diabetes Care* 1999; 22(8):1245–51.

39. Vorhaus MG et al. Crystalline vitamin B1: observations in diabetes. *Am J Dig Dis Nutr* 1935; 2(9):541–57.

40. Anonymous. Nicotinic acid in NIDDM. *JAMA* 1990; 264(23):2994–5.

41. Passariello N et al. Effects of pyridoxine alpha-glutarate on blood glucose and lactate in type I and II diabetics. *Int J Clin Pharmacol Ther Toxicol* 1983; 21(5):252–6.

42. Yaqub BA et al. Effects of methylcobalamin on diabetic neuropathy. *Clin Neurol Neurosurg* 1992; 94(1):105–11.

43. Maebashi M et al. Therapeutic evaluation of the effect of biotin on hyperglycemia in patients with non-insulin dependent diabetes mellitus. *J Clin Biochem Nutr* 1993; 14(3):211–18.

44. Salway J et al. Effect of myo-inositol on peripheral nerve function in diabetes. *Lancet* 1978; 2(8103):1282–4.

45. Paolisso G et al. Daily magnesium supplements improve glucose handling in elderly subjects. *Am J Clin Nutr* 1992; 55(6):1161–7.

46. Solomon SJ et al. Effect of low zinc intake on carbohydrate and fat metabolism in men. *Fed Proc* 1983; 42:391.

47. Anderson RA et al. Elevated intakes of supplemental chromium improve glucose and insulin variables in individuals with type II diabetes. *Diabetes* 1997; 46(11):1786–91.

48. Ravina A et al. Clinical use of the trace element chromium (III) in the treatment of diabetes mellitus. *J Trace Elem Exp Med* 1995; 8(3):183–90.

49. Fox GN et al. Chromium picolinate supplementation for diabetes mellitus. *J Fam Pract* 1998; 46(1):83–6.

50. Cutler P et al. Deferoxamine therapy in high-ferritin diabetes. *Diabetes* 1989; 38(10):1207–10.

51. Boden G et al. Effects of vanadyl sulfate in carbohydrate metabolism in patients with non-insulin-dependent diabetes mellitus. *Metabolism* 1996; 45(9):1130–5.

52. Kamada T et al. Dietary sardine oil increases erythrocyte membrane fluidity in diabetic patients. *Diabetes* 1986; 35(5):604–11.

53. Keen H et al. Treatment of diabetic neuropathy with gamma-linolenic acid. *Diabetes Care* 1993; 16(1):8–15.

54. Konrad T et al. Alpha-lipoic acid treatment decreases serum lactate and pyruvate concentrations and improves glucose effectiveness in lean and obese patients with type II diabetes. *Diabetes Care* 1999; 22(2):280–7.

55. Mingrone G et al. L-carnitine improves glucose disposal in type 2 diabetic patients. *J Am Coll Nutr* 1999; 18(1):77–82.

56. Franconi F et al. Plasma and platelet taurine are reduced in subjects with insulin-dependent diabetes mellitus: effects of taurine supplementation. *Am J Clin Nutr* 1995; 61(5):1115–19.

57. Backonjia M et al. Gabapentin for the symptomatic treatment of painful neuropathy in patients with diabetes mellitus: a randomized controlled trial. *JAMA* 1998; 280(21):1831–6.

58. Rogers MA et al. Improvement in glucose tolerance after one week of exercise in patients with mild NIDDM. *Diabetes Care* 1988; 11(8):613–18.

59. Chakravarthy BK et al. Antidiabetic effect of (−)-epicatechin. *Lancet* 1982; 2(8292):272–3.

60. Nagata H et al. Antioxidation action of flavonoids, quercitin and catechin, mediated by the activation of glutathione peroxidase. *Tokai J Exp Clin Med* 1999; 24(1):1–11.
61. Ghannam N et al. The antidiabetic activity of aloes: preliminary clinical and experimental observations. *Horm Res* 1986; 24(4):288–94.
62. Soltaniemi EA et al. Ginseng treatment in non-insulin-dependent diabetic patients. *Diabetes Care* 1995; 18(10):1373–5.
63. Sharma RD et al. Effect of fenugreek seeds on blood glucose and serum lipids in type I diabetes. *Eur J Clin Nutr* 1990; 44(4): 301–6.
64. Welihinda J et al. Effect of *Mormordica charantia* in maturity onset diabetes. *J Ethnopharmacol* 1986; 17(3):277–82.
65. Baskaran K et al. Antidiabetic effect of a leaf extract from Gymnema sylvestre in non-insulin-dependent diabetes mellitus patients. *J Ethnopharmacol* 1990; 30(3):295–300.
66. Velussi M et al. Long-term (12 months) treatment with an anti-oxidant drug (silymarin) is effective on hyperinsulinemia, exogenous insulin need and malondialdehyde levels in cirrhotic patients. *J Hepatol* 1996; 26(4):871–9.
67. Shulimson AD et al. Diabetic ulcers: the effects of thermal biofeedback-mediated relaxation training on healing. *Biofeedback Self Regul* 1987; 11(4):311–19.
68. Jain SC et al. A study of response pattern of non-insulin dependent diabetics to yoga therapy. *Diabetes Res Clin Pract* 1993; 19(1):69–74.
69. Lustman PJ et al. Cognitive behavior therapy for depression in type 2 diabetes mellitus. *Ann Intern Med* 1998; 129(8):613–21.
70. Lustman PJ et al. Effects of nortriptyline on depression and glycemic control in diabetes: results of a double-blind, placebo-controlled trial. *Psychosom Med* 1997; 59(3):241–50.
71. McCord H. Hypnotherapy in diabetes: a brief note. *Am J Clin Hypn* 1968; 10(4):309–10.
72. Kornerup L et al. Vitamin B12 and retinopathy in juvenile diabetics. *Acta Paediatr* 1958; 47(6):646–51.
73. Hii CS et al. Effects of epicatechin on rat islets of Langerhans. *Diabetes* 1984; 33(3):291–6.
74. Barnes BO. Hypertension and the thyroid gland. *Clin Exp Pharmacol Physiol* 1975; Suppl 2:167–70.

75. Gaby AR. Treatment with thyroid hormone. *JAMA* 1989; 262(13):1774.
76. Bennett JC, Plum F. (eds.) *Cecil Textbook of Medicine*, 20th ed. Philadephia: W.B. Saunders, 1996.
77. Cushing GW. Subclinical hypothyroidism. Understanding is the key to decision making. *Postgrad Med* 1993; 94(1):95–107.
78. Escobar-Morreale HF et al. Only the combined treatment with thyroxine and triiodothyronine ensures euthyroidism in all tissues of the rat. *Endocrinology* 1996; 137(6):2490–2502.
79. Campbell NR et al. Ferrous sulfate reduces thyroxine efficacy in patients with hypothyroidism. *Ann Intern Med* 1992; 117(12):1010.
80. Liel Y et al. Evidence for a clinically important adverse effect of fiber-enriched diet on the bioavailability of levothyroxine in adult hypothyroid patients. *J Clin Endocrinol Metab* 1996; 81(2):857–9.
81. Arthur JR et al. The role of selenium in thyroid hormone metabolism and effects of selenium deficiency on thyroid hormone and iodine metabolism. *Biol Trace Elem Res* 1992; 33:37–42.
82. Padmanabhan V et al. Does time of exposure to estradiol and LHRH affect LH release from bovine pituitary cells? *Proc Soc Exp Biol Med.* 1978;159(1):157–60.
83. Goichot B et al. Thyroid hormone status and nutrient intake in the free-living elderly. Interest of reverse triiodothyronine assessment. *Eur J Endocrinol* 1994; 130(3):244–52.

7

Chapter Seven

Women's Diseases

Premenstrual Syndrome...

■ DESCRIPTION

Premenstrual syndrome describes the array of distressing symptoms occurring within 2 weeks prior to the onset of menstruation
in many women. The symptoms include tension, anxiety, irritability, depression, mood swings, food cravings, depleted energy,
headache, backache, abdominal bloating, edema of hands and
feet, altered sex drive, and tenderness and swelling of the breasts.
Endocrine, reproductive, gastrointestinal and psychological systems are involved in premenstrual syndrome (PMS). The diagnosis is strongly suspected on the basis of the history, and hormone
abnormalities (see following) can be confirmed by blood tests,
including thyroid profile, progesterone, estrogen, and prolactin
levels. Red blood cell magnesium or magnesium loading test, ferritin, red blood cell transketolase, vitamin D level, and aldosterone
tests may also be of help.

■ PREVALENCE

An estimated 30–60 percent of women experience unpleasant
premenstrual symptoms. Ten percent of women experience
severe degrees of disturbance that interfere with activities of daily
living. The greatest incidence occurs in women in their 30s and
40s.

■ ETIOLOGY AND RISK FACTORS

The most important contributing factors in PMS appear to be:

1. stress, endorphin deficiency,
2. depression—decreased brain levels of neurotransmitters serotonin, and gamma butyric acid,[1,2]
3. decreased vitamin B_6 levels,[3]
4. deficient exposure to natural light, with a predisposition to seasonal affective depression,
5. hypothyroidism—a high percentage of PMS patients exhibit evidence of overt or subclinical deficient thyroid function. Several studies have found a 70–90 percent incidence of low thyroid status in women with PMS versus 0–20 percent in controls without PMS.[4]
6. elevated prolactin contributes to breast tenderness,
7. obesity—body fat synthesizes estrone, contributing to higher estrogen/progesterone ratio, with increased estrogen and deficient progesterone; an increased estrogen/progesterone ratio, which is common,[5] tends to lead to:

   - decreased endorphin production, tending to produce anxiety, depression, insomnia,[6]
   - mildly increased aldosterone secretion, contributing to fluid retention,[7]
   - increased prolactin production, contributing to breast tenderness and swelling,[8]
   - diminished liver function with decreased bile flow,
   - probable depleted vitamin B_6 levels, impairing neurotransmitter and prostaglandin synthesis,

8. history of having been raised in an alcoholic family system in which women have experienced abuse and are scripted to take care of every situation—a "relationship" addiction,[9]
9. association with candidiasis.[10]

Compared to women without PMS, the nutritional fare of women with PMS is made up of[6]

- up to 2-fold greater consumption of dairy products,
- up to $2\frac{1}{2}$ times greater consumption of sugar,[11]
- half-again the amounts of refined carbohydrate intake,[12]
- noticeable deficiency of manganese and zinc intake,
- deficiency of dietary magnesium,[13]
- greater intake of caffeine (soft drinks, coffee, tea, chocolate),[14]
- excess amounts of dietary fat,[15]
- deficient intake of tryptophan.

Precipitating events associated with onset or aggravation of PMS include[9]

- onset of menses with puberty,
- the 1–2 years before menopause,
- after stopping oral contraceptives,
- after a pregnancy complicated by toxemia,
- after a period of amenorrhea,
- after tubal ligation for contraception,
- following intense stressful psychological trauma (post-traumatic stress disorder).

■ CONVENTIONAL TREATMENT

Some physicians still think that premenstrual symptoms are a variant of depression and patients are too often told "Its all in your head." This may stem from the fact that there is no simple, definitive laboratory test. Conventional initiatives include:

- Suppression of ovulation with oral contraceptive medications. This temporarily relieves symptoms, but underlying problems remain.
- Antidepressant prescriptions are commonly used, either tricyclics or selective serotonin reuptake inhibitors (SSRIs).
- Anxiolytic medications such as buspirone for associated anxiety.
- Severe water retention has been treated with diuretics, preferably of the potassium sparing variety.

- Analgesics including aspirin and tylenol for headache and cramps.
- NSAIDs for associated dysmenorrhea.
- Spironolactone during the last half of the menstrual cycle for hormonal predilection for acneiform changes, oily skin, and hirsutism.
- Bromocryptine in the last half of the menstrual cycle for extreme breast tenderness (suppresses prolactin).

■ HOLISTIC TREATMENT

Nutrition

The following choices are therapeutic.

- Progressing toward a whole foods, vegetarian diet.
- Reduction of fat intake.[16]
- Reduction and elimination of as much of the dietary sugar as possible.
- Reduction of foods contaminated with hormone disruptors—estrogen-mimicking pesticides DDE, PCB, dieldrin, and chlordane. These so-called hormone disruptors are much higher in animal meats, eggs and milk products.
- Increase phytoestrogen-containing foods (soy, seeds, nuts, apples, parsley, alfalfa).
- Omitting beverages and food with caffeine diminishes anxiety and reduces breast sensitivity.
- Limiting salt intake to less than 2 g daily reduces the disposition to fluid retention.

Suggested essential daily *supplements* include:

- vitamin B_6—100 mg,[17]
- vitamin E—400–800 IU,[18]
- calcium—1 g,[19]
- magnesium—800 mg,[19]
- manganese—15 mg,[20]
- the majority of, but by no means all studies suggest benefit from omega-oils: fish oil 4–6 g daily (EPA content 1 g

daily and DHA 0.75 g daily) or flaxseed oil—1 tsp b.i.d., although the main focus of treatment has been on dysmenorrhea.[21] The results of studies of gamma linolenic acid treatment with evening primrose oil have predominantly shown no benefit.

- tryptophan—2 g: available from compounding pharmacists by prescription.[22]

A high potency vitamin–mineral supplement will supply most of the above and simplifies the dosing schedule. See Chapter 1.

Exercise

Aerobic workouts 30–45 minutes 3 times weekly have been shown to greatly reduce breast tenderness, water retention, tension, and depression compared to non-exercising women. Consistent exercise also markedly improves mood and reduces irritability.[23]

Biomolecular Options

- Treatment with progesterone vaginal suppositories is also used with mild to moderate benefit reported (dosage 200–800 mg daily, available by prescription).[24] Other studies report no benefit with 200 mg doses.
- A report in 1982 detailed the highly successful treatment of PMS with subdermal injections of tiny, sub-pharmacological, desensitizing doses of dilute aqueous progesterone which gave substantial and sometimes dramatic relief in 85 percent of cases.[25] In spite of the successful use of this protocol in the hands of many physicians, its use has not become commonplace.
- Small, uncontrolled studies have highlighted improvement in symptoms when standard treatment for intestinal candidiasis was undertaken, suggesting the possible contribution of this much-debated syndrome to PMS. Empirically trying a sugar-restricted diet and treatment with nystatin (1 tablet, or $\frac{1}{4}$ tsp of the powder if available, q.i.d. for 1–2 months) is an option with little risk.

- If subclinical hypothyroidism is shown by either sophisticated thyrotropin-releasing hormone (TRH) tests or the finding of a low basal body temperature, a trial of small amounts of thyroxin or Armour whole thyroid will often bring great or complete relief.[4] Small doses of thyroid supplements, even in women who had normal thyroid tests, gave prompt relief, "sometimes dramatic," in 3 of every 4 women in this study.
- If a pattern of deterioration during wintertime decreased sunlight exposure in northern latitudes is present, exposure to full-spectrum bright light for at least 2 hours daily (light boxes or full-spectrum lighting) can be a significant contribution to better management of the syndrome.[26]

Botanical Choices

- Black cohosh (*Cimicifuga racemosa*) 100–600 mg daily in divided doses,[27] particularly for symptoms accompanied by the presence of uterine fibroids.
- Chasteberry (*Vitex agnus castus*) 175 mg daily.[28]
- Dong Quai (*Angelica sinensis*) 1–2 g t.i.d.[29] especially for symptoms followed by marked dysmenorrhea.[29]
- Licorice root (*Glycyrrhiza glabra*) 250–500 mg t.i.d., especially when marked fluid retention is a prominent symptom.[30]

Homeopathy

An individualized, constitutional homeopathic prescription is complicated and requires a knowledgeable practitioner. Common acute remedies utilized in 12X to 30C potencies are:[31]

- Pulsatilla for PMS with irregular periods, headaches, and weepiness.
- Kreosotum for headache, nausea and irritability, especially with severe vaginitis.
- *Calcarea carbonica* for marked mastodynia, fatigue, and early profuse menstrual flow.
- Borax for irritability, insomnia, and headache.

- *Nux vomica* for extreme irritability, crampy pain, and cravings for food and alcohol.

Manual Medicine

Weekly ear, hand and foot reflexology treatments of 30 minutes each have been shown in a controlled study to reduce physical and emotional symptoms 40 percent.[32] Significant fall in resting EMG-recorded electrical activity of lumbar muscles and great relief in cramping and pain followed low-amplitude, high-velocity spinal manipulation in women with a prominent low back pain component and dysmenorrhea as part of their symptoms.[33] Other studies, however, show equivalent improvement in sham manipulation.[34] Cranial osteopathy in PMS also has particularly good results.

Acupuncture

The benefits of acupuncture in research have emphasized the treatment of dysmenorrhea more than premenstrual distress. Controlled studies demonstrate very significant benefits in pain relief.[35]

Psychological Treatments

It is essential to acknowledge negative patterns of coping with stress and PMS symptoms and to take steps to move them in a positive direction. Elements of post-traumatic stress issues often require extensive psychological work for resolution. Self-destructive responses which worsen the cycle of symptoms include overeating, becoming sedentary, becoming an observer instead of a participant (e.g., television), and lapsing into habits of overspending and dependence on prescription and illicit drugs. Cognitive therapy with skilled counselors, supplemented with behavioral approaches is often necessary. Biofeedback and relaxation practices are also highly therapeutic and empowering options.[36,37]

Menopause

■ DESCRIPTION

Menopause is the phenomenon experienced by women with cessation of menstrual cycles. Menopause is thought to occur when the supply of ova is exhausted and the ovaries can no longer participate in ovulatory hormone cycles. Some 400,000 ova are present at puberty, about 400 of which will mature during the menstrual years. The cessation of normal hormonal reproductive cycles occurs between the ages of 45 and 55 in American women, with an average of 52 years.

As the ovaries become unresponsive, the pituitary gland secretes larger amounts of the gonadotropins follicle-stimulating hormone (FSH) and lutcinizing hormone (LH). The ovaries respond with androgenic hormone secretion, which is converted into estrogen in the fat cells of the hips and thighs. This source of estrogen is the major contributor to the low levels of circulating estrogen present in menopausal women. The decrease in estrogen levels is responsible for the vasomotor changes and other associated symptoms experienced by a great majority of women in the United States.

In the 1960s, menopause was transformed from a simple, natural life phenomenon to the status of a disease. Conventional medical authorities began to regard menopause as a treatable illness in which estrogen replacement therapy was emphasized. Symptoms of this change in hormonal and reproductive status in women vary tremendously from culture to culture. The symptoms most commonly experienced by women in America are:

- Amenorrhea, with sudden cessation of menses, or more gradual onset taking up to four years for complete cessation.
- Vasomotor symptoms: hot flashes with or without heavy soaking perspiration, often worse at night, cold extremities, tachycardia, headaches, and dizziness.
- Weight gain.

- Insomnia.
- Fatigue.
- Atrophic vaginitis and periurethritis (the outer third of the urethra is estrogen-sensitive), with drying and thinning of the vaginal mucosa.
- Moodiness, depression, and irritability.
- Mental fogginess with forgetfulness and inability to concentrate.
- Dermatological changes with thinning and wrinkling of the skin (decreased estrogen) and a tendency toward facial hirsutism.

Libido may be decreased, and increased urinary frequency with susceptibility to bladder infections is often encountered. Other accompanying phenomena include acceleration in the incidence of coronary heart disease and osteoporosis following menopause.

Premature menopause occurs if a hysterectomy for any reason is accompanied by removal of both ovaries. Hormone replacement (see following) is a very important consideration in this circumstance.

The diagnosis of menopause is made with a typical history of symptoms. Laboratory evidence of increased FSH blood levels above 40 mIU/ml is confirmatory.

■ PREVALENCE

The numbers of women experiencing menopausal symptoms vary considerably from culture to culture. Research shows that Mayan Indian women experience neither osteoporosis nor any menopausal symptoms.[38] In the American culture, however, between 65 and 85 percent of women experience symptoms during onset of menopause.

■ ETIOLOGY AND RISK FACTORS

The direct cause of menopausal symptoms is the cessation of high levels of estrogen production from the ovaries. Women who smoke double the likelihood of an early menopause before the age of 50. Japanese women, who have far less severe menopausal symptoms compared to American women, also have much higher body levels of phytoestrogens. Soy is a major source of these compounds.

■ CONVENTIONAL TREATMENT

Menopause is an occasion for a health re-evaluation including examination of the genital organs and breasts, assessment of blood chemistry, cholesterol, thyroid and adrenal function, and determination of bone density.

Estrogen replacement therapy is almost universally recommended. Estrogen vaginal cream can be prescribed when vaginal symptoms predominate. Oral estrogen is prescribed for peri-menopausal and menopausal women for its properties of relieving hot flashes, vaginal dryness, retarding the progression of osteoporosis, reducing risks of dementia, and for its apparent benefits in reducing risks of heart disease.[39] However, recent studies have carefully separated out other confusing variables and have shown no significant benefits for heart disease prevention.[40]

Hazards of hormone replacement therapy (HRT) include:

- Estrogen-only replacement is associated with a marked increase in the incidence of uterine cancer and a modest increase in breast cancer. The majority of the increased risk for breast cancer arises from the cohort of women who also use alcohol.[41] If a patient has high risk factors for uterine or breast cancer, the benefits and risks of this therapy require extra consideration. Smaller doses of 0.6 mg daily of Premarin, the most commonly prescribed drug, appear to be as sufficient as higher doses. Estrogen patches are also satisfactory. Conventional prescriptions for estrogen are often accompanied by a prescription for the progestin drug Provera, which reduces the risks for uterine cancer from estrogen, but does not appear to affect breast cancer risk. Women users of postmenopausal estrogen replacement therapy tend to fall into the poorer risk categories if breast cancer ensues.[42] The use of raloxifine may perhaps be a conventional answer since it spares mammary tissue from its generalized estrogenic effects. Authoritative opinions regarding hormone replacement therapy are widely disparate and not totally resolved at this time.

- The incidence of adult-onset bronchial asthma in postmenopausal women using HRT for 10 years or more is double that of never-users.[43]
- Clotting problems and phlebitis incidence are increased in HRT users.[44]
- The incidence of gallstones and gall bladder inflammation increases noticeably in users of hormone replacement therapy, with double the risk for cholecystectomy.[45]
- Complaints of breast tenderness, fluid retention, headaches, and depression are bothersome to many users, leading to a decision to quit hormone therapy by up to one-half of women for whom it is prescribed.
- Liver abnormalities, exaggeration of blood sugar variations, and growth of uterine fibroids are also problems for some women.

Estrogen replacement therapy is contraindicated in uterine and breast cancer, clotting disorders, obesity, diabetes, acute liver disease and not-yet-diagnosed vaginal bleeding.

■ HOLISTIC TREATMENT

Physical Treatment

Nutrition. Phytoestrogens from food have weak but detectable estrogenic activity. Phytoestrogens are attracted to the same receptor sites as pharmaceutical estrogens, preventing occupation by these more powerful hormones and therefore reducing total estrogenic influence in the body; this may explain the lower incidence of estrogen-dependent cancers such as breast cancer in women who consume high amounts of phytoestrogens from soy, flaxseed and its oil, nuts, whole grains, apples, parsley and alfalfa. Consumption of high amounts of phytoestrogens by Japanese women may explain their very low incidence of hot flashes, hormone-related cancers, and osteoporosis.[46]

Supplements. Gamma-oryzanol, a rice bran oil derivative, 300 mg daily, totally or partially relieved hot flashes and other menopausal symptoms in over 85 percent of users.[42]

A combination of vitamin C (1,200 mg), hesperidin (a citrus bioflavonoid, 900 mg), and hesperidin methyl chalcone (900 mg) daily has been shown to give near total relief from hot flashes in over 55 percent and partial relief in 35 percent of users.[48]

Vitamin E in 400–800 IU daily amounts totally relieves distressing menopausal symptoms in over one-quarter of menopausal women, and affords partial relief in another 25 percent. Effects are equivalent to the use of estrogen.[49] Women with higher calcium intake experience a later menopause.

A high dose multivitamin–mineral combination is good insurance for meeting all micronutrient needs in aging women whose intestinal assimilation tends to decline each decade (see Chapter 1).

Habits. Caffeine and alcohol consumption tend to aggravate hot flashes. Maintaining regular sexual activity, with or without a partner, promotes the healthy condition of the vagina.

Exercise. Women exercising half an hour daily have significantly fewer hot flashes and much less mood distortion. Most exercising women in one study were able to negotiate the menopause without hormone replacement treatment. Regular exercise fosters all aspects of health.[50]

Biomolecular Options

Estriol in doses of 8 mg daily improved hot flashes and improved vaginal lubrication 90 percent within 6 months without detectable endometrial buildup.[51]

Natural forms of estrogen can be prescribed for menopausal symptoms with less risk and fewer side effects. A formula consisting of estriol, estrone, and estradiol in an 80/10/10 ratio can be obtained through compounding pharmacists on prescription. These three estrogens roughly approximate the ratio of the same estrogens elaborated during a woman's menstrual years. Cancer risks stem mainly from the estrone and estradiol fractions; this formula therefore is assumed to reduce the risk of cancerous stimulation. Appropriate doses of this "tri-est" formula are 2.5–5 mg daily.

Estriol vaginal cream prepared by a compounding pharmacist (0.5 mg/g) can be used in $\frac{1}{4}$ tsp doses daily for a week followed by one dose 3 times a week for maintenance. This improves vaginal dryness and prevents thinning and atrophy. It is also helpful in breaking the cycle of recurrent bladder infections (see following).

Progesterone from plant sources is readily absorbed through the skin when applied regularly or can be taken by mouth. Appropriate doses of the progesterone cream are $\frac{1}{4}$ to $\frac{1}{2}$ level measuring tsp daily, rotated over 7 different sites of the body, avoiding thicker skin—1 site for each day of the week. Oral micronized progesterone capsules need to supply 10–15 mg in a daily dose. Both can be formulated by a compounding pharmacist. Progesterone has a potent effect in promoting osteoblastosis. Osteoporosis is a major consideration and is discussed in Chapter 10. Progesterone carries no known hazard of stimulating either uterine or breast cancer. In fact, women with higher levels of progesterone at the time of biopsy for breast cancer have a better prognosis.[52]

If laboratory tests have shown low thyroid function, or if basal temperatures are low (see Chapter 6), thyroid hormone replacement is in order. If adrenal (DHEA) function is low, replacement doses of 15–25 mg daily are reasonable.

If diminished libido is a problem, consideration should be given to cautious supplementation with testosterone. Testosterone can be prescribed as a skin cream or as a capsule. The usual beginning test dose is 5–10 mg daily.[53]

If depression is a persisting problem, treatment can be initiated with exercise and botanical, or, if necessary, with pharmaceutical prescriptions.

Herbs

- Black cohosh (*Cimicifuga racemosa*) enjoys wide use in relieving hot flashes, depression and vaginal atrophy, modulating symptoms in 80 percent of users in 6–8 weeks (100–600 mg daily in divided doses).
- Dong quai (*Angelica sinensis*) is widely used in Asia for menopausal symptoms, dysmenorrhea, and menorrhagia. It has demonstrable estrogenic properties (1–2 g t.i.d.).
- Licorice (*Glycyrrhiza glabra*) tends to raise progesterone levels (250–500 mg t.i.d.). Prolonged use can raise blood pressures.
- Chasteberry (*Vitex agnus castus*) has effects on pituitary hormone function (175 mg daily).
- *Ginkgo biloba* improves circulation, giving relief to cold hands and feet, and improving memory (40 mg t.i.d.).

Homeopathy

Homeopathic physicians frequently work with women to evolve a satisfactory remedy for relief. The commonest remedies used are Lachesis and Sulphur (hot flashes), pulsatilla, Mulimen (a German combination of chasteberry, black cohosh, St. John's wort, and cuttlefish ink), bryonia, *Ferrum phosphoricum* and *Lycopodium* (dyspareunia), and Sepia.[54]

Mental and Emotional Elements

It is extremely helpful to focus on menopause as the opportunity for the beginning of a creative, expressive, freer time of life rather than the end the reproductive years. The less menopause is seen as a problem, the better. It is helpful to encourage patients to affirm their trust in their bodies' ability to remain healthy through this natural change.

Relaxation and Mental Imagery

The vasomotor blood vessel instability of hot flashes improves with regular practice of relaxation and meditation. Helpful accompanying imagery can picture the vaginal walls as healthy, pink, and lubricated.

Cystitis

■ DESCRIPTION

Cystitis is a state of infection or inflammation of the bladder. The bladder can accommodate up to 500 mL of urine before an elimination signal is triggered, and the female urethra is much shorter than the urethra in the male, possibly explaining why cystitis is much more common in women. Bacteria reach the bladder by retrograde passage up the urethra from the external environment. By far the most common pathogen is *E. coli*, an organism with permanent residence in the bowel.

Cystitis presents with urinary frequency and urgency, and, particularly if the urethra is involved, marked dysuria during micturition. The volume of urine passed is frequently small, and the urine may be foul-smelling, cloudy, or bloody. Severe infections are accompanied by fever and chills. The diagnosis is confirmed by a positive urinalysis; the urine may also be cultured in the laboratory for identification of the offending bacterium, used for guidance in antibiotic treatment.

Symptoms of a bladder infection may be present with the urine relatively or completely sterile. This appears to happen relatively frequently. Other pelvic, neurological, and systemic causes then need to be considered.

■ PREVALENCE

Ten to 20 percent of all adult women in the United States have at least one bladder infection each year, triggering 6–9 million physician visits annually. Two to 4 percent of asymptomatic women have bacteria in any random urine specimen. Women subject to recurring infections average over one episode each year and 20 percent of women having one episode will have another. Thirty-seven percent have at least one urinary tract infection in a decade.[55] Recurrences of infection are of particular concern, since they frequently involve infection of the kidney as well, due to unrecognized ureteral reflux. Repeated pyelonephritis episodes can cause permanent and progressive degrees of kidney failure. Bladder infections in men are much less common, and are usually associated with some anatomical abnormality.

■ ETIOLOGY AND RISK FACTORS

The propensity for women to have a bladder infection on becoming sexually active is well known. Bladder infection is likewise common in pregnancy. Women in menopause and approaching menopause are more susceptible to infections as well, apparently due to some weakening of pelvic structures with decreases in estrogen. Diaphragms used for contraception also increase risk for infection. Spermacidal creams containing nonoxynol-9 alter the vaginal flora and encourage the proliferation of *E. coli*. Feminine hygiene sprays and douching are also hazards. Recurring or persistent vaginal infections (see following) also predispose to bladder infections.

Resistance against infection depends partially on the flushing action of urine in both the ureters and the urethra. If this flushing activity becomes sluggish, the hazard of infection increases. Contributors to this problem are diseases that interfere with regular urination (e.g., spinal cord injury), partial obstruction by spasm or urethral stenosis, or underhydration. Compromised immune resistance to any infection is present in hypothyroidism.

Some foods tend to be bladder irritants, including caffeine in coffee, tea and colas; alcohol on occasion; and specific sensitizing foods in susceptible people.[56]

Excessive sympathetic nervous system activity due to the tension of unmanaged stress predisposes to spasm and incomplete emptying of the bladder.

■ CONVENTIONAL TREATMENT

Conventional precautions to prevent episodes and recurrences emphasize adequate hydration, with 6–8 glasses of water daily as a common standard. This usually keeps the urine a pale yellow color. Particularly in patients with recurrent infections, risks are reduced by cultivating a habit of more frequent voidings, and by making a conscious effort to pay attend to the bladder's signals without ignoring them. What women were commonly taught about wiping from the front to the back after urination may also be relevant. Although some authorities disagree, many think that urinating after sexual intercourse makes real sense and recommend it for those with susceptibility to recurrences. Cranberry juice reduces the frequency of infections; it has been documented to make it more difficult for bacteria to adhere to the bladder wall.[57]

Medical treatment usually involves the prescribing of antibiotics. The commonest ones used include sulfa drugs, broad-spectrum penicillins, fluoroquinolones (Cipro, Noroxin) and nitrofurantoins (Macrodantin). The former standard was a 10-day prescription; 3–5 days has been found to work just as well in uncomplicated infections. For frequently recurring episodes, some physicians recommend low antibiotic dosage daily for several weeks or months.

A common hazard with any antibiotic treatment is the destruction of normal friendly bacteria in the intestine and overgrowth of other organisms including candida (see Chapter 13). Occasionally, when a tight urethral opening is a contributing factor in recurring infections, urological dilation of the urethral meatus may help the emptying process.

■ HOLISTIC TREATMENT

Nutrition

Sugar inhibits phagocytosis and should be avoided.[58] Blueberry juice, although harder to find than cranberry juice, also contains the inhibitory factor that prevents adherence of bacteria to the bladder wall. Since most cranberry juices on the market are sweetened with sugar, and unsweetened cranberry juice is not very palatable, blueberry juice is probably preferable: a reasonable intake is 8 ounces a day.

Alkalinizing the urine also is beneficial; one study showed 80 percent relief in symptoms of cystitis after 48 hours of treatment with sodium citrate.[57] The most desirable forms are calcium, potassium, or magnesium citrate, in doses of 250 mg t.i.d. of elemental Ca, K, or Mg.

Vitamin C is also effective in bladder and urethral infections. Vitamin C has distinct antimicrobial properties and taken in large doses (1–2 g q.i.d.) is quickly hyperconcentrated in the urine. Calcium, magnesium, and potassium ascorbate will simultaneously alkalinize the urine.[60]

Vitamin A, which helps with many infections, can be taken in doses of 50,000 units daily for up to a week in adults and for 2 days in a row in children and infants. Do not recommend if pregnancy is a possibility.

Food Sensitivities

The urine specimens of up to 40 percent of women with typical symptoms of bladder or urethral infection have no detectable bacteria. Chronic interstitial cystitis is a chronic bladder irritation without bacterial infection. Food sensitivities can cause urinary frequency and urgency and may be a cause for interstitial cystitis. If a patient with recurring or chronic dysuria has negative urinalyses and cultures, a food elimination trial and rechallenge is well worth doing.

Herbs

Uva ursi (*Arctostaphylos uva ursi*) is an herb with a long history of use in preventing and treating bladder infections, recently documented with research; dosage 250–500 mg t.i.d.[61] Goldenseal (*Hydrastis canadensis*), containing berberine, 250–500 mg t.i.d. is also efficacious against many of the bacteria commonly involved.[62] *Centella asiatica* (gotu kola) has been used with success in interstitial cystitis; use an extract supplying 120 mg daily of triterpenic acids.[63]

Biomolecular Options

Capitalizing on the known increase in recurrent infections in menopausal women, astute observers found in one study that that use of estriol in an intravaginal cream, used nightly for 2 weeks each month, *reduced recurrences 92 percent*. A compounding pharmacist can prepare an intravaginal cream delivering 0.5 mg daily,[64] and oral supplementation with 2 mg daily doses of estriol appears to also reduce recurrences of bladder and vaginal infections.

Homeopathy

Classical homeopathic diagnosis and treatment may be curative for recurrent cystitis. Symptomatic homeopathic remedies to use for treatment include Apis Mel or Cantharis. *Acupuncture* also can be of help with recurrent infections.

Mental and Emotional Treatment Options

If stress and consequent tension are prominent in the history of the recurrent cystitis patient, incorporating some measure of regular relaxation practice will tend to improve bladder emptying and reduce the frequency of recurrences. Meditation, biofeedback, and other techniques all decrease sympathetic nervous system activity, reducing the contribution made by urethral spasm and poor bladder emptying. Immune responses also improve with the practice of these skills.

Vaginitis

■ DESCRIPTION

Infections of the vagina[65] may be:

- limited to superficial invasion of the outer layer of the vaginal mucosa;
- part of a more serious generalized infection including the cervix; or
- part of a total pelvic inflammatory disease process involving the uterus and Fallopian tubes as well. The pH of the vagina is normally mildly acidic.

Three organisms—*Trichomonas vaginalis, Candida albicans,* and *Gardnerella vaginalis*—cause the vast majority of vaginal infections. Other pathogenic invaders include *Chlamydia trachomatis, Neisseria gonorrhea,* and *Herpes simplex.*

- Trichomoniasis is caused by a unicellular parasite transmitted by sexual intercourse and manifests as an odoriferous greenish discharge, with pruritis and burning. The diagnosis is made by finding the organism in a microscopic wet mount of vaginal secretions, the pH of which is usually between 5.5 and 5.8.
- *Candida albicans,* the most common cause of vaginal discharge in women today, is a normal fungal resident in the vagina and overgrows due to a variety of factors, giving intense itching, and a white cottage-cheesy discharge.
- *Gardnerella vaginalis* (formerly *Hemophilus vaginalis*) is found in over 90 percent of non-trichomonas, non-yeast infections, usually called "non-specific vaginitis."[66] Minimal itching and a more profuse odorous discharge are clues to this infection. Gardnerella is an opportunistic invader that is found in 40 percent of asymptomatic women, and contributes to non-specific infection when the vaginal medium is compromised. Other anaerobic bacteria are

more likely the causative organisms in non-specific vaginitis.

- *Chlamydia trachomatis* is a sexually transmitted parasitic infection, which is a major cause of serious deep pelvic inflammatory disease and consequent infertility.
- Gonorrhea is a sexually transmitted, bacterial disease often cultured in serious deep pelvic inflammatory infections and often manifests as a bloody, pussy discharge.
- *Herpes simplex* infection is the most common sexually transmitted infection in the United States today. Both herpes type 1 and type 2 viruses may be involved. Vulvo-vaginal herpes manifests as localized, vesicular lesions which usually ulcerate, often becoming painful, sometimes excruciatingly so, and taking about 2–3 weeks to completely heal. Vaginal herpetic infections are commonly transmitted by genital, manual, or oral contact.

■ PREVALENCE

Thirty-five to 50 percent of American women will deal with a vaginal infection sooner or later. Three out of 4 young sexually active women have had one or more types of infection, and vaginal infections have now been shown to be 6 times more common than bladder infections.[67]

Vaginitis, particularly the variety caused by Candidiasis, is extremely common and is on the increase. About 1.3 million women are treated or treat themselves for vaginal candidiasis infections each year; the number of yearly antifungal prescriptions has risen over 50 percent in the last decade. Antibody studies indicate that 30 to 100 percent of adults have been infected with both varieties of herpes organisms which can cause infections in the vulvo-vaginal tissues as well as elsewhere. Chlamydia infection is found in 5–10 percent of young sexually active women.[68]

■ ETIOLOGY AND RISK FACTORS

Vaginitis involves the invasion of infecting organisms from the reservoir of organisms in the colon and rectum or transmitted through sexual contact. Infection can also arise from multiplication of normal organisms resident in the vagina which proliferate or overgrow due to changes in the vaginal medium—including the pH, the presence of blood with menstruation, the population and balance of micro-organisms, the level of sugar in the blood and vaginal tissues, the adequacy of the natural flushing action of vaginal fluids, and the presence of immunity-determined resistance factors.

Predisposing factors favorable to these infections include:

1. diabetes—elevated blood and tissue sugar levels encourage growth of candida and diminish immune resistance;
2. pregnancy and oral contraceptive agents change the hormone balance, encouraging candida growth;
3. treatment with immune suppressants, chemotherapeutic anti-cancer agents or cortisone compromises immune resistance;
4. poor nutritional habits—high sugar and low antioxidant intake—compromise immune resistance;
5. anemia reduces resistance and increases susceptibility to infection;
6. hypothyroidism reduces metabolism of all systems including cellular immunity;
7. obesity increases the frequency of vaginitis, probably due to trapping of greater amounts of moisture in skin folds and the genitalia;
8. antibiotics markedly reduce the population of normal organisms (*L. acidophilus*), promoting proliferation of candida;
9. wearing panty hose with synthetic materials triples the incidence of yeast infections compared to the wearing of cotton underclothing;[69]
10. scented and perfumed toilet paper, and tampons containing deodorants are often irritating and sensitizing, and predispose to invasion by infecting organisms;

11. multiple sex partners increase risk of sexually transmitted organisms including trichomonas and herpes;
12. failure to use barrier contraceptive methods (which reduce transmission of organisms) with sexual intercourse increases risk;
13. stress which is not managed well results in tension, high levels of which compromise immunity and resistance to infection in the vagina as well as elsewhere;
14. semen has a pH of about 9; it takes about 8 hours for the normally mildly acidic vagina to return to normal. Sexual intercourse several times in 24 hours alters the normally acidic pH, tending to support abnormal organisms.[70]

Studies have shown that in women with recurrent vaginal candida infections, a majority have the same yeast strains in the gastrointestinal tract. As most women know, yeast infections are highly associated with the use of broad-spectrum antibiotics. Candida infections tend to aggravate or evoke more frequent generalized allergic reactions.

The onset of vaginitis may have a psychosocial implication as well. In *Women's Bodies, Women's Wisdom*, Dr. Christiane Northrup says "Chronic vaginitis is a socially acceptable way for a woman to say no to sex."

■ CONVENTIONAL TREATMENT

Standard advice includes avoiding routine douching, ceasing use of scented toilet paper and tampons, and removing tampons after no more than 8 hours. Trichomoniasis is treated with Flagyl, prescribed in a large single dose or in smaller amounts over 5–7 days. Sexual partners need to be treated at the same time. Nausea is a significant side effect, metallic taste is common, and, occasionally, seizures and persistent neuropathy have been reported.

Candida infection is treated by prescription and over-the-counter vaginal creams and suppositories; the most popular are Gyne-Lotrimin and Monistat; generic OTC preparations are also available. When vaginal yeast overgrowth is present, overgrowth in the intestine is also likely, since the predisposing factors favoring yeast multiplication affect the entire body. There is evidence that treating the intestinal candidiasis at the same time as the vaginal infection reduces the rate of recurrences. The mechanism by which intestinal infection affects the vaginal manifestations is not completely clear, but may occur through an allergic phenomenon or by transmission of organisms from anorectal surfaces. Conventional treatment of the intestinal infection utilizes nystatin 500,000-unit tablets q.i.d.

For herpetic outbreaks, acyclovir (Zovirax) and similar drugs are used effectively in ointment form, orally (200 mg q 4 h, 5 doses daily), and even intravenously, injected over an hour, t.i.d. for 2–5 days. It should not be given intravenously in those who are pregnant or who have any degree of renal failure, and it can produce nausea, headache and malaise. Long-term daily prophylactic use is also prescribed for patients with a history of frequent recurrences.

Non-specific vaginitis, gonorrhea, and chlamydia infections are all treated with antibiotics. Some strains of Neisseria gonorrhea are now resistant to the usual treatment with penicillin and common broad-spectrum antibiotics. Antibacterial prescription creams (Cleomycin, Metrogel) are also used for bacterial vaginitis. *Antibiotics do not alter the circumstances predisposing to the infections in the first place.*

■ HOLISTIC TREATMENT

Candida

Nutrition

- Abate sugar intake.
- Avoid milk and milk products including cheese.
- Avoid foods with high yeast or mold content: nuts, melons, dried fruits, alcohol.

- Augment fluid intake. Women subject to candidiasis have a higher rate of sensitive and insensitive fluid loss through the skin.
- Omit any known food allergens.
- Add plain yogurt to regular nutritional intake.[71]

Supplements

- Suggest a high-potency multivitamin, multimineral supplement with megadose antioxidants.
- Orally ingested *L. acidophillus* re-establishes normal intestinal populations.[72]
- Nutritional agents which address intestinal candidiasis simultaneously with vaginal treatment include garlic, short-chain fatty acids (e.g., caprylic acid), and herbs containing berberine.

Local treatment

- Re-establish normal vaginal flora by douching daily with a solution of *L. acidophillus*, prepared from a high-quality supplement with live organisms, or an active-culture yogurt (most live-organism preparations have to be refrigerated).[73] Use preparations supplying 1 billion organisms per dose and mix with 10 cc of water and inject into the vagina with a syringe b.i.d.
- A vast majority of women using yogurt instilled into the vagina in 15 cc amounts b.i.d. become asymptomatic within 1–3 months.[74]
- Boric acid capsules or suppositories (600 mg twice daily) have a higher treatment success rate than antifungal prescription creams and suppositories. Persistent treatment for several months achieves the greatest success in re-establishing totally normal vaginal flora. Side effects of minor burning sensations are usually not severe enough to trigger discontinuation of treatment.[75]
- Positive results have also been reported with insertion of a gentian-violet-soaked tampon into the vagina daily for 7–14 days. The hazard of this approach is the irrevocable

staining of clothing exposed to this intensely potent violet dye.[76]

- Betadine, available in pharmacies, contains iodine which has broad spectrum antibacterial, antifungal, and antiparasitic activity. Iodine is, after all, used to treat water to render it potable. A solution of one part Betadine to 100 parts water can be used as a douche on a daily basis for 2 weeks. Studies have shown *100 percent effectiveness* in vaginal candidiasis.[77]

Homeopathy. Symptomatic prescribing includes *Calcarea carbonica* for cases with intense premenstrual pruritis and thick whitish discharge. Borax is prescribed for mid-cycle egg-white-like discharge.

Trichomonas

Iodine douche is 80 percent successful.[78] Homeopathic *Arsenicum album* for a discharge with offensive odor is an option.

Non-specific Vaginitis

Iodine douche is 93 percent effective in mixed infections.[79] Oxaluria can also be responsible for intractable vulvovaginal symptomatology, and can be treated with supplemental calcium and a low-oxalate diet.[80]

Homeopathic Sepia for the milky, white discharge and burning pain is another option.

Herpes

Treatment options in herpes vaginalis include:

Nutritional

- Low arginine intake (avoid chocolate, peanuts, seeds, almonds, nuts).
- Increase in lysine foods (most vegetables, legumes, fish, turkey, chicken).

Supplements

- Oral vitamin C 2 g daily.

- Zinc 50–75 mg daily.
- Lysine 1,000 mg t.i.d.
- Mixed bioflavonoids 1,000 mg daily.

These oral supplements help assist with healing lesions as well as being highly effective in prevention of recurrences.

Topical nutrients

- Vitamin C solution (Ascoxal) significantly accelerates rate of healing.[81] It is applied with a cotton pad soaked in the solution and pressed to the lesions for 2 minutes on three occasions 30 minutes apart. Ascoxal is listed in the *Physicians' Desk Reference* (PDR).
- Zinc sulfate solution 0.025 percent markedly accelerates healing, and prevents outbreaks.[82] A compounded prescription is written for "$ZnSO_4$ 0.25% in saturated solution of camphor water; sig: apply q 30–90 minutes at outbreak. Disp 30 cc." The solution can be daubed on lesions and allowed to dry each time. When the solution is applied immediately at the outset of the tingly prodrome which heralds an outbreak, it will abort the outbreak up to 90 percent of the time. If an outbreak does occur, it is attended with much less pain.

Biomolecular agents. Bovine thymus extracts improve cellular immunity. Prescribe 500 mg of crude polypeptide fraction daily (or 120 mg of purified polypeptides).[83]

Herbal treatment

- Topical application of 70 : 1 concentrated extract of lemon balm (*Melissa officinalis*) b.i.d. to q.i.d. in cream form has been shown to prevent recurrences of herpes simplex 100 percent of the time when used continuously.[84] It also works well in genital herpes.
- Glycyrrhetinic acid (licorice root) applied topically b.i.d. speeds healing and reduces pain.[85]

Homeopathy. Symptomatic treatment with 12X to 30C potency remedies *Apis mellifica* for stinging herpetic pain, Petrolatum for spreading lesions, and Graphites for intense itching is part of the armamentarium. Yeast-gard is a well-tolerated combination homeopathic remedy.

Biofeedback, relaxation skills, and meditation. Regular practice of meditation and relaxation skills improves immunity. A high portion of the outbreaks and recurrences of herpes, candida, and other infections follow times of acute stress.

Social health parameters. Insightful observers discern a positive relationship between immune strength, and a clear sense of internal power and clarity in sexual relationships. If patients exhibit ambivalence in regard to sexual relationships; cannot state what they want in regard to sexual relations at a given time; and seem to need to have excuses, they will probably benefit from brief counseling. Greater self-esteem enables patients to be clear about their wants and feel self-assured about negotiating comfortable solutions regarding sexual choices. The psychological growth which ensues will enhance their comfort levels and benefit immunity.

Fibrocystic Breast Disease

■ DESCRIPTION

The fibrous masses that cause the palpable breast nodularity in this disease are most commonly cystic and may contain up to 60 cc of fluid and be 5 cm or more in diameter. The involved areas are often tender due to inflammation, and may be confusing enough that a biopsy is undertaken to rule out malignancy. The tendency for fibrocystic masses to manifest cyclic changes, becoming more prominent during the premenstrual days, is a prominent factor in making the diagnosis. The finding of clear amber fluid on needling a possibly cystic mass almost completely rules out its non-malignant nature.

■ PREVALENCE

Estimates of the portion of women who have some degree of fibrocystic breast disease involvement go as high as 80 percent. The disease disappears at menopause as strong hormonal influences disappear.

■ ETIOLOGY AND RISK FACTORS

Genetic

There is evidence that women with cystic breast disease have a hereditary predisposition to greater sensitivity to methylxanthines.

Nutritional Factors

Consistently low iodine levels are found in animals with fibrocystic breast disease.[86] This is thought to render the breast tissues more sensitive to estrogen effects. Essential fatty acid levels are low in fibrocystic breast disease.[87]

Habit Factors

Cystic breast changes are associated with constipation; women having less than 3 bowel movements per week have a significantly greater incidence of fibrocystic breast disease compared to women with a daily bowel habit. This association is probably due to greater intestinal reabsorption of estrogenic steroids or absorption of toxic metabolites of estrogenic steroids formed by bacteria in the large bowel.[88,89]

Environmental Factors

Consumption of coffee is strongly associated with PMS symptoms. The incidence and severity of symptoms is 7-fold greater in those drinking 8–10 cups of coffee daily compared to non-coffee drinkers. Caffeine and methyl xanthines have been shown to contribute to cystic breast disease in a number of studies.[90] In those which have not come to this conclusion, total elimination of all caffeine was apparently not achieved during treatment, as evidenced by the presence of methylxanthine metabolites in cystic breast fluid.

Biomolecular Factors

Since cystic breast disease regresses permanently at menopause, hormone factors loom large in the list of potential causes. Fibrocystic breast disease (FBD) is apparently the result of hormonal imbalances, with a higher-than-normal estrogen to progesterone ratio, and elevated levels of prolactin, which itself may be related to the higher estrogen/progesterone ratio.[91] It is commonly present in women who have prominent pre-menstrual symptoms, in which estrogen/progesterone ratios are also elevated.

■ CONVENTIONAL TREATMENT

Conventional physicians accept major responsibility for monitoring breast masses, which if persistent may need to be biopsied. Medications for pain are usually made available.

■ HOLISTIC TREATMENT

Nutrition

Patients should avoid chocolate, caffeinated beverages, and OTC caffeine medicines. Elimination of caffeine must be 100 percent, since even small amounts of caffeine can be problematic, such as the 3 percent caffeine content in decaffeinated coffee. Significant improvement in over 95 percent of patients who totally eliminate caffeine has been reported.[92]

High fiber intake is associated with a 50 percent lower incidence of FBD as well as a lower rate of breast cancer. Nutritional intake should minimize animal meat, dairy products, and processed sugars.[93]

Supplements

- Vitamin E has a researched record for reducing symptoms and findings in 2/3 of patients with FBD (600 IU daily).[94]

Some studies have subsequently found it less useful. Vitamin E appears to reduce pituitary LH and FSH production, reducing estrogen stimulation.

- Vitamin A, although less researched, brought about partial or full disease remission in 50 percent of those treated in one study (150,000 IU daily).[95] This is a high dose and needs to be used when other measures fail; monitoring by a physician is essential; it should not be used if there is any possibility of pregnancy.
- The liver metabolizes estrogen to glucuronic acid for elimination into the intestine. Adequate B complex vitamins are necessary to accomplish the task ("B-50," one daily).
- Other daily antioxidant intake should include vitamin C 1–2 g, 1 beta-carotene 25,000 IU, zinc 30 mg, and selenium 200 μg.
- Because of its effect on reducing inflammatory factors in the body, flaxseed oil 1 tbsp daily, or fish oil, two 1,000 mg capsules b.i.d. are important.
- In a study of 140 women with painful fibrocystic breast disease, 72 percent became totally asymptomatic after treatment with iodized casein.[96] Lugol's solution or elemental iodine, 2–8 drops daily, can be used but should be monitored carefully; excess doses can alter thyroid function and lead to toxic iodism. Five to 12 drops per day of SSKI, a prescription expectorant, will also suffice.
- Probiotics *L. acidophillus* and *Bifidus* also appear to increase estrogen excretion and are worth trying for at least a 6-month trial. Preparations should supply 1–5 billion live organisms a day.

Biomolecular Options

A 1981 study achieved partial or total relief in 3 of every 4 FBD patients by using Synthroid 0.1 mg daily for 2 months, in spite of the fact that the thyroid blood tests were normal in all but one patient.[97]

Biofeedback and Stress Management

Observers of women with fibrocystic breast disease consistently see patterns of exacerbation during times of stress. Regular practice of biofeedback, deep relaxation or meditation techniques are of considerable help in evoking healing energies. Imagery and repetition of positive affirmations regarding the health of the body and breasts supplements other healing initiatives.

Addressing Psychoenergetic Issues

The pain of cystic breast disease may be intertwined with residual blocked energy from past painful experiences involving the breasts. Calling to mind repressed memories of childhood and early adulthood experiences and psychological traumas, especially those with a sexual connotation, may be part of the therapy of resolving those memories as well as painful manifestations in the breast or genital organs. It is important for patients to be gentle and forgiving of themselves in allowing past issues be acknowledged, resolved and then dispatched into the past where they belong. We are whole beings with bodies, feelings, thoughts, and spiritual beliefs. All aspects need to be integrated into the opportunity for optimal health.

REFERENCES

1. Halbreich U et al. Low plasma gamma-aminobutyric acid levels during the late luteal phase of women with premenstrual dysphoric disorder. *Am J Psychiatry* 1996; 153(5):718–20.
2. Ericksson E et al. Cerebrospinal fluid levels of monoamine metabolites. A preliminary study of their relation to menstrual cycle phase, sex steroids, and pituitary hormones in healthy women and in women with premenstrual syndrome. *Neuropsychopharmacology* 1994; 11(3):201–13.
3. Bermond P. Therapy of side effects of oral contraceptive agents with vitamin B6. *Acta Vitaminol Enzymol* 1982; 4(1–2): 45–54.

4. Brayshaw ND et al. Thyroid hypofunction in premenstrual syndrome. *N Engl J Med* 1986; 315(23):1486–7.
5. Facchinetti F et al. Oestradiol/progesterone imbalance and the premenstrual syndrome. *Lancet* 1983; 2(8362):1302.
6. Abraham GE. Nutritional factors in the etiology of the premenstrual tension syndromes. *J Reprod Med* 1983; 8(7):446–64.
7. Chuong CJ et al. Periovulatory beta-endorphin levels in premenstrual syndrome. *Obstet Gynecol* 1994; 83(5 Pt 1): 755–60.
8. Cerin A et al. Hormonal and biochemical profiles of premenstrual syndrome. Treatment with essential fatty acids. *Acta Obstet Gynecol Scand* 1993; 72(5):337–43.
9. O'Brien PM et al. Prolactin levels in the premenstrual syndrome. *Br J Obstet Gynaecol* 1982; 89(4):306–8.
10. Northrup C. *Women's Bodies, Women's Wisdom.* New York: Bantam, 1994.
11. Crook WG. PMS and yeasts: an etiological connection? *Hosp Pract* 1983; 18(9):21–24.
12. Abraham GE. Nutritional factors in the etiology of the premenstrual tension syndromes. *J Reprod Med* 1983;28(7):446–64.
13. Johnson WG et al. Macronutrient intake, eating habits, and exercise as moderators of menstrual distress in healthy women. *Psychosom Med* 1995; 57(4):324–30.
14. Abraham GE et al. Serum and red cell magnesium levels in patients with premenstrual tension. *Am J Clin Nutr* 1981; 34(11):2364–6.
15. Rossignol AM et al. Do women with premenstrual symptoms self-medicate with caffeine? *Epidemiology* 1991; 2(6):403–8.
16. Longcope C et al. The effect of a low fat diet on estrogen metabolism. *J Clin Endocrinol Metab* 1987; 64(6):1246–50.
17. Kendall KE et al. The effects of vitamin B6 supplementation on premenstrual symptoms. *Obstet Gynecol* 1987; 70(2):145–9.
18. London RA et al. The effect of alpha-tocopherol on premenstrual symptomatology: a double-blind study. II. Endocrine correlates. *J Am Coll Nutr* 1984; 3(4):351–6.
19. Parker PD. Premenstrual syndrome. *Am Fam Physician* 1994; 50(6):1309–17, 1323–4.
20. Penland JG et al. Dietary calcium and manganese effects on menstrual cycle symptoms. *Am J Obstet Gynecol* 1993; 168(5): 1417–23.

21. Harel Z et al. Supplementation with omega-3 polyunsaturated fatty acids in the management of dysmenorrhea in adolescents. *Am J Obstet Gynecol* 1996; 174(4):1335–8.
22. Menkes DB et al. Acute tryptophan depletion aggravates premenstrual syndrome. *J Affect Disord* 1994; 32(1):37–44.
23. Steege JF et al. The effects of aerobic exercise on premenstrual symptoms in middle-aged women: a preliminary study. *J Psychosom Res* 1993; 37(2):127–33.
24. Mackenzie N et al. Premenstrual syndrome and progesterone suppositories. *JAMA* 1991; 265(1):26.
25. Mabray CR et al. Treatment of common gynecologic-endocrinologic symptoms by allergy management procedures. *Obstet Gynecol* 1982; 59(5):560–4.
26. Parry BL et al. Light therapy of late luteal phase dysphoric disorder: an extended study. *Am J Psychiatry* 1993; 150(9):1417–19.
27. Schlidge E. Essay on the treatment of premenstrual and menopausal mood swings and depressive states. *Rigelh Biol Umsch* 1964; 19(2):18–22.
28. Milewicz A et al. Vitex agnus castus extract in the treatment of luteal phase defects due to latent hyperprolactinemia. Results of a randomized placebo-controlled double-blind study. *Arzneimittelforschung* 1993; 43(7):752–6.
29. Mei QB et al. Advances in the pharmacological studies of radix *Angelica sinensis* (Oliv) Diels (Chinese Danggui). *Chin Med J (Engl)* 1991; 104(9):776–81.
30. Kumagai A et al. Effect of Glycyrrharrizin on estrogen action. *Endocrinol Jpn* 1967; 14(1):34–8.
31. Blumenthal M (ed.). *The Complete German Commission E Monographs*. Boston: Integrative Medicine Communications, 1998:90, 108, 119–20, 226–7.
32. Oleson T et al. Randomized controlled study of premenstrual symptoms treated with ear, hand, and foot reflexology. *Obstet Gynecol* 1993 ; 82(6):906–11.
33. Boesler D et al. Efficacy of high-velocity low-amplitude manipulative technique in subjects with low-back pain during menstrual cramping. *J Am Osteopath Assoc* 1993; 93(2):203–8, 213–14.
34. Kokjohn K et al. The effect of spinal manipulation on pain and prostaglandin levels in women with primary dysmenorrhea. *J Manipulative Physiol Ther* 1992; 15(5):279–85.

35. Helms JM. Acupuncture for the management of primary dysmenorrhea. *Obstet Gynecol* 1987; 69(1):51–6.
36. Benson H et al. Relaxation and other alternative therapies. *Patient Care* 1993; 15:75–80.
37. Goodale IL et al. Alleviation of premenstrual syndrome symptoms with the relaxation response. *Obstet Gynecol* 1990; 75(4): 649–55.
38. Martin MC et al. Menopause without symptoms: the endocrinology of menopause among rural Mayan Indians. *Am J Obstet Gynecol* 1993; 168(6 pt 1):1839–43.
39. Ginsburg GS et al. Why cardiologists should be interested in estrogen. *Am J Cardiol* 1996; 78(5):559–61.
40. Sidney S et al. Myocardial infarction and the use of estrogen-progesterone in postmenopausal women. *Ann Intern Med* 1997; 127(7):501–8.
41. Ginsburg ES. Estrogen, alcohol and breast cancer risk. *J Steroid Biochem Mol Biol* 1999; 69(1–6):299–306.
42. LeBlanc ES et al. Postmenopausal estrogen replacement therapy is associated with adverse breast cancer prognostic indices. *J Womens Health Gend Based Med* 1999; 8(6):815–23.
43. Troisi RJ et al. Menopause, postmenopausal estrogen preparations, and the risk of adult-onset asthma. A prospective cohort study. *Am J Respir Crit Care Med* 1995; 152(4 Pt 1):1183–8.
44. Levi M et al. Oral contraceptives and hormonal replacement therapy cause an imbalance in coagulation and fibrinolysis which may explain the increased risk of venous thromboembolism. *Cardiovasc Res* 1999; 41(1):21–4.
45. Grodstein F et al. Postmenopausal hormone use and cholecystectomy in a large prospective study. *Obstet Gynecol* 1994; 83(1): 5–11.
46. Adlercreutz H et al. Dietary phyto-oestrogens and the menopause in Japan. *Lancet* 1992; 339(8803):1233.
47. Murase Y et al. Clinical studies of oral administration of gamma-oryzanol on climacteric complaints and its syndrome. *Obstet Gynecol Prac* 1963; 12:147–9.
48. Smith CJ. Non-hormonal control of vasomotor flushing in menopausal patients. *Chic Med* 1964; 67:193–5.
49. Koh KK et al. Vascular effects of estrogen and vitamin E therapies in postmenopausal women. *Circulation* 1999; 100(18):1851–7.

50. Slaven L et al. Mood and symptom reporting among middle-aged women: the relationship between menopausal status, hormone replacement therapy, and exercise participation. *Health Psychol* 1997; 16(3):203–8.
51. Tzingounis VA et al. Estriol in the management of the menopause. *JAMA* 1978; 239(16):1638–41.
52. Mohr PE et al. Serum progesterone and prognosis in operable breast cancer. *Br J Cancer* 1996; 73(12):1552–3.
53. Basson R. Androgen replacement for women. *Can Fam Physician* 1999; 45:2100–7.
54. Blumenthal M (ed.). *The Complete German Commission E Monographs*. Boston: Integrative Medicine Communications, 1998:108–466.
55. Branch WT. *Office Practice of Medicine*. Philadelphia: W. B. Saunders, 1982:488–504, 679–85.
56. Marshall FF et al. Eosinophilic cystitis. *J Urol* 1974; 112(3): 335–7.
57. Sobota AE. Inhibition of bacterial adherence by cranberry juice: potential use for the treatment of urinary tract infections. *J Urol* 1984; 131(5):1013–16.
58. Sanchez A et al. Role of sugars in human neutrophilic phagocytosis. *Am J Clin Nutr* 1973; 26(11):1180–4.
59. Spooner JB. Alkalinisation in the management of cystitis. *J Int Med Res* 1984; 12(1):30–4.
60. Lundberg JO et al. Urinary nitrite: more than a marker of infection. *Urology* 1997; 50(2):189–91.
61. Larsson B et al. Prophylactic effect of UVA-E in women with recurrent cystitis: a preliminary report. *Curr Ther Res* 1993; 53:441–3.
62. Amin AH et al. Berberine sulfate: antimicrobial activity, bioassay, and mode of action. *Can J Microbiol* 1969; 15(9):1067–76.
63. Fam A. Use of titrated extract of *Centella asiatica* in Bilharzial bladder lesions. *Int Surg* 1973; 58(7):451–2.
64. Raz R et al. A controlled trial of intravaginal estriol in postmenopausal women with recurrent urinary tract infections. *N Engl J Med* 1993; 329(11):753–6.
65. Fauci AS et al (eds.). *Harrison's Principles of Internal Medicine*, 14th ed. New York: McGraw-Hill, 1998.
66. Eschenbach DA. Vaginal infection. *Clin Obstet Gynecol* 1983; 26(1):186–202.

67. McCue JD et al. Strategies for diagnosing vaginitis. *J Fam Pract* 1979; 9(3):395–402.
68. Holmes KK. The Chlamydia epidemic. *JAMA* 1981; 245(17): 1718–23.
69. Heidrich FE et al. Clothing factors and vaginitis. *J Fam Pract* 1984; 19(4):491–4.
70. Northrup C. *Women's Bodies, Women's Wisdom.* New York: Bantam, 1994.
71. Hilton E et al. Ingestion of yogurt containing *Lactobacillus acidophilus* as prophylaxis for candidal vaginitis. *Ann Intern Med* 1992; 116(5):353–7.
72. Shalev E et al. Ingestion of yogurt containing *Lactobacillus acidophilus* compared with pasteurized yogurt as prophylaxis for recurrent candidal vaginitis and bacterial vaginosis. *Arch Fam Med* 1996; 5(10):593–6.
73. Friedlander A et al. *Lactobacillus acidophillus* and vitamin B complex in the treatment of vaginal infection. *Panminerva Med* 1986; 28(1):51–3.
74. Neri A et al. Bacterial vaginosis in pregnancy treated with yoghurt. *Acta Obstet Gynecol Scand* 1993; 72(1):17–19.
75. Van Slyke KK et al. Treatment of vulvovaginal candidiasis with boric acid powder. *Am J Obstet Gynecol* 1981; 141(2):145–8.
76. Karnaky KJ. A stainless washable gentian violet specific for *Candida albicans* (monilia) and other vaginal pathogens. One medication for all vaginal infections. *Southwest Med* 1970; 51(12):271–2.
77. Reeve P. The inactivation of *Chlamydia trachomatis* by povidone–iodine. *J Antimicrob Chemother* 1976; 2(1):77–80.
78. Ratzan JJ. Monilial and trichomonal vaginitis. Topical treatment with povidone–iodine preparations. *Calif Med* 1969; 110(1):24–7.
79. Mayhew SR. Vaginitis: a study of the efficacy of povidone–iodine in unselected cases. *J Int Med Res*; 9(2):157–9.
80. Solomons CC et al. Calcium citrate for vulvar vestibulitis. A case report. *J Reprod Med* 1991; 36(12):879–82.
81. Hovi T et al. Topical treatment of recurrent mucocutaneous herpes with ascorbic acid-containing solution. *Antiviral Res* 1995; 27(3):263–70.
82. Finnerty EF. Topical zinc in the treatment of herpes simplex. *Cutis* 1986; 37(2):130–1.

83. Aiuti F et al. A placebo-controlled trial of thymic hormone treatment of recurrent *herpes simplex labialis* infection in immunodeficient hosts. *Int J Clin Pharmacol Ther Toxicol* 1983; 21(2):81–6.

84. Wolbling RH et al. Local therapy of herpes simplex with dried extract from *Melissa officinalis. Phytomed* 1994; 1:25–31.

85. Csonka GW et al. Treatment of herpes genitalis with carbenoxolone and cicloxolone creams: a double blind placebo controlled clinical trial. *Br J Vener Dis* 1984; 60(3):178–81.

86. Eskin BA et al. Mammary gland dysplasia in iodine deficiency. Studies in rats. *JAMA* 1967; 200(8):691–5.

87. Gately CA et al. Plasma fatty acid profiles in benign breast disorders. *Br J Surg* 1992; 79(5):407–9.

88. Hentges DJ. Does diet influence human fecal microflora composition? *Nutr Rev* 1980; 38(10):329–36.

89. Goldin BNR et al. Effect of diet on excretion of estrogens in pre- and postmenopausal women. *Cancer Res* 1981; 41(9 Pt 2):3771–3.

90. Ernster VL et al. Effects of caffeine-free diet on benign breast disease: a randomized trial. *Surgery* 1982; 91(3):263–7.

91. Peters F et al. Serum prolactin levels in patients with fibrocystic breast disease. *Obstet Gynecol* 1984; 64(3):381–5.

92. Minton JP et al. Clinical and biochemical studies on methylxanthine-related fibrocystic breast disease. *Surgery* 1981; 90(2):299–304.

93. Baghurst PA et al. Dietary fiber and risk of benign proliferative epithelial disorders of the breast. *Int J Cancer* 1995; 63(4):481–5.

94. Abrams AA. The use of vitamin E in chronic cystic mastitis. *N Engl J Med* 1965; 272:1080.

95. Band PR et al. Treatment of benign breast disease with vitamin A. *Prev Med* 1984; 13(5):549–54.

96. Ghent WR et al. Iodine replacement in fibrocystic disease of the breast. *Can J Surg* 1993; 36(5):453–60.

97. Estes NC. Mastodynia due to fibrocystic disease of the breast controlled with thyroid hormone. *Am J Surg* 1981; 142(6):764–6.

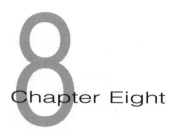

Chapter Eight

Psychological Diseases

Depression

■ DESCRIPTION

Depression is a psychological mood state which varies from occasional and mild (adjustment problems, sadness, feelings of being blue and morose) to severe states of psychotic unipolar and bipolar melancholy associated with threatened suicide and requiring hospitalization. A definitive diagnosis of depression should not be made until physical conditions have been surveyed by physical examination and laboratory assessment including a complete blood cell (CBC) count, chemistries, thyroid and adrenal function tests, and a stool examination for candida overgrowth. Other conditions ruled out, the diagnosis can be made reflecting at least 4 of the following 9 recognized criteria, present for at least 2 weeks:

1. depressed, hopeless mood for most of the day,
2. markedly diminished interest in usual activities,
3. insomnia or excessive sleep nearly every day,
4. significant loss of weight or appetite,
5. agitated or markedly slowed movements,
6. fatigue or lack of energy nearly every day,
7. feelings of worthlessness or inappropriate guilt,
8. diminished ability to think or concentrate,
9. recurrent suicidal thoughts or suicidal planning.

Depression is also often accompanied by diminished sense of self-esteem, decreased libido, crying spells, self-deprecation, irritability, and thoughts of futility and death. Impaired functionality for normal activities of daily living, accelerated loss of joy and happiness, and decreased social contacts are also common. Mild depression is often self-limited and does not come to the attention of the health professional. It is estimated that 40 percent of people with depression are never diagnosed or treated.

■ PREVALENCE

Depression, in its broadest definition, afflicts 11 million people in the United States each year. This disorder does not distinguish between age, race, culture, or occupation—it pervades all stations of society. According to the World Health Organization, depression is presently the fourth leading cause of disability in the world, and major depression occurs in 10–20 percent of the world's population in the course of a lifetime. More than twice as many women are treated for depression than men, but it is not known whether this is only because more women seek treatment. Suicide, especially in younger age groups, is on the rise. Some studies of high school children have concluded that up to 30 percent commonly think of suicide and feel hopeless. Depressed people are much more likely to die from a second heart attack,[1,2] develop cancer,[3] and prematurely die.

■ ETIOLOGY AND RISK FACTORS

The following are believed to be the most significant risk factors contributing to depression. Physical factors include heredity; about 50 percent of depressed persons have a positive family history. A disproportionate percentage of persons with candidiasis, chronic fatigue syndrome, and chemical sensitivity syndrome experience depression. Depression can be triggered by inhalant and food allergies and sensitivities, hypothyroidism, hypoglycemia, folic acid deficiency, deficiency of vitamins B_2, B_6, and B_{12}, the postpartum state, physical deconditioning, biochemical states of low serotonin and norepinephrine, air pollution, increased concentrations of positive air ions, insufficient sunlight (seasonal depression), overcrowding, and during treatment with certain drugs (including but not limited to Tagamet, Inderal, narcotics, benzodiazepines, oral contraceptives, hypnotics, corticosteroids, alcohol, marijuana).

Mental and emotional risk factors for depression include distorted thinking, grief and bereavement following loss of relationships and material possessions, divorce, retirement, feelings of failure, lack of stimulation, addiction to work, sense of helplessness, powerlessness, or being overwhelmed, lack of self-expression, and emotional traumas as a child including a history of abuse or violence.

Spiritual and social risk factors include lack of purpose or meaning in life, feelings of isolation, lack of compassion or a committed loving relationship, or feeling disconnected from God or divine consciousness.

■ CONVENTIONAL MEDICAL TREATMENT

The most common treatments for depression are medications and psychotherapy. The first major class of antidepressants is the tricyclics (Pamelor, Norpramin, Tofranil, Elavil, Anafranil, Sinequan). The advantages of this group are benefits in insomnia, mild anti-anxiety effect, and improved general functioning. The disadvantageous side effects include dryness of the mouth, constipation, drowsiness, impotence, longer time for onset of effectiveness, and occasional cardiac arrhythmias.

Monoamine oxidase (MAO) inhibitors now less used include Nardil, Parnate, and Marplan. Side effects include headache, hypotension, mild increase in suicidal ideation and psychosis, impotence, and untoward interactions with many drugs and high tyramine foods.

Selective serotonin uptake inhibitors (SSRIs) comprise a popular, newer generation of drugs (Prozac, Zoloft, Paxil, Luvox, Celexa). The advantages of this group include a low profile of side effects, and onset of action in about 10–14 days. The disadvantages are: frequent sexual dysfunction, insomnia, headache, increased anxiety, and occasional gastrointestinal symptoms.

Effexor inhibits reuptake of both norepinephrine and serotonin; advantages include wider spectrum because of its dual action; disadvantages include headache, insomnia, nausea, and impotence. Wellbutrin SR is an aminoketone which works well in some patients when other classes of drugs have not; it is contraindicated in seizure disorders, and side effects include decreased libido, anxiety, rash, and gastrointestinal effects. Serzone, a phenylpiperazine, is another choice with a modest profile of side effects including adverse interaction with statin drugs, insomnia, dry mouth, and dizziness. Desyrel and Ludiomil are lesser used drugs in other chemical classes which may be used.

None of the antidepressant medications are addicting, but they can become psychologically habituating. Drug classes should be mixed with great caution, particularly providing a 2-week window before switching to or from the MAO inhibitors. Antidepresssant drugs generally have very few withdrawal effects. *As sole treatment, of course, they do nothing to deal with underlying causes of the mood disorder.*

Psychotherapy literally means treating the mind and includes all forms of psychological therapy approaches. Conventional psychotherapy usually means talk therapy. In the era of managed care, drug treatment is increasingly favored because it is seen as more cost-effective. Most psychiatric care is actually provided by primary care physicians, not psychiatrists. The combination of medication and conventional psychotherapy alone, without treatment of the body and spirit, is often insufficient to effectively treat moderate to severe depression.

Still occasionally used in intractable depression is electroconvulsive therapy, the results of which are still lauded by some psychiatrists. Many others seriously question its appropriateness.

■ HOLISTIC MEDICAL TREATMENT

Severe depression will usually require antidepressant medication, but can be combined with many of the following recommendations to enhance the therapeutic result. The following initiatives often meet with marked success in mild to moderate depression.

Nutritional and environmental treatment. Spending time in nature with exposure to plants, beauty, clean optimal air with negative air ion concentrations over 3,000 ions/cc, and sunlight are substantial treatment options. A diet that is high in complex carbohydrates, including whole grains (whole wheat, brown rice, barley, millet, oats, and corn), vegetables, beans, lentils, and fruits tends to increase serotonin and promote feelings of well being. Included should be generous amounts of protein, spices of red pepper, garlic, and ginger, and reduced amounts of fat. One to 2 weekly servings of cold-water fish, such as salmon or sardines, supply helpful amounts of essential fatty acids. Caffeine, alcohol, and sugar evoke potential problems and should be avoided. A food elimination diet can identify any food allergens, should they be contributing.

Supplements. In many situations, natural supplements have mood effects as great as the effect of drugs. Every patient should be considered in the light of biochemical individuality, with variable needs for amino acids, vitamins, minerals, and essential fatty acids.

D-L-phenylalanine is an amino acid precursor of catecholamines, major neurotransmitters affecting mood. Supplemental doses which improve mood are 500 mg b.i.d. to 1,000 mg t.i.d.[4] Vitamins B_6 and B_3 enhance utilization of D-L- phenylalanine, and 1 g of vitamin C consumed at the same time is helpful. Vitamin B_6 is particularly important in regulating the absorption, metabolism, and utilization of many amino acids.

L-tyrosine is converted from phenylalanine, and is one step closer to catecholamine formation. Dosing is similar to phenylalanine.[5] Glutamine is an amino acid that seems to work synergistically with L-tyrosine. A single product is available, combining the two together in a satisfactory ratio, given as 6 capsules daily in divided doses.

Taurine is an amino acid synthesized by the body, with lesser amounts being obtained from food. Complementary medical physicians have noted antidepressant effects with 500 mg t.i.d.[6]

Phenylalanine and tyrosine can raise blood pressure, cause headaches, and aggravate insomnia; they should not be combined with antidepressants, especially MAO inhibitors. These amino acids are contraindicated in patients with phenylketonuria (PKU), hepatic cirrhosis, or malignant melanoma.

Because L-tryptophan is an essential amino acid, it must be obtained from food and/or supplements. It is the substrate for synthesis of serotonin, a critical neuropeptide in stabilizing mood. When properly taken, tryptophan is extremely useful as a natural antidepressant as well as a sleep aid. The FDA ban on tryptophan, dating from the early 1990s, has recently been relaxed to permit its prescription filled through compounding pharmacies. Decades of previous use have already proven this amino acid's broad therapeutic effectiveness.[7,8] For depression, prescribe 2 g of tryptophan b.i.d. or t.i.d. between meals to improve absorption. It should not be combined with protein foods, since all amino acids compete with each other for both absorption and passage across the blood-brain barrier. To convert tryptophan to serotonin, adequate levels of folic acid, vitamin B_6, magnesium, niacin, and glutamine must be present.

The tryptophan metabolite 5-hydroxytryptophan has potent antidepressant and hypnotic properties and is available in most health food stores. Dosage 1–200 mg b.i.d. between meals or 200 mg h.s. The foregoing amino acids, if being tried empirically, should be tried one at a time. If the higher doses do not bring improvement in about 6 weeks, a trial of a different amino acid is in order. Determination of amino acid levels is available in reference laboratories, and involves considerable expense.

A B-complex combination containing individual B vitamins in 50 mg amounts, taken b.i.d., is an important eclectic trial.[9] Postpartum depression may result primarily from a deficiency of vitamin B_6.

Vitamin B_{12}, 1 mg/day, along with a weekly injection of B_{12}, 1 mg combined with up to 5 mg of folic acid, is helpful in cognitive disorders associated with depression. It appears to be most helpful in the elderly and those with digestive disorders.[10] Post-partum depression may result from a deficiency of B_{12} and folic acid.

Folic acid doses should approximate 5 mg daily for 1 month, followed by 800 µg daily. Niacinamide (a form of vitamin B_3) 500 mg b.i.d. may also be useful, especially in depression accompanied by anxiety and/or phobias.

For patients who give evidence of higher histamine levels (tendency for seasonal allergies, sneezing in sunlight, tolerate a lot of alcohol), extra calcium 500 mg b.i.d., methionine 500 mg b.i.d. and avoiding extra folic acid are indicated.[11] Vitamin C, 1 g daily, vitamin E 400 IU daily and zinc 30–50 mg daily yield empirically observed benefits. Magnesium is a cofactor in many neurotransmitter enzymatic conversions, is often deficient, and often needs repletion with 500–1,000 mg daily. Essential fatty acids (omega-3 fatty acids) are helpful in depression, including the bipolar variety. Appropriate doses used have been 8–10 grams/day.[12] Flaxseed oil 1 tsp t.i.d. also yields significant amounts of omega-3 oils.

Herbs. A disadvantage of treatment of depression with herbs is the longer time required to reach the point of effectiveness compared to SSRIs. Advantages include greater safety in long-term use because of the non-concentrated aspects of the herbs themselves and the common absence of reported serious side effects.

St. John's Wort (*Hypericum perforatum*) has been shown in a number of clinical studies to be as effective as pharmaceutical antidepressants.[13] Hypericum also appears to have far fewer side effects, the most prominent of which is occasional increased susceptibility to the effects of the sun. The dose is 300 mg t.i.d. of a standard extract containing 0.3 percent hypericin, the active ingredient. A trial of 1 month is needed to assess its effects. St. John's Wort should not be taken with antidepressant drugs. It is acceptable to start hypericum after being on phenylalanine or tyrosine for 6 weeks.

Ginkgo biloba improves cerebral circulation, improving memory and often benefiting depression. Ginkgo is usually not as effective as St. John's Wort for depression, but can be taken along with other nutrients and botanicals improve overall mood. *Ginkgo biloba* dosage of a standardized extract of 24 percent ginkgolides is 80–120 mg b.i.d.

Yohimbine, an herb from West Africa, has been used for decades to treat impotence and diminished libido. Recent research has indicated that yohimbine can also improve the overall effectiveness of standard antidepressant medications. In some cases, yohimbine can be used by itself to both stimulate sexual functioning in men and relieve mild depression. The dosage is 5.4 mg of standardized yohimbine extract t.i.d., with a trial lasting a minimum of 3 weeks. Yohimbine can increase anxiety and stimulate cardiac activity and must be carefully monitored.

Biomolecular treatment. Dessicated thyroid (Armour) or a combination of Synthroid and Cytomel can often elicit a dramatic improvement, especially in middle-aged women. This can be true even when TSH levels are within normal limits. Lethargy, sensitivity to cold, fatigue and inability to control weight in the face of normal caloric intake are often symptoms of subclinical hypothyroidism. Thirty mg of Armour thyroid is a reasonable starting daily dosage, and Synthroid/Cytomel in a 4 : 1 ratio (50/12.5 µg daily) may also yield significant improvement. DHEA can also be effective in treating depression, but the dosage should be chosen after blood levels have been determined to be low.

Exercise. The beneficial effects of regular aerobic exercise in the treatment of depression are well documented. One-third of all depressed patients may need no other intervention beyond aerobic exercise.[14] Many authorities consider exercise as effective as most pharmacological and cognitive approaches to depression. It certainly takes the prize for being the most cost effective. Getting depressed patients to exercise is often difficult. Encouraging patients to join groups for exercise will help overcome resistance.

Other initiatives. Traditional Chinese Medicine including herbs and acupuncture, and classical homeopathic prescribing in the hands of skilled practitioners can also be quite effective in depression.

Regular exposure to sunlight and filtered sun 20–30 minutes daily or installation of full-spectrum fluorescent tubes that simulate sunshine are especially important for patients who experience wintertime seasonal affective disorder (SAD).

Mental and emotional treatment. The holistic approach to depression devotes attention to presenting psychological symptoms and problems, as well as the lifestyle, social relationships, spiritual beliefs and value system, sense of life purpose, and dynamics of life force energy of the patient. This orientation could also be described as personal growth psychotherapy. Providing encouragement and motivation to change in a comfortable milieu are the hallmarks of a skilled therapist. This requires working in ways that evoke the assets and gifts in each person, as well as focusing on proactive solutions to current problems.

Although this trusted connection between therapist and client is more important than the treatment model utilized, several options in addition to cognitive psychotherapy are helpful in treating depression. They include:

1. Affirmations and imagery as part of the therapeutic approach. Every image is an action in a latent state.[15]
2. Psychosynthesis—a holistic type of spiritual psychotherapy.
3. Hakomi therapy—a body-centered form of psychotherapy.
4. Solution-focused/brief therapy—a goal-oriented form of psychotherapy.

Stress and tension are an integral part of the experience of depression. Stress reduction techniques offer enormous adjunctive help in managing depression. They include meditation, breathing techniques, relaxation techniques, biofeedback training, and journaling.

Meditation is a sitting technique for calming the mind. The elements of meditation incorporate (1) the use of a quiet environment with decreased environmental stimuli; (2) a comfortable position with decreased muscle tone; (3) adoption of a passive attitude returning the focus of concentration gently from distractions as they occur; and (4) use of a mental device such as a repeated word, mantra, phrase, thought or image; a repeated sound; or gazing at an object. The stages of skill development are (1) identification of the relaxed state; (2) recognition of the achievement path; (3) ongoing practice; and (4) habit development. Once the stage of habituation is reached, the patient is able to manage daily activities with a lower baseline of arousal and catecholamine response, offering not only a decreased level of depression, but also a score of biochemical and physiological benefits.

Many meditative approaches are therapeutic; they include Transcendental Meditation, Raja yoga, Vipassana, and Zen techniques, to name a few. Qi Gong is a moving meditation practiced by over 300 million Chinese on a daily basis that strengthens life force energy, or chi. It is relatively easy to learn and can be used to both treat and prevent depression and anxiety.

Progressive muscle relaxation training utilizes the perception of a state of physical relaxation through a series of progressively tensing muscular contractions followed by sudden relaxation of different muscle groups in the body. This produces a "letting go" effect that can then be enhanced by focusing on counting down from 5 to 1, picturing each number in a different color. Unlike meditation, this method emphasizes physical relaxation. Since this process deters the mind from focussing on depressive cognitions while relaxing, it is effective for calming the mind as well.

Breathing techniques include several breathing methods derived from yoga and various forms of meditation. These methods enhance psychotherapy by calming the mind and body. During the process, repressed emotions often surface and can be dealt with and released. These approaches are also enhanced with imagery and music.

Biofeedback is a systematized approach for learning relaxation which furnishes feedback evidence of reaching a calmer level of brainwave activity and physiological response. By allowing a re-focussing of energy in a self-empowering way, a greater sense of control over autonomic ("involuntary") nervous system reactions, including those triggered by stress is achieved. As with meditation, depression is often greatly attenuated.

Journaling is a technique for recording of emotions and gaining insight into patterns of behavior and interactions with feelings. It is an effective type of assignment or homework which can be incorporated into cognitive therapy and has numerous physiological benefits as well as contributing to lessening of tension, anxiety and depression.[16,17] Patients may benefit by starting to consciously focus on positive events by asking themselves "What do I have gratitude for?" This tends to neutralize the mind-set that focuses on only negative events, inducing the cycle of depression and hopelessness.

Therapies such as therapeutic touch, healing touch, and Reiki are hands-on energetic techniques that have been shown in research and practice to benefit both depression and anxiety. Still very much rejected by the conventional community,[18] clinical experience is overwhelmingly positive.

Hypnosis can be quite effective with milder types of depression and anxiety. Hypnosis evokes an altered state of consciousness in which certain senses are heightened, and others seem to fade into the background. It is not a state of sleep. While in a hypnotic state, patients become more aware of words and suggestions that develop a greater intensity. Calm and relaxing images are often suggested for clients with anxiety. Hypnotherapy can be used to introduce, while in a heightened state of suggestibility, more hopeful options and better methods of dealing with painful issues associated with the depression. While in a hypnotic state, patients can also rehearse new ways of perceiving themselves. Much of the benefit from hypnosis is achieved through the simple act of learning to relax. Self-hypnosis, which can easily be learned from a skilled counselor, provides simple and effective methods for patients to train themselves to achieve hypnotic states. Audiotapes can be an excellent source of training in self-hypnosis and relaxation. They are especially effective when individualized by a therapist with whom the patient has already established a strong rapport.

Bodywork therapies which can help to release deeply repressed emotions related to depression include deep-tissue bodywork, such as Rolfing, with types of body movement, such as yoga or Feldenkrais. Depression and anxiety are frequently more amenable to physical touch than verbal cognitive therapies. These therapies are particularly important for patients with a history of physical and sexual abuse or poor body image.

Patients who agree to engage in altruistic service often do much better in dealing with their depression. Lastly, connection to an appropriately facilitated support group is usually helpful for depressed people by the strengthening of their social contacts and relationships. Working on strengthening a committed relationship with a spouse or partner can often mitigate depression.

Anxiety

■ DESCRIPTION

Anxiety is a state of fear or worry in the face of perceived threat of danger or potential injury that lacks a realistic basis. It is a spectrum of emotional discomfort ranging from appropriate concern to being overwhelmed by an excessive continuous state of worry. Anxiety almost always accompanies depression, and is the distinguishing emotion in obsessive compulsive disorder, post-traumatic stress disorder, panic disorder, and agoraphobia. It is often referred to as anxiety neurosis, or generalized anxiety disorder, characterized by excessive or unwarranted worry concerning work, finances, relationships, or health, and diagnosed when lasting for at least 6 months.

Anxiety is often accompanied by physiological symptoms of sympathetic arousal preparing the body for action, including extrasystoles and tachycardia, dyspnea, diaphoresis, dry mouth, ataxia, muscle tension, and urinary and bowel urgency. When no physical action is undertaken, the unexpressed nervous energy triggers a complex of additional symptoms, including restlessness, irritability, fatigue, difficulty concentrating, insomnia, tremulousness, headaches, and anorexia.

■ PREVALENCE

Anxiety is a universally experienced emotion. It is thought that 15 million Americans experience a medically significant degree of anxiety. This disorder of mood affects twice as many women as men. About 15 percent of the population experience at least one panic attack in a lifetime.

■ ETIOLOGY AND RISK FACTORS

Contributory causes and risk factors for anxiety include uncertainties in relationships and stressful life situations, excess caffeine, sugar, chocolate, aspartame, excess of highly acidic foods (tomatoes, eggplant, peppers), stimulant medicines and substances (decongestants, NoDoze, nicotine, sympathomimetics), hyperthyroidism, hyperadrenalism, hypoglycemia, nutritional deficiencies of B-vitamins, calcium, and magnesium,[19] and a history of trauma in the form of physical, sexual, or emotional abuse.

■ CONVENTIONAL MEDICAL TREATMENT

Conventional medical management of anxiety is centered in anxiolytic medications and psychotherapy. The benzodiazepines are the most frequently prescribed medications. They include Valium (diazepam), Xanax (alprozalam), Klonopin (clonazepam), Ativan (lorazepam), Librium, and Tranxene. Benzodiazepines act rapidly and are extremely effective in relieving panic attacks and general anxiety. They can be addictive, impair memory, increase tiredness and when stopped can manifest withdrawal effects, including lowering of the seizure threshold. When carefully used over the short term, these drugs can be quite helpful. Other medications which are used with benefit include Buspar, Atarax (hydroxyzine), and the selective serotonin reuptake inhibitors used most often for depression.

Psychotherapy for anxiety includes many of the same initiatives described in the treatment of depression.

■ **HOLISTIC MEDICAL TREATMENT**

Nutritional and environmental treatment. Recommendations include a diet which emphasizes complex carbohydrates (whole grains—brown rice, barley, millet, corn, wheat), whole wheat pasta, vegetables, seaweed, kasha, and foods containing L–tryptophan (sunflower seeds, bananas, milk). The diet is low in protein, fat, and strong spices. Caffeine, chocolate, alcohol, sugar, and highly acidic foods contribute to production of lactate, higher levels of which are associated with anxiety and panic disorder, and should be minimized.

Nutritional supplements. Gamma amino butyric acid (GABA) is a neurotransmitter in the brain that exerts a calming effect on mood. Benzodiazepine drugs stimulate the GABA receptors in the brain. Unlike Valium, GABA taken p.o. cannot pass the blood-brain barrier and is not effective in calming mood. However, it is very helpful in relieving anxiety symptoms originating in the digestive tract and adjacent organs, including diarrhea, "butterflies," heart palpitations, and hyperventilation. This appears to stem from its effect on what has been referred to as the "second, or GI brain." Gamma aminobutyric acid dosage is 750 mg t.i.d. for daytime relaxation, and 1,500 mg at h.s. for improved sleep. Several weeks are required to assess full therapeutic effectiveness.

Tryptophan is often quite effective in dealing with anxiety as well as depression. It is converted into serotonin, with calming and antidepressant effects. It is more readily and selectively absorbed and converted to serotonin in the presence of carbohydrate (fruit juice works nicely), and conversion is catalyzed by vitamins B_3 and B_6. Tryptophan prescribed 500 mg b.i.d. between meals is often sufficient. Two to 3 g at h.s. assists in achieving better sleep. 5-HT discussed under depression may be even better as a means to increase serotonin. Doses are

100 mg b.i.d. for daytime anxiety and 200 mg at h.s. for improved sleep.

Vitamin C, at least 1,000 mg t.i.d., vitamin B complex 50 mg b.i.d., with extra niacinamide (500 mg t.i.d.), vitamin B_1 (up to 100 mg t.i.d.), vitamin B_{12} (sublingual tablets 2 mg/day), and vitamin E, 1,200 IU/day, can all contribute to reduction of anxiety. A small number of patients have *increased* anxiety with B-complex supplements.

Magnesium, calcium, and essential fatty acids[20] are all helpful in treating anxiety. Daily requirements are the same as for depression.

Inositol is a simple polyol, classified as a B vitamin, that serves as a precursor to second messenger compounds. Evidence for reduction of anxiety when taken in high doses of 6 g daily has been published.[21] The dose can be titrated upwards until benefit is obtained. There is no known toxicity to inositol in doses up to 50 g daily.

Herbs. Kava kava (*Piper methysticum*) is an herb with a centuries-long tradition of use by indigenous peoples. It has anxiolytic and hypnotic effects in doses of 250 mg t.i.d. for daytime anxiety and 1 g at h.s. for sleep (standardized to 30 percent kavalactone content). Numerous controlled trials have been published.[22] Trials have not determined long-term effects and continuous use should consequently be limited to 4 months at a time.

Extracts of valerian have also been widely used in numerous cultures for centuries as a favored treatment for anxiety and insomnia. Again, although it is quite safe to take for short-term use, long-term effects are not well researched.[23] For daytime anxiety, the dose is 150 mg t.i.d. (standardized extract of 0.8 percent valerenic acid). For sleep onset delay, the dose is 150 mg 45 minutes before h.s., titrated upwards to 600 mg as necessary. Other less researched herbs that can be used for treating anxiety include lemon balm and skullcap.

Other options. Food elimination diets may pinpoint offending foods that make a marked contribution to anxiety, and should be considered with failure of other approaches.[24] Longer, low intensity, aerobic exercise regimens building greater endurance (brisk walking, jogging, swimming, and hiking) are excellent for relief of anxiety as well as depression. Traditional Chinese Medicine and Homeopathy in the hands of skilled practitioners meet with considerable success in managing anxiety. Cranial electrical stimulation, utilizing subliminal 2-second bursts of 100 Hz current applied to the temples, has been shown to significantly reduce anxiety levels in controlled studies.[25]

Mental and emotional treatment. Nearly all the initiatives used in depression are also effective in anxiety, including cognitive psychotherapy, stress-management techniques (meditation, relaxation training, breath therapy, and biofeedback), journaling, energy therapies (healing and Therapeutic Touch, Reiki, Qi Gong), hypnosis, and bodywork therapies.

Spiritual and social health treatment. Recommendations are similar to those discussed under depression. Prayer appears to reap significant benefits in this condition[26] and can be especially beneficial. Neurolinguistic programming, shown to be extremely successful with intractable phobias and certain types of anxiety, utilizes transformational imagery to reframe emotional issues and modify behavior.

Insomnia

■ DESCRIPTION

Insomnia describes the condition of disordered sleep in which one or more types of disturbances are present. These include sleep onset delay, nighttime awakening, lack of deep stage 3 and 4 sleep, early awakening, and sleep apnea. Primary insomnias refer to those disorders with no apparent psychiatric, medical, or environmental cause. Secondary insomnias are those spawned by psychological and medical conditions and therapies. Sleep apnea is one of the better known examples of secondary insomnias. Ninety years ago, Americans averaged 9 hours of sleep per night; in the late 1990s, one-third of adults sleep just over 6 hours during the week. Most authorities believe the vast majority of people require 7–8 hours of sleep to function optimally. Insomnia is commonly accompanied by fatigue, immunodeficiency, headaches, weight gain, irritability, depression, increased substance abuse, diminished short-term memory, decreased libido, prolonged reaction times, and substandard job performance.

The two identifiable physiological phases of sleep are non-rapid-eye-movement (NREM), with stages 1–4 distinguished by EEG, and REM sleep, characterized by episodic bursts of rapid eye movements, muscle relaxation, and dream activity. Commonly, NREM and REM sleep periods last about 90 minutes, alternating 3–6 times each night. It appears that REM sleep enables the body to replenish energy cycles, accelerate healing and increase the synthesis of a number of important hormones during REM sleep. Studies also show that REM sleep is essential for proper mental and emotional function.

■ PREVALENCE

Insomnia, the most common type of sleep disorder, has become a rapidly increasing crisis of the 1990s. Forty-nine percent of Americans reported sleep difficulty in 1995 in contrast to 36 percent in 1991. Insomnia as the chief complaint generates 10 million physician office visits each year. Most of the 70 million Americans who experience insomnia are unaware of the severity of the widespread effects accruing from years of accumulated sleep debt. Estimated loss of work productivity due to insomnia is about 70 billion dollars yearly. An estimated 38,000 people die each year from sleep apnea which can precipitate myocardial infarction or stroke. Twenty-four thousand are estimated to die in accidents occurring secondary to sleep deprivation.

■ ETIOLOGY AND RISK FACTORS

Physical and environmental factors related to insomnia include advancing age (over 40), menopause, intake of caffeine, drugs (sympathomimetics, thyroid medications, oral contraceptives, beta blockers, marijuana and hallucinogens, and overuse of sedatives), stimulating herbs (ephedra, ginger, ginseng, kola nut), sugar (in some sensitive individuals), alcohol (sedative at h.s. with opposite effects in early morning hours), distorted environment (noise, light, temperature, humidity, uncomfortable mattress), insufficient exercise, nocturia, hypo- and hyperthroidism, hyperadrenalism, chemical hypersensitivity, and deficiency of calcium, magnesium, and B-vitamins.

Mental and emotional factors include anxiety, the fear of not sleeping, depression, grief, excitement, and the manic phase of bipolar disease. Societal causes include the overworked and overstimulated nature of modern culture in which people are continually pressured to accomplish more in less time.

■ CONVENTIONAL MEDICAL TREATMENT

Conventional therapy focuses on treatment of the underlying causes if known, habit re-formation, and symptomatic medications. Benzodiazepine hypnotics are commonly used, including Halcion (triazolam), Dalmane (flurazepam) and Restoril (temazepam). They are most effective for the short-term management of insomnia, and nicely decrease the time to sleep onset while improving the quality of sleep. The sedative effects of the longer-acting drugs can linger into the following morning, resulting in daytime drowsiness and impairment in cognitive function. Habituation develops quite easily, and when short-acting forms are discontinued abruptly, they may decrease the seizure threshold and cause rebound insomnia. All hypnotic drugs should be slowly tapered before being terminated.

Ambien (zolpidem) is the newest effective short-acting medication for insomnia with fewer side effects and less potential for rebound than the benzodiazepines. If the insomnia is caused by depression, then a sedating antidepressant such as Desyrel or Elavil is often prescribed. The antidepressants do not promote the dependence or the addiction often caused by the hypnotics. Most over-the-counter sleeping pills are antihistamines which may also cause morning drowsiness. If urinary frequency from prostatic hypertrophy contributes to frequent awakening, pharmacological and surgical interventions are often considered.

■ HOLISTIC MEDICAL TREATMENT

Nutritional initiatives. All caffeine intake should be eliminated from the diet, including coffee, tea, chocolate, cola soft drinks, and over-the-counter (OTC) caffeine-containing drugs. Other stimulants also need to be omitted, including cigarettes, stimulant prescriptions (if possible) and botanicals, hot spicy foods (especially cayenne), sugar, refined carbohydrates (deplete the B vitamins), alcohol, and food additives. Insomnia is occasionally due to food sensitivities. The most common offending foods are dairy products, wheat, corn, and chocolate. A food elimination and reintroduction trial may be warranted. Heavy meals should not be consumed close to bedtime. Encouraging regular meals entrains improved circadian rhythms.

Foods that enhance sleep have high tryptophan/tyrosine and tryptophan/phenylalanine ratios: pumpkins, potatoes, bananas, onions, spinach, broccoli, cauliflower, eggs, fish, liver, milk, peanuts, cheddar cheese, whole grains (especially whole wheat, brown rice, and oats), cottage cheese, and beans. Eating tryptophan-rich foods for the evening meal or an evening snack may help induce sleep: milk products, turkey, chicken, beef, soy products, nuts and nut butters, bananas, papayas, and figs. If hypoglycemia is suspected, a diet that is higher in protein and avoids sugar and high glycemic foods is essential. High carbohydrate foods raise the level of serotonin in the brain by enhancing selective tryptophan assimilation and passage across the blood-brain barrier. A small amount of pasta or toast at h.s. often suffices.

Supplements. A number of supplements encourage better sleep. Vitamin B-complex, 50–100 mg/day of each constituent with meals maximizes catalysis of enzymatic conversions of neurotransmitters. High food sources of the B vitamins include liver, tuna, whole grains, wheat germ, walnuts, peanuts, bananas, sunflower seeds, and blackstrap molasses.

Other helpful options are: niacinamide (vitamin B_3) up to 1 g at h.s. for those who experience night awakening; calcium and magnesium, 500–1000 mg of each within 45 minutes of bedtime; chromium, 250 μg b.i.d., especially for people with hypoglycemia; tryptophan, 3–5 g 45 minutes before h.s., and at least $1\frac{1}{2}$ hours after eating protein, taken with vitamin B_6 25–50 mg; 5-hydroxy tryptophan 150–200 mg at h.s.; phosphatidylserine, up to 300 mg daily (an amino acid for those whose insomnia is due to elevated nighttime cortisol, usually induced by stress).

Biomolecular treatment. Melatonin is the hormone synthesized and released by the pineal gland in response to darkness. Doses of 1–3 mg 45–90 minutes before h.s. is most effective for sleep-onset delay insomnia. Melatonin can also be used for sleep maintenance with a sustained-release of 1 mg preparation. There is also documentation of benefit with insomnia associated with jet lag. Melatonin does not increase the length of sleep. Natural progesterone has been used with good results for insomnia associated with menopause and premenstrual syndrome (PMS). Progesterone restores hormonal balance and has a calming effect.

Herbs. Herbs which aid in treatment include valerian, passionflower, Kava kava, hypericum, chamomile, lemon balm, and skullcap.[27] Chamomile tea has a mild calming effect and can be used in children.

Valeriana officinalis, 150–300 mg of extract of 0.8 percent valerenic acid content offers substantial sedative potency. Effects tend to diminish with continued uninterrupted use. Passionflower 300–450 mg at h.s (extract containing 2.6 percent flavonoids) is also effective, especially taken with 5-HT, discussed above. Kava kava, discussed under anxiety, is helpful in insomnia in doses containing 135–210 mg of kavalactones, an hour before bedtime.

St. John's wort is used primarily for depression, but also is effective for insomnia. Recommended dosage is 300 mg, t.i.d. of an extract standardized to contain 0.3 percent hypericin.

Chinese herbs and acupuncture often produce dramatic and long-lasting relief from insomnia, when coordinated by a qualified Chinese medicine practitioner (OMD).

Exercise. Exercising 5–6 hours before h.s. appears to be an optimal time. Outdoor activity also brings the advantage of filtered or direct sunlight for those who have a seasonal component with depression contributing to insomnia. A warm tub bath an hour or two before h.s. is helpful for many. Suggest that patients experiment with the nighttime bedroom temperature to determine what works best.

Prostatic hypertrophy with nocturia is treated with the approach discussed in Chapter 11.

Principles of optimal bedroom preparation include the acquisition of a mattress that feels right; restricting the bedroom to sleeping and sexual activity only; prohibiting television; avoiding naps if possible; setting a consistent hour for getting into bed; avoiding bright lights after 9 p.m; overriding unavoidable noise with a white-noise generator; creating a relaxing ritual before bed—reading, listening to quiet music; and meditating or utilizing breathing exercises at bedtime.

For night awakening problems, ask patients to affirm at bedtime that they will remember the thoughts of the unconscious mind as they awaken, and provide pen and paper on their bedside table. If night awakening occurs, they should allow themselves to awaken sufficiently to turn on the light and record a sentence or 2 about the first thoughts that were present on awakening. Surprisingly often, the thoughts will relate to issues being processed in the unconscious which led to the awakening. Once the awareness is recorded, the awakening tends to rapidly taper off.

Addictions and Alcoholism

■ DESCRIPTION

An addiction is an overwhelming craving for or dependence on a mind-altering substance or activity, without regard for its health and social consequences. Addictions are either psychological or physiological, or both. The most common addictions in America are to drugs, alcohol, nicotine, caffeine, food, work, gambling, and sex. The most studied drug is alcohol, which can serve as a model for the less studied drugs. Drugs with the greatest addictive potential are: narcotics, including morphine, opium, heroin, and methadone; depressants such as alcohol, barbiturates, and sedatives; stimulants such as cocaine and amphetamines; hallucinogens; and marijuana.

Symptoms indicative of addiction are loss of control over the use of a drug or a behavior; mood swings and irrational behavior; and acceptance of significant health, legal, or social risks associated with use of a substance. Specific symptoms of drug addiction include sore or inflamed eyes, dilated or constricted pupils, irregular breathing, tremulous extremities, itchy or runny nose, and nausea. Drug withdrawal manifests as craving, depression, anxiety, restlessness, yawning, diaphoresis, abdominal pain, anorexia, emesis, and diarrhea.

Specific symptoms of alcohol addiction are depression, social isolation, arrests for DWI, drinking before breakfast, unexplained work absences, frequent accidents, and failure to meet obligations.

■ PREVALENCE

Drug usage in the United States has, in the true sense of the word, become an epidemic. Alcoholism among men is 5 times greater than it is for women, and for illicit drugs, the prevalence rate for men is 3 times greater than for women. The disparity probably lies in a combination of emotional, societal and conditioning factors. The national cost of abuse of alcohol and other drugs in terms of health care, absenteeism, and lost productivity is approximately $166 billion per year. Over 15 million people are estimated to experience significant health problems as a direct result of their alcohol use and abuse, and 100,000 people die every year from alcoholism. The diseases most often associated with alcohol abuse are cirrhosis, cancer, and heart disease. Among young alcoholics, the death rates from suicide, accidents, and cirrhosis are 10 times higher than normal. Alcoholics shorten their life expectancy by about 20 years, and nearly half of the violent deaths from accidents, suicide, and homicide are alcohol-related, as well as half of all automobile fatalities. One-third of all suicides and one-third of all mental health disorders are associated with serious alcohol abuse. At least 40 million spouses, children, and close relatives suffer from the destruction associated with alcohol abuse.

Sixty-three percent of all persons arrested for all reasons have illegal drugs in their urine. Legal drugs also are destructive: tobacco use takes the lives of 420,000 Americans each year. Food addiction, especially to sugar, has been a significant contributor to the dramatic increase in obesity in this country. Workalcoholism is a common problem seen in offices of primary-care physicians, and the prevalence of sex addiction has been estimated at 3–6 percent of the population.

■ ETIOLOGY AND RISK FACTORS

Predisposition to addictions involves strong genetic factors. Studies find that alcoholism is 4–6 times more common in biological children of alcoholics compared to children of non-alcoholic parents.[28] In identical twins separated at birth, if one twin becomes alcoholic, the chance of the second twin being alcoholic is 4 times greater than the likelihood in fraternal twins. These studies suggest that the genetically addiction-prone brain is biochemically altered so that the individual is more susceptible to craving a wide range of substances and activities. Hundreds of studies conclude that irresistible cravings (alcohol, drug, and food addictions) and compulsive behavior disorders (sex and gambling addictions) are associated with an abnormality in the functioning of the reward-pleasure centers of the hypothalamus, involving serotonin, opioids, and dopamine and their receptors. Some researchers now believe that the root cause of addictive and compulsive diseases may be a defect in the gene that regulates the function of the dopamine D2 receptors in the limbic-hypothalamic brain. Addictive substances such as morphine, cocaine, amphetamines, alcohol, and possibly sugar provoke the brief release of abnormal amounts of dopamine which temporarily offsets the diminished pleasurable experience created by these genetic defects. Although the malfunction may begin with a gene, it can be modified by controllable factors in the physical and psychosocial environment. Some authorities postulate that alcohol and drug abuse actually cause a relatively permanent disruption in the normal neurotransmitter pathways that mimics the defects that were thought to be purely genetic. For example, habitual use of cocaine can cause these neurotransmitter changes in just a few weeks or months, after which they become difficult to reverse.

Hypoglycemia is a strong risk factor which may be present in 90 percent of alcoholics. With a rapid fall in blood sugar, a number of symptoms often occur—rapid heart rate, hunger, excessive sweating, craving for sweets, headaches, loss of concentration, and anxiety—all of which can be relieved by drinking alcohol, which works powerfully as a sugar. Marijuana, amphetamines, cocaine, nicotine, and caffeine all tend to produce hypoglycemia. It is not uncommon for users of these drugs to frequently drink alcohol as well. Hypoglycemia can be a significant cause of depression, anxiety, and mental confusion. Suboptimal function of the pancreas, adrenal, thyroid, and pituitary glands contributes to hypoglycemia. Alcohol relieves the symptoms of this vicious cycle.

Nutritional deficiencies can both contribute to and result from addictive behaviors. This further aggravates the altered brain biochemistry, reinforcing the vicious cycle. The secondary loss of nutrients includes zinc, chromium, manganese, magnesium, calcium, copper, and iron and the B-vitamins.

Food allergy is also a cause of alcoholism. Some people are allergic to the foods from which the alcohol is extracted, such as wheat or potatoes in beer; grapes in wine; or corn in bourbon. Brewer's yeast, found in most alcoholic beverages, is another potential allergen. One of the responses of the nervous and immune systems to the allergenic foods to which they are exposed is the production of their own addictive opioid endorphins. These create feelings of euphoria, followed by withdrawal or hangover, which is then relieved with more alcohol.

By altering brain chemistry, environmental pollutants such as gasoline, cleaning solvents, and formaldehyde, a common indoor toxin found in many building materials, can also contribute to causing alcoholism.

An excess of sugar and alcohol fuels an overgrowth of candida organisms (see Chapter 13). This condition weakens the immune system, contributing to further overgrowth of candida. Candidiasis shares many of the symptoms of hypoglycemia (e.g., fatigue and anxiety), the awareness of which can temporarily be abolished by drugs and alcohol.

Regardless of genetic predisposition, emotions and belief systems can have a profound effect on creating addictive behavior. The emotional causes contributing to alcohol abuse include feelings of anger and rage, self-deprecation, guilt, hopelessness, or inadequacy. Emotional factors with drug abuse probably include fear of taking responsibility and an inability to accept and love oneself.

■ CONVENTIONAL MEDICAL TREATMENT

Conventional alcohol and drug addiction rehabilitation programs usually involve detoxification, drug withdrawal, and counseling in both in-patient and out-patient settings. Through the 1980s many insurance companies were covering the costs of 4-week stays at expensive residential alcohol and rehabilitation centers. Studies, however, have shown that the outcomes of expensive inpatient care are no better than outpatient care. Some outpatient programs reach a 50 percent rate of abstinence and rehabilitation to productivity.

■ HOLISTIC MEDICAL TREATMENT

Successful programs emphasize avoiding alcohol, illegal drugs, sugar, nicotine, and caffeine; and the repletion of protein, vitamin, mineral, and neurotransmitter deficiencies. The neurotransmitter pathways are maintained with a vegetarian diet, supplements, herbs, psychological work, and spiritual support.

Nutrition. A diet for hypoglycemia is moderately low in protein and high in complex carbohydrate (beans, lentils, and vegetables). Healthy snacks (nuts, seeds, organic fruit, or vegetables) between meals prevent drops in blood sugar, which could trigger alcohol cravings. The first step in this process of biochemical repair is to avoid all hypoglycemic activators, including sugar products, caffeine, nicotine, and chewing tobacco. These substances produce hypoglycemic symptoms through an overstimulation of the adrenals that reinforces the addictive cycle. The dietary emphasis for treating addictions is on whole and organic foods, free of additives, chemicals, and hormones. As mentioned elsewhere, it is also important to identify and avoid any allergy-triggering foods or inhalants.

Supplements. The following nutrients are an integral part of a holistic alcohol and drug addiction program, primarily because they help to relieve hypoglycemia, which contributes significantly to the cycle of addiction. They include: chromium picolinate 4–600 µg daily to equilibrate sugar metabolism; glutamine ≥ 1,000 mg q.i.d.—to reduce the craving for alcohol, drugs, and sugar and enhance GABA production to improve sleep and relaxation; calcium and magnesium—to aid in detoxification, and relax the system to diminish irritability, anxiety, unstable emotions, muscle spasm, and insomnia; pantothenic acid—to enhance production of all the adrenal hormones, and to extinguish sugar cravings; niacin—to stabilize blood sugar; vitamins C and B-complex—to help neutralize oxidative stress and fully catalyze neurotransmitter synthesis; vitamins B_6, B_3, copper, iron, zinc, folic acid, phenylalanine, and tyrosine to treat depression (refer to "Depression," earlier in this chapter for discussion and dosage of the latter two amino acids) and to aid in biochemical repair of the dopamine neurotransmitter system; and gamma linolenic acid from borage or black currant seed oil to compensate for the interference with essential fatty acid synthesis which occurs with alcohol.

Supplements needed to prevent deterioration and stimulate healing of the liver include: N-acetylcysteine (NAC)—500 mg t.i.d.; lipoic acid—300 mg b.i.d.; L-carnitine—500 mg t.i.d.; choline—1,000 mg t.i.d.; and inositol—5–9 g b.i.d.

Herbs. Herbs have utility in preventing liver deterioration and relieving nervousness during withdrawal. Detoxifying the liver and tending to reverse the rise in liver enzymes are milk thistle extract (*Silybum marianum*) one or two 70 mg capsules t.i.d. (standardized to 80 percent silymarin) and dandelion root (*Taraxacum officinale*) 200 mg t.i.d.

Valerian (refer to "Insomnia," earlier in this chapter), passionflower, and chamomile relieve the tension experienced during withdrawal. Feverfew provides relief from the headache of caffeine withdrawal. Lobelia is well suited to reduce cravings for nicotine, by virtue of its long duration of action. It can be advantageously combined with Avena (1 : 1, 20 drops q.i.d.). Lobelia use should be limited to a month. Oatstraw, long used in India for opium addiction, has also been shown to help reduce cigarette smoking, apparently by rebalancing endorphin levels in the brain.

Exercise. The full oxygenation of aerobic exercise contributes to revitalization of the body debilitated by drug and alcohol addiction and nutrient depletion. It also improves the likelihood of maintaining abstinence by reducing anxiety and depression and is particularly important in withdrawal from nicotine.[29] Yoga is also an effective form of exercise in treating alcohol and drug addiction.

Homeopathy. Constitutional homeopathic treatment is effective in treating most addictions, requiring a competent and experienced practitioner. *Nux vomica* is a homeopathic remedy that works well for alcoholism and cigarette smoking. Candida treatment is often indicated (see Chapter 13). In alcohol addiction it is preferable to use a homeopathic remedy to kill the candida, along with replacement of normal flora with an acidophilus/bifidus preparation.

Acupuncture. Acupuncture has been extremely successfully in treating withdrawal symptoms from addictive substances including heroin and cocaine, at Lincoln Hospital in New York City for over 20 years.[30]

Mental and emotional treatment. Since addictions typically accompany depression and vice-versa, many of the following therapies are effective for both conditions: cognitive psychotherapy; stress-reduction techniques (meditation works well in alcoholism); biofeedback can be very effective in managing the craving for nicotine; journaling; Qi gong helps with nicotine addiction; hypnosis; and bodywork therapies.

Twelve-Step programs with a spiritual orientation are helpful in overcoming addictions, offering social support in early withdrawal. Alcoholics Anonymous (A.A.) is quite helpful in treating alcoholism by providing group reinforcement for abstinence and behavioral modification. The holistic spiritual and social recommendations are similar to those discussed under depression.

An independent study of a biochemical approach to alcohol addiction done by Joan Matthews Larson, PhD, at the Health Recovery Center in Minneapolis, MN, published in the *International Journal of Biosocial and Medical Research,* documented the following results: Alcohol cravings from the outset to discharge had dropped from 84 to 9 percent; anxiety dropped from 64 to 11 percent; poor memory dropped from 69 to 11 percent; insomnia dropped from 44 to 6 percent; tremors and shakiness dropped from 44 to 2 percent; depression dropped from 61 to 5 percent. With the biochemical approach alone, research at the Health Recovery Center showed that 92 percent of the clients were abstinent after six months, and 74 percent remained abstinent $3\frac{1}{2}$ years later. This compares to an average abstinence rate of 25 percent for clients using other drug treatment programs at one year, and the same as that of patients who tried to break their drug addiction without using any program.

REFERENCES

1. Penninx BW et al. Cardiovascular events and mortality in newly and chronically depressed persons >70 years of age. *Am J Cardiol* 1998; 81(8):988–94.
2. Barefoot JC et al. Symptoms of acute myocardial infarction, and total mortality in a community sample. *Circulation* 1996; 93(11): 1976–80.
3. Penninx BW et al. Chronically depressed mood and cancer risk in older persons. *J Natl Cancer Inst* 1998; 90(24):1888–93.
4. Beckmann H et al. DL-phenylalanine in depressed patients: an open study. *J Neural Trans* 1977; 41:123–4.
5. Goldberg IK. L-tyrosine in depression. *Lancet* 1980; 1(8190): 364–5.
6. Tachiki KH et al. A rapid column chromatographic procedure for the routine measurement of taurine in plasma of normals and depressed patients. *Clin Chim Acta* 1977; 75(3):455–65.
7. Thomson J et al. The treatment of depression in general practice: a comparison of L-tryptophan, amitriptyline, and a combination of L-tryptophan and amitriptyline with placebo. *Psychol Med* 1982; 12(4):741–51.
8. Young SN et al. Tryptophan in the treatment of depression. *Adv Exp Med Biol* 1981; 133:727–37.
9. Bell IR et al. B complex vitamin patterns in geriatric and young adult populations with major depression. *J Am Geriatr Soc* 1991; 39(3):252–7.
10. Nilsson K et al. Plasma homocysteine in relation to serum cobalamin and blood folate in a psychogeriatric population. *Eur J Clin Invest* 1994; 24(9):600–6.
11. Pfeiffer C. *Nutrition and Mental Illness* Rochester. VT: Healing Arts Press, 1987.
12. Stoll AL et al. *Arch Gen Psychiatry* 1999; 56(5):407–12.
13. Harrer G et al. Clinical investigation of the antidepressant effectiveness of hypericum. *J Geriatr Psychiatry Neurol* 1994; 7(Suppl 1):S6–S8.
14. Weyerer S et al. Physical inactivity and depression in the community: evidence from the upper Bavarian field study. *Int J Sports Med* 1992; 13(6):492–6.
15. Assagioli R. *The Act of Will*. New York: Viking, 1973.

16. Smyth JM et al. Effects of writing about stressful experiences on symptom reduction in patients with asthma or rheumatoid arthritis: a randomized trial. *JAMA* 1999; 281(14):1304–9.

17. Pennebaker JW et al. Disclosure of traumas and immune function: health implications for psychotherapy. *J Consult Clin Psychol* 1988; 56(2):239–45.

18. Rosa L et al. A close look at Therapeutic Touch. *JAMA* 1998; 279(13):1005–10.

19. Werbach M. *Nutritional Influences of Mental Illness: A Sourcebook of Clinical Research.* Tarzana, CA: Third Line Press, 1991

20. Rudin DO. The major psychoses and neuroses as Omega-3 essential fatty acid deficiency syndrome: substrate pellagra. *Biol Psychiatry* 1981; 16(9):837–50.

21. Cohen H et al. Inositol has behavioral effects with adaptation after chronic administration. *J Neural Transm* 1997; 104(2–3):299–305.

22. Volz HP et al. Kava-kava extract WS 1490 versus placebo in anxiety disorders—a randomized placebo-controlled 25-week outpatient trial. *Pharmacopsychiatry* 1997; 30(1):1–5.

23. Leathwood PD et al. Aqueous extract of valerian root (*Valeriana officinalis* L.) improves sleep quality in man. *Pharmacol Biochem Behav* 1982; 17(1):65–71.

24. Hedges H. The elimination diet as a diagnostic tool. *AFP Journal* 1992; 46(5):77s–85s.

25. Ryan JJ et al. Effects of transcerebral electrotherapy (electrosleep) on state anxiety according to suggestibility levels. *Biol Psychiatry* 1976; 11(2):233–7.

26. O'Laoire S. An experimental study of the effects of distant, intercessory prayer on self-esteem, anxiety, and depression. *Alt Ther Health Med* 1997; 3(6):38–53.

27. Leung A. *Encyclopedia of Common Natural Ingredients used in Food, Drugs and Cosmetics.* New York: Wiley, 1980.

28. Cruz-Coke R. Genetics and alcoholism. *Neurobehav Toxicol Teratol* 1983; 5(2):179–80.

29. Koplan JP et al. An epidemiologic study of the benefits and risks of running. *JAMA* 1982; 248(23):3118–21.

30. Brumbaugh AG et al. Acupuncture: new perspectives in chemical dependency treatment. *J Subst Abuse Treat* 1993; 10(1):35–43.

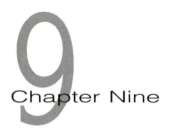

Chapter Nine

Respiratory Disease

■ DESCRIPTION

The respiratory tract is comprised of the nose, throat, sinuses, middle ears, and lungs. The nose and sinuses function to filter inspired air, humidify dry air, warm cold air, and cool hot air. The lining of the respiratory tract is one continuous mucous membrane extending from the nostrils to the alveoli. The alveolar sacs exchange gases across a membrane the size of one-half of a tennis court. The lungs respire about 22,000 times a day in exchanging air through the respiratory passages. Inspired air is laden with bacteria, viruses, molds, yeasts, pollens, smoke, dust, animal danders, and pollutants. As a result of widespread air pollution, most urbanites breathe unhealthy air. These airborne particulates constantly assault the respiratory tract, leaving a trail of infectious, allergic, inflammatory, and malignant diseases.

■ PREVALENCE

Diseases of the respiratory tract are the most common illnesses experienced by Americans. Some 90 million patients experience chronic respiratory illness or at least one episode of acute illness each year. Fifty thousand deaths a year are attributed to particulate air pollution, and it has been estimated that those living in highly polluted cities die 10 years prematurely.

■ ETIOLOGY AND RISK FACTORS

Air pollution is the leading cause of respiratory disease. Every chronic respiratory condition is impacted by air quality, and the condition of our indoor and outdoor air. Particulates appear to be the most unhealthy outdoor pollutant. These tiny particles of dust, sand, cinders, soot, smoke, and liquid droplets come from a variety of sources, including roads, cultivated fields, wind-blown dust, manufacturing plants, construction sites, fossil fuel power plants, fireplaces, wood-burning stoves, and diesel and vehicular exhaust.

Persistent mucous membrane and tissue edema from infections and allergies often blocks sinus drainage, leading to a sinus infection. Sinus infection can lead to acute bronchitis or episodes of bronchospasm in susceptible persons.

Those with an allergic diathesis are vulnerable to the effects of indoor smoke from cigarettes and cigars. This indoor air pollution is a significant contributing factor to all respiratory tract disease. In addition to indoor and outdoor pollution, significant risk factors for respiratory disease include:

1. diminished immune function,
2. emotional stress,
3. food allergies and sensitivities,
4. dysbiosis and altered assimilation of small intestinal proteins, carbohydrates, fats and foreign substances.

CHRONIC RESPIRATORY DISEASES
Chronic Sinusitus

■ DESCRIPTION

Acute sinusitis is an infection or inflammation of one or more of the eight sinuses. Early symptoms include head congestion, headache or facial pain, postnasal drainage, green or yellow mucus, and fatigue. The symptoms of the common cold may be similar.

The condition in which symptoms become continuous, or recur 3 or more times within 6 months, is usually diagnosed as chronic sinusitis. Although the diagnosis can usually be made clinically, the definitive medical diagnosis of sinusitis is determined with a CT scan of the sinuses.

■ PREVALENCE

Acute sinusitis is very common, rivaling the common cold in frequency. Indeed, distinguishing the two may sometimes be difficult.

■ ETIOLOGY AND RISK FACTORS

The etiology of chronic sinusitis has its roots in indoor and outdoor air pollution; cigarette smoke; overuse of antibiotics with attendant antibiotic-resistant infection; yeast (candida) overgrowth with dysbiosis and distorted intestinal assimilation; dental problems (especially with the upper teeth); poorly managed emotional stress, especially accompanied with repressed anger and sadness ("unshed tears"); dry air; cold air; pollen, dust mite, animal dander, mold and food allergies; and occupational hazards (auto mechanics, construction workers, airport employees, airline personnel, farm workers).

■ CONVENTIONAL MEDICAL TREATMENT

The most common treatment for acute or recurrent sinusitis is the prescribing of broad-spectrum antibiotics, with amoxicillin being most commonly selected. Cultures can be done, but often do not reveal pathogenic bacteria. Often additional antibiotics are prescribed if symptoms are not largely clear within 10 days to 2 weeks. If *H. influenza* or *S. pneumoniae* are suspected, Augmentin, cephalosporins, biaxin, Bactrim/Septra, and vibramycin are commonly used. If staphylococci are suspected, the choices usually include macrolides (clarithromycin), cephalosporins, Augmentin, and Bactrim/Septra. Decongestants, including pseudoephedrine, phenylpropanolamine, or phenylephrine are commonly suggested or prescribed. Phenylpropanolamine has now been linked to a small but noticeable increased risk for strokes, especially in younger people. Nasal decongestant sprays including Afrin, Sinex, Dristan or Neosynephrine give temporary relief, but may also induce rebound effects. Analgesics, expectorants, and antitussives may also give relief.

If repeated courses of antibiotic do not terminate the constant or recurrent symptoms, endoscopic surgery may be a last resort. This procedure enlarges the ostia of the sinuses, promoting better drainage. Up to half a million such procedures are performed yearly in the United States. Short-term improvement is common, but exacerbation of the recurrent symptom cycle is also common. *None of these approaches, however, alters the underlying causes spawning the symptoms in the first place.*

The frequent use of antibiotics, the mainstay of conventional treatment, fosters development of resistant bacterial strains, also alters the balance of intestinal micro-organisms, destroying reservoirs of friendly bacteria and promoting overgrowth of other normal residents of the gut, especially the candida organisms. In sinusitis, as well as many other chronic conditions, repressed emotions contribute to compromised immunity. Repressed anger is common enough in the pattern that it should receive consideration among other etiological factors.

■ HOLISTIC MEDICAL TREATMENT

See pages 283–288 below.

Chronic Bronchitis

■ DESCRIPTION

Bronchitis refers to infection or inflammation of the bronchi. The typical bronchitis patient has smoked for 2–3 decades. Acute bronchitis is often associated with acute sinusitis, in which bacteria in infected mucus draining postnasally from the sinuses invades the trachea. Acute bronchitis is heralded by a pervasive, mucousy cough productive of green and yellow sputum. In chronic bronchitis, excess mucus is secreted by the inflamed bronchial mucosa. A cough producing thick gray/white mucus for at least 3 months, and recurring for at least two consecutive years meets the technical definition for chronic bronchitis. The cough is most often accompanied by dyspnea and wheezing, reminiscent of asthma. In advanced chronic disease, recurrent episodes of acute bronchitis, weakness and loss of weight are common. The bronchial walls gradually thicken, the bronchial mucosa becomes more inflamed and secretes a higher volume of thicker mucus from increased numbers of mucus-bearing glands. Chronic bronchitis may become incapacitating, often leading to emphysema and premature death.

■ PREVALENCE

Chronic lung disease (bronchitis, emphysema, and asthma) is the fourth leading cause of death in the United States. With decreasing incidence of coronary artery disease and stroke, and the stabilizing of cancer incidence, it is gaining ground on these three leading causes of mortality.

■ ETIOLOGY AND RISK FACTORS

Cigarette smoking is by far the most important etiological factor in chronic bronchitis. Many smokers with chronic bronchitis experience nocturnal cough. Smoke from a single cigarette poisons the cilia of the respiratory tract for 1–2 hours; several cigarettes per day limits effective cough to nighttime hours only. The additional contributors include all factors mentioned under chronic sinusitis.

■ CONVENTIONAL MEDICAL TREATMENT

All treatment will ultimately fail without the first critical step: smoking cessation. Macrolides (erythromycin, clarithromycin) are commonly used as first-line antibiotics. Steam, delivered in the shower, a steam room, or by a Steam Inhaler, is often helpful for improving the drainage of tenacious, infected mucus from the bronchi and trachea. Postural drainage should follow to enhance removal. Additional physical techniques include avoiding highly polluted, dry or cold air, drinking adequate liquids, using a warm-moisture humidifier and avoiding cough suppressants. Avoiding allergenic triggers during acute exacerbations is important. The conventional medical treatment mitigates chronic symptoms, but progression is the rule.

■ **HOLISTIC MEDICAL TREATMENT**

See pages 283–288 below.

Allergic Rhinitis (Hay Fever)

■ **DESCRIPTION**

The response to allergens such as pollen or mold triggers a strong immune response in the mucous membrane lining the nose. IgE antibodies and eosinophils flood the nasal membranes accompanied by a marked release of inflammatory chemicals including histamine, prostaglandins, and leukotrienes. This results in dramatic nasal congestion and watery drainage, sneezing, and itching of the nasal and conjunctival tissues.

■ **PREVALENCE**

Thirty to 35 million people are thought to experience some degree of chronic or seasonal hay fever symptoms.

■ **ETIOLOGY AND RISK FACTORS**

Allergic rhinitis has a strong genetic component. Evidence of allergic rhinitis, asthma or eczema is frequently obtained in the family history. Airborne allergens (pollen, mold, animal dander, dust mites, chemical exposures) are common triggers for onset of symptoms. Ragweed is the most common pollen offender in central and eastern regions of the United States. Emotional factors, also, may trigger allergic symptoms. Chronic exposure to excessively dry, cold or polluted air can act as an irritant which causes nasal mucous membranes to become extremely sensitive and hyperreactive to airborne allergens. Although not commonly considered in adults, foods may make major contributions to symptoms, most commonly cow's milk and dairy products, wheat and other grains, corn, processed sugar (sucrose), chocolate, soy, yeast (brewer's and baker's), oranges, tomatoes, bell peppers, white potatoes, eggs, fish, shellfish, cocoa, onions, nuts, garlic, peanuts, black pepper, red meat, artificial food coloring, coffee, black tea, beer, wine, and champagne.[1] Milk proteins are by far the most common food allergen contributing to hay fever. Aged cheeses, cottage cheese, and yogurt all are partially digested, and may provoke milder symptoms. Aspirin, and occasionally other medications may be contributing factors as well.

The emotion most often identified in patients with allergic rhinitis is fear. It may be more important to determine the people, situations or circumstances provoking fear in the lives of patients than it is to determine the inhalant or ingestant triggers.

■ CONVENTIONAL MEDICAL TREATMENT

Medical treatment emphasizes elimination of all offending allergens, as much as possible, allergic desensitization with intradermal and subcutaneous injections of dilute desensitizing doses of the offending allergen, and the prescribing of medications. Complete elimination of all allergens is usually impossible, but the following are often helpful: removal of carpets, upholstered furniture, heavy curtains, venetian blinds, fuzzy wool blankets, and comforters stuffed with wool or feathers; meticulous frequent cleaning of the home, especially the bedroom, laundering curtains weekly; utilizing wood or metal furniture; keeping clothing in plastic-zippered bags and shoes in closed boxes off the floor. Removing family pets may be a challenging problem. Placing electronic or HEPA filters in the bedroom, or equipping a forced-air furnace with these devices can be quite helpful. Reducing humidity to the 40 percent range will greatly reduce dust mite and mold populations.

For temporary relief of mild allergies, antihistamines are commonly prescribed or recommended. The newer generation of prescription drugs (Claritin, Allegra, Hismanal) are non-sedating, but many OTC preparations carry the drowsiness hazard.

Cromolyn sodium often works well for relief of nasal symptoms (Nasalcrom spray) and eye symptoms (Opticrom eye drops), but must be used on a continuing regular schedule. Prescription corticosteroid nasal sprays (Vancenase, Beconase, Nasalide, and Nasacort) bring great relief for many. For patients who are prone to sinus infections during seasonal allergic rhinitis, controlling nasal congestion may be critical. Long-term use of these corticosteroid sprays over 3 months, can cause chronic irritation, and increased mucus secretion, and adrenal suppression with overuse has been reported. Desensitization injections, based on dermal skin testing, may be helpful for pollen allergy, but generally work less well for those with allergy to dust mites, mold, and animal danders. Skin tests for food offenders yield inconsistent results, and appear to be a poor guide for therapy.

■ **HOLISTIC MEDICAL TREATMENT**

See pages 283–288 below.

Asthma

■ **DESCRIPTION**

Asthma is the most dramatic of the respiratory diseases, and is heralded by difficulty breathing (with or without audible wheezing), cough, constricted chest, or congested lungs. Asthma affects the bronchioles, involving inflammation and swelling of the respiratory mucosa, increased secretion of thicker mucus into the airway, and constriction of the smooth muscle of the airway. Over time, the bronchiolar mucosa develops a heightened sensitivity to airborne allergens, particulates, and cold and dry air.

Auscultation of the chest reveals wheezes, commonly expiratory. When physical signs are not definitive, the diagnosis can be made by breathing function tests. The diagnosis is more difficult in subtle asthma in children up to 6–8 years of age because they are unable to follow directions for the tests. Asthmatics commonly give a history of dyspnea, coughing, wheezing, and chest congestion, often associated with a cold, sinusitis, hay fever, emotional stress, or exercise. In fact, exercise can trigger wheezing and shortness of breath in up to 80 percent of individuals who have been diagnosed with asthma, most of whom require treatment.

■ PREVALENCE

The incidence of asthma in the United States has doubled in the last 2 decades to now include 15 million people. One-half of all cases are initially diagnosed under the age of 10. It is thought that many asthmatics are never diagnosed and treated. The mortality from advanced, severe disease has doubled since 1980. Mortality strikes most often children who are urban, male or black.

■ ETIOLOGY AND RISK FACTORS

The most common contributors to bouts of asthma include upper respiratory infections and colds, sinus infections, exposure to inhalant allergens, exercise, cold air, and emotional stress. Studies in metropolitan areas have revealed a strong association between asthma severity and ozone pollution in smog. Ozone appears to enhance reactivity to ragweed and grass pollens. Asthmatics exercising outdoors in urban zones of high air pollution, in cold temperatures, or on days with high pollen counts incur an increased risk for triggering an episode.

Ingestant allergens also play important etiological roles in children and adults with so-called intrinsic asthma. Some studies have suggested that foods may be a contributing factor in 40–70 percent of children and adults with perennial asthma.[2] Milk, eggs, wheat and other grains, fish, shellfish, peanuts, cocoa, corn, nuts, wheat, onion, and garlic are the most common offenders. Aspirin, and tartrazine dyes are also problematic. Asthmatic children have a 25 percent higher intake of high fat foods and a 23 percent higher intake of sugar.[3]

Low intake of magnesium is significantly related to increased risk of asthma.[4] Research has strongly implicated asthma as a free-radical-mediated process with a marked oxidant/antioxidant imbalance[5] and increased need for antioxidants. Asthmatics also have lower vitamin B_6 levels.[6]

Questions have arisen related to a higher observed incidence of asthma in children receiving DPT and polio immunizations compared to un-immunized children.[7] Emotional and stress factors also play roles in asthma. Observations of patients with multiple personality disorder have demonstrated asthma reactivity to cats and foods in one personality state but not in others.[8] In children, there is often enmeshment, a smothering love between parent and child which can create a feeling of being stifled, with a degree of dependence that is symbolically equivalent to children's inability to breathe for themselves. Emotional factors rank high on the list of associations increasing the risk of mortality with this disease.[9] In other children there may be a lack of healthy bonding between the parents. Asthma is also often associated with suppressed crying, sometimes related to a lack of nurturing, sufficient touching and affection, commonly seen within asthmatic families. In asthma-prone subjects, recurrent bouts of asthma are often clearly associated with episodes of emotional stress.

■ CONVENTIONAL MEDICAL TREATMENT

The NIH "Guidelines for the Diagnosis and Management of Asthma" describe four aspects of effective management of asthma. They include objective pulmonary function tests to diagnose and monitor the status of the asthma; pharmacological treatment; control of environmental factors; and patient education.

Initial therapy is directed at preventing and controlling the inflammation of the bronciolar mucosa. During periods of high ozone alerts, asthmatics should reduce activity, stay indoors, and use air conditioners. Exposure to known allergens and irritants must be reduced or eliminated; triggering factors (colds, sinusitis, otitis media, allergic rhinitis) must be treated. Influenza vaccinations and pneumococcal vaccines are often indicated for those with frequent recurrences. Consultation with an allergist for evaluation of allergic factors may be indicated.

A pharmacological step-care approach involves frequent monitoring and use of medications, including anti-inflammatory, bronchodilator, and expectorant drugs. Anti-inflammatory medications include inhaled corticosteroids such as Azmacort, Beclovent, AeroBid, Vanceril, Decadron, and oral corticosteroids (prednisone, prednisolone, Medrol). Bronchodilators include beta-agonist metered-dose inhalers (Alupent, Brethaire, Bronkometer, Isuprel Mistometer, Maxair, Metaprel, Proventil, and Ventolin). Theophylline is the principal oral methylxanthine bronchodilator in Aerolate, Bronkodyl, Choledyl, Dilor, Elixophyllin, Lufyllin, Marax, Quibron, Respbid, Slo-bid, Slophyllin, Tedral, Theo-Dur, Theo-24, Theolair, and Uniphyl. Popular over-the-counter agents include Primatene Mist and Sudafed. Primatene contains ephedrine as well as theophylline. Anticholinergic agents (Atrovent), delivered by inhaler, inhibit the parasympathetic nervous system. Expectorants to liquefy and mobilize secretions contain guaifenesin or iodinated glycerol. Agents includes Fenesin, Humibid, Organidin, Sinumist, and SSKI. A profusion of OTC products containing guaifenesin includes Anti-Tuss, Guiatuss, Glycotuss, Halotussin, Hytuss 2X, Naldecon Senior EX, Robitussin, and Uni-tussin.

■ HOLISTIC MEDICAL TREATMENT

The complementary treatment of each of the four chronic respiratory diseases is similar and is summarized here. There are two objectives of treatment for chronic respiratory disease: healing the damaged mucous membrane of the respiratory tract, and enhancing the activity of the immune system. The following delineates the steps involved.

Environmental treatment. Outdoor air quality has been slightly improved with public health measures in the past two decades. The quality of indoor air, however, is more amenable to immediate control. The quintessential step in improving indoor air quality requires the cessation of personal or secondary exposure to cigarette and cigar smoke. Optimal indoor air is clean, 35–60 percent relative humidity, between 65 and 85°F, and containing 3–6,000 negative air ions/cc. EPA reports indicate that average indoor environment in the United States contains only 200 ions/cc. Negative air ions are generated outdoors in forests, mountains, and areas with moving water. Negative-ion generators used indoors attract dust, pollen, mold, animal dander, and some bacteria and viruses, precipitating these particles from circulating air.[10] They also help repair damaged mucous membranes by stimulating cilial action. Negative-ion generators are easily commercially available.

Air cleaners with HEPA filters placed in bedrooms have beneficial effects. High efficiency (HEPA) filters can be installed in furnace heating systems as well. Humidifiers are often essential to combat the drying effect of constant winter heating. Many plants add moisture as well as oxygen to the atmosphere; spider plants, aloe vera, pothos, philodendrons, and chrysanthemums all function as effective air filters. Avoiding times of smog alerts, good ventilation can enhance indoor air quality. Air duct cleaning and non-toxic carpet cleaning are helpful. Adequate hydration from an adequate intake of drinking water is necessary for proper liquefaction of mucus secretions. Dried, thickened secretions promote obstruction. Water and herbal teas are probably the best maintenance liquids. The entire respiratory-tract benefits from exposure to the moisture of hot showers or a Steam Inhaler. Nasal irrigation with saline, using a rubber ear syringe, a porcelain Neti pot or a Grossan nasal attachment to a Water Pik, is extremely useful in reducing nasal swelling and flushing infected sinuses. Irrigating solutions can be easily prepared by adding $\frac{1}{3}$ tsp of salt in an 8 ounce glass of water with a pinch of baking soda.

Nutritional treatment. Cow's milk and milk derivatives, wheat, corn (corn starch and corn syrup), eggs and soy are leading contributors to respiratory allergies and should be avoided or greatly reduced.[11] Elimination of offenders must be tried for at least a month before effects may be fully apparent. A food elimination trial for a month is an inexpensive clinical approach to diagnosis for cooperative patients. Each food must then be reintroduced one at a time in a pure form, at 3-day intervals (see Chapter 1). For patients dependent on milk as a calcium source, long-term elimination must be accompanied with calcium supplementation. Sucrose compromises immune function[12] and intake should likewise be very limited. Sucrose also contributes to proliferation of candidiasis, which may also be problematic. Caffeine also has numerous detrimental effects.

Supplements. Daily doses of supplements helpful in these four respiratory-tract problems include antioxidants—vitamin C 1–3 g, vitamin E 400 IU, beta carotene 2–5 mg, vitamin B_6 25–50 mg, B_{12} 500 μg, grape seed extract 80–160 mg, zinc 30–60 mg, and selenium 200 μg. Botanical remedies discussed below are also helpful in asthma. Magnesium deserves special attention. Intravenous infusion of 1 g of $MgSO_4$ over 7–20 min often has a dramatic effect in status asthmaticus,[13] as well as significantly improving FEV_1 up to 75 percent in 2 h in patients experiencing acute exacerbations.[14] Suggested magnesium daily oral intake is 300–700 mg, through foods and/or supplements. Excess sodium contributes to the deterioration of FEV_1 and peak expiratory flow rates in asthmatics.[15]

For allergies, supplements that are most effective are quercitin (t.i.d. a.c.), which inhibits leukotriene synthesis and histamine release from mast cells,[16,17] and grapeseed extracts containing procyanidines, which exert potent effects including antioxidation, inhibition of loss of capillary integrity, and reduction in swelling.[18] For chronic bronchitis, the amino acid *N*-acetylcysteine 500 mg t.i.d. is useful in reducing mucus viscosity. The herbal bronchodilator ephedra can be used if wheezing accompanies the bronchitis. However, its use should be limited to a few days, and should be avoided by anyone with heart disease, high blood pressure, thyroid disease, diabetes, or an enlarged prostate.

Botanical treatment. Botanical remedies which have been shown to be helpful in asthma and respiratory allergies include ephedra sinica, 500–1,000 mg t.i.d. (each dose containing ephedrine content of 1.2–25 mg), used with the precautions mentioned earlier. Licorice root (*Glycyrrhiza glabra*) 250–500 mg t.i.d. has expectorant properties and anti-inflammatory activity, inhibiting leukotrienes and proinflammatory prostaglandins.[19] Its tendency to elevate blood pressures with long-term use requires careful monitoring. *Tylophora indica* is an herb long used in Ayurvedic medicine for asthma, valued for its antihistaminic action and ability to inhibit mast cell prostaglandins (200 mg b.i.d.).[20,21] Herbal teas in liberal amounts 3–5 times daily are helpful, particularly those containing *Prunus serotina* (cherry bark), *plantago major* (plaintain), and *Scutellaria laterifolia* (skullcap). Other herbs mixed in a tincture, taken 5–10 drops every 15 minutes up to eight doses, include *Lobelia inflata* (Indian tobacco) 2 parts, *Thymus vulgaris* (Thyme) 1 part, *Zingiber officinalis* (ginger root) 1 part, *Gelsemium sempiverens* 1 part, *Ephedra sinica* $\frac{1}{2}$ part, and belladonna $\frac{1}{2}$ part. The combination has antispasmodic effects.

Homeopathic treatment. Homeopathic prescribing in 12-X to 30C dilutions for acute symptoms utilizes *Arsenicum album* for wheezing with restlessness and anxiety, Ipecac for chest constriction with cough, *Pulsatilla* with chest pressure and air hunger, and *Sambucus* for wheezing awakening the patient at night.

Exercise. Physical exercise, requiring increased pulmonary air exchange, is problematic for many with chronic respiratory disease. Exercise out of doors in polluted air increases risk for bronchospasm. When the proper precautions are taken, however, walking can be one of the most beneficial of all forms of exercise. An outdoor program, or walking indoors on a treadmill with very modest increases in exertion can determine manageable thresholds of activity which can often be slowly increased. Ozone levels in most homes, gyms, and pools are about half those of the outdoors, and even less with a good air-conditioning system. Two grams of vitamin C taken before exercise has been shown to significantly reduce the incidence of exercise-induced asthma.[22] If tolerated, patients should engage in aerobic exercise consisting of three 30-minute workouts each week, while reaching their target heart rate (220 minus age multiplied by 0.6 to 0.85 depending on conditioning). A variety of activities can accomplish this; it is important for patients to find an activity they enjoy.

Acupuncture. This is particularly effective for mild asthma, with at least 6 sessions needed to demonstrate any positive effects and more for long-lasting results.[23] Other therapies of help in treating respiratory diseases are massage, reflexology, Shiatsu, chiropractic, and craniosacral therapy.

Mental and emotional treatment. Treatment options in managing respiratory disease include the use of imagery, affirmations, suggestion, hypnosis, biofeedback, relaxation exercises, meditation, modification of beliefs, and counseling. Images have powerful effects on immunological and neurological function, often as powerful as observations from reality.[24] Positive affirmations tend to create positive images, and many of them have appeared to be beneficial in respiratory disease patients. An example would be "My sinuses (lungs or allergies) are getting better every day."

Suggestion alone has been shown to induce bronchospasm in asthmatic subjects.[25] Asthmatics given a bronchodilator with a positive suggestion get twice the benefit compared to taking the same medication with a negative suggestion.[26] Hypnosis has been effectively used in treating asthma.[27] Suppressed emotions (anger, fear, and sadness) seem to be a common theme in respiratory disease. Counseling settings in which patients express feelings verbally or in writing are therapeutic. Asthmatics writing about their most distressing emotional trauma for 20 minutes on each of 4 consecutive days, tested 4 months later, improved their FEV_1 12 percent compared to baseline, versus no change in asthmatics writing about their daily schedules.[28] Regular practice of biofeedback,[29] yoga,[30] and programmed breathing[31] significantly improves function, sometimes dramatically. Meditation, also, can have profound effects on immunity[32] and consequently on respiratory disease.

Though large-scale research studies have yet to be reported, energy medicine techniques including therapeutic or healing touch, Reiki, and Qi gong can be beneficial in modifying immune responses and treating and preventing respiratory diseases.[33] For instance, the perfectionism and strong need for control often seen in people with chronic sinusitis can be modified through these techniques with benefit.

ACUTE RESPIRATORY DISEASES

Upper respiratory infections, influenza, otitis media, acute respiratory illnesses, rank among the 10 most common acute ailments in the United States.

Upper Respiratory Infections (Colds)

■ DESCRIPTION

Upper respiratory infections are viral infections of the membranes of the nose and throat. Over 200 cold viruses have been identified. Commonest symptoms include sore throat, weakness, fatigue, malaise, clear mucous nasal drainage, nasal congestion, sneezing, and sometimes fever and lacrimation. Upper respiratory infections typically last 3–10 days, and resolve spontaneously.

■ PREVALENCE

Americans are subject to an estimated one billion upper respiratory infections each year. The average adult has 2–4 colds a year, usually in the winter, and children average 6–10 colds per year. Those over 60 commonly have less than one cold a year. Upper respiratory infections are the leading cause of work absenteeism, accounting for 7 lost workdays per person per year.

■ ETIOLOGY AND RISK FACTORS

In the late fall and winter, colds are usually caused by either parain-fluenza and respiratory syncytial viruses; in spring, summer, and fall the predominant virus is one of the 100 or more rhinoviruses. Patients become infected when exposed to the virus, either by inhaling it as an air-borne vector, or from contact with an infected surface, usually the hand of an infected person. Rhinoviruses survive up to 3 hours outside the nasal passages.

As with most diseases, the degree of immune resistance exhibited by a patient at any given moment plays a major role in the risk of clinical illness when exposed to cold viruses. Emotional tension, time pressures and unresolved psychological conflicts are among the most prevalent stress-related risk factors for colds. Lack of restful sleep is a significant risk factor; the immune system is at the peak of its activity during the nighttime hours when corticosteroid synthesis is at its nadir. Any of the previously mentioned environmental risks—cigarette smoke, heavy air pollution, or extremely dry or cold air —can irritate the mucous membrane of the nose or throat sufficiently to allow viruses to invade weakened cells.

■ CONVENTIONAL MEDICAL TREATMENT FOR COLDS

Conventional treatment consists of treatment of symptoms. Most conventional physicians believe that vitamin C, chicken soup, rest, liquids, gargling, and most multi-ingredient OTC cold tablets offer little benefit. Decongestants are recommended for nasal congestion, antihistamines for rhinorrhea, anti-tussives for cough, expectorants to loosen secretions and acetaminophen or aspirin (not in children) for aching. Antihistamines may dry secretions and should be used carefully.

■ HOLISTIC MEDICAL TREATMENT

The common cold is usually the trigger for causing acute sinusitis, acute bronchitis, exacerbations of asthma. Prevention of colds, and attenuation of their worst symptoms, is therefore quite important, and also feasible if the immune system can be strengthened. A healthy immune system also facilitates quicker recovery with fewer complications.

At the earliest hints of a cold, patients will benefit from immediately taking steps to get extra rest, rather then "keep on going." Saline gargles reduce swelling and nasal sprays with anti-viral herbs may be of benefit. Warm and hot liquids, ginger root tea, with or without honey and lemon also appear anecdotally to have benefit. A hot bath and steam, adding a few drops of eucalyptus, peppermint, and/or tea tree oil is also highly touted although studies are lacking.

Nutritional Factors

Although widely debated, extra doses of vitamin C have been shown at the very least to reduce the total recovery time from colds by 50 percent.[34] Anecdotal evidence compiled from the experience of many holistic practitioners concludes that vitamin C taken in very large amounts to the limit of bowel tolerance (usually 15–24 g in the first 24 hours after symptom onset) often aborts the process, leading to total clearing of symptoms in 12–24 hours. Ester C is more completely absorbed than standard preparations, allowing a larger dose to be taken before bowel tolerance (onset of rectal gas and extra-soft stools) is reached. After an initial dose of 4–5 g, 1–2 g can be taken every 1–2 hours while awake, tapering the dose once symptoms disappear. Vitamin A 50,000 IU t.i.d. for 2–3 days, then gradually tapered over 4–5 days, is impressive in its benefit with many viruses; rubeola is probably the best example.[35] Zinc gluconate lozenges (13–22 mg) have been shown to lead to complete recovery in about $4\frac{1}{2}$ days, versus 8 in those using placebo lozenges.[36] Effective formulations are sweetened with glycine rather than with mannitol, sorbitol, or citric acid.

The diet should eliminate dairy products and sugar and eat small meals with easily digested foods and less protein. Warm and hot foods often serve to loosen secretions.

Botanical Options

Yin Chiao, a Chinese herb, 5 tablets q.i.d. for the first 2 days; garlic, eaten raw (1 or 2 cloves a day) or in liquid or capsule form, 4 g daily;[37] and echinacea, 1 dropperful in water q.i.d. for 3–5 days, or 900 mg capsules, one q.i.d.[38] (avoid echinacea in pregnancy or autoimmune disease) have demonstrated benefits.

Homeopathic Remedies

Homeopathic remedies with experiential reputations for benefit include Aconitum (monkshood) and Ferrum phos. Controlled studies have accorded benefit to treatment by *Eupatorium perfoliatum* D_2[39] and Engystol-N,[40] a combination product. Acupuncture and acupressure, especially points #3, 4, and 8, is also used.

Influenza

■ DESCRIPTION

Influenza is a highly contagious and debilitating viral infection of the respiratory tract that can potentially be fatal. Type A influenza causes the most severe disease and frequently lasts up to 2 weeks. In contrast to type B disease, the type A virus undergoes frequent mutations, negating the effect of community immunity.

Influenza most commonly presents with abrupt onset of dry cough, severe muscle aching, fever, chills, sore throat, marked fatigue, rhinorrhea, and headache. Other symptoms may include anorexia, abdominal pain, diarrhea, and ataxia. The contagious period lasts about 4 days from the earliest onset of symptoms.

■ PREVALENCE

The incidence of influenza viral infections reaches a peak through the winter months, causing about 20,000 deaths each year in the United States. A severe outbreak affects 20–25 percent of the population. An outbreak typically begins abruptly, accelerating for about 3 weeks and diminishing for another 3 weeks, leaving behind about 20–50 percent of a community population affected. Children aged 5–14 are most often among the more seriously ill. Influenza A illness has caused hundreds of thousands of deaths in the United States in the past century, with major pandemics in 1918, 1957 and 1968. Pandemics of the type A strain have tended to appear at about 10-year intervals in contrast to type B outbreaks appearing about every 4–5 years.

■ ETIOLOGY AND RISK FACTORS

Influenza is a viral illness, spread easily via droplet contamination from an infected person or skin contact with dried, infected material on objects handled by the infected person. Those whose immunity is compromised are at greater risk. Physicians practicing complementary medicine often note that those whose immunity is strengthened by physical exercise, better management of stress, the best macro- and micro-nutrient food and supplement intake, and positive attitudes are most often resistant, or experience mild forms of the disease.

■ CONVENTIONAL MEDICAL TREATMENT

As with most viral illnesses, there is little to be offered for this potentially serious disease beyond mitigation of symptoms. Bed rest and liquids, analgesics (aspirin in children is contraindicated because of risk of Reye's syndrome), cough suppressants, expectorants and decongestants can ease the symptoms of the afflicted patient.

Amantidine (Symmetrel), 200 mg daily, can be effective with attenuating the effects of influenza A if used within a day or two of earliest onset of symptoms. It can shorten both the intensity and duration of the symptoms. Antibiotics are sometimes prescribed to prevent bacterial pneumonia in the elderly.

Public health emphasis has been placed on prevention by urging immunization for those over age 65, those with heart and lung disease, pregnant women and health personnel in contact with the public. The latest flu vaccines are reported to be 60–90 percent effective for at least 6 months against either type A or B.

■ HOLISTIC MEDICAL TREATMENT

Influenza prophylaxis incorporates recommendations for adequate rest, optimal air, water, exercise, food, supplements, and regular periods of relaxation to maintain high levels of wellness with resistant immunity. For patients succumbing to illness, earliest treatment reaps the greatest benefits. The recommended regimen is similar to that outlined under upper respiratory infections, above: rest, increased intake of warm or hot liquids, vitamins C and A, Yin Chiao, garlic, and echinacea. Chicken soup has recently been shown to inhibit neutrophil chemotaxis in vitro, explaining its folk-wisdom popularity in respiratory viral infections. *N*-acetylcysteine, 500 mg q.i.d. for cough, bronchitis, or pneumonia[41] has demonstrated benefit. The odds ratio for early recovery from aching, chills, and fever in patients taking oscillococcinum, a homeopathic remedy, was 1.9 compared to those on placebo in a British study.[42] Ginger, taken as a tea or in capsules relieves nausea and elimination of milk and sugar is recommended for reasons listed under upper respiratory infections.

Otitis Media

■ DESCRIPTION

Upper respiratory infections often lead to otitis media because of the anatomical proximity of the eustachian tube to the nasopharynx. Infection in the middle ear space is not uncommonly relieved by rupture of the eardrum and external drainage, with relief of pain and clearing of the acute episode of infection. Occasionally, however, the eardrum does not heal and requires surgical repair. Other rare complications include mastoiditis or meningitis. Chronic and recurrent serous otitis media can also lead to scarring of the middle ear structures, causing hearing loss.

As a result of the build-up of pressure from the secretions trapped in the middle ear, acute otitis media presents with pain, often with fever, diminished hearing, and upper respiratory infection. Children usually experience about 2 days of pain and fever, whether treated with antibiotics or not. In infants, symptoms may be non-specific, presenting as runny nose, fever, irritability, pulling at the affected ear, and unwillingness to nurse or suck on a bottle. Otoscopic examination confirms an inflamed or bulging eardrum.

■ PREVALENCE

Acute otitis media accounts for 35 percent of all preschoolers' visits to physicians. One-half of all children have at least one episode.

■ ETIOLOGY AND RISK FACTORS

Exposure to second-hand smoke is a significant risk factor, with a 40 percent greater incidence in those who are consistently exposed compared to those who are not.[43] Children who are breast fed until age one or older have a much lower incidence of otitis media.[44]

Allergies play major roles in otitis media. Dust mites, pets, and molds are the most common inhalant offenders.[45] Food allergies and sensitivities are also commonly related in many children.[46] The most common offender is cow's milk, with most hard cheeses and some yogurts less likely to be problematic. Other potential food allergens for otitis media are wheat, corn, eggs, soy, chocolate, peanuts, and chicken. Sugar compromises phagocytosis[12] and is a problem in many cases.

■ CONVENTIONAL MEDICAL TREATMENT

Antibiotics are nearly always prescribed for otitis media, in spite of research published by the National Academy of Sciences' Institute of Medicine which concluded that antibiotics were no more effective than placebos in treating middle ear infections. Many ear infections are viral in nature, beyond the benefits of antibiotics. Analgesics and decongestants are also usually prescribed. Nasal decongestant sprays and drops are often difficult to use properly in the very young. With the common use of antibiotics, mastoiditis and meningitis have become quite uncommon.

In Europe, physicians usually adopt an approach of watchful waiting, reserving antibiotics for the few children who do not resolve the infection quickly. Repeated infections are common, often prompting referral to an otolaryngologist. Over a million tympanostomies with ear tube placement are performed yearly in the United States. Some studies, however, have shown that this surgery results in a greater incidence of hearing loss than non-surgical treatment, and many authorities believe a significant portion of tympanostomies are inappropriate.[47] The Scandinavians have a much lower rate of surgery and an equivalent complication rate.

■ HOLISTIC MEDICAL TREATMENT

Alternating wet compresses to the outer ear, using 3 minutes of hot up to tolerance followed by 30 seconds of a cold pack often relieves pain. Instilled early, with an intact ear drum, drops containing warm garlic oil with St. John's wort and mullein often bring relief. Parents can buy the liquid form of each of the 3 herbs at health food stores, mixing 2 : 1 : 1 portions of the 3 ingredients.

Following antibiotic treatment, children should also be given bifidus (age 1–5) and acidophilus bacteria (age 6 and over) to replace the resident bacteria in the bowel. Refrigerated or lyophilized brands are preferable.

Allergies need to be addressed. In children with recurrent episodes, inhalant offenders should be considered and eliminated or controlled if warranted. Ingestant food allergens play a surprisingly prominent role. It is relatively simple to eliminate cow's milk, and a blind trial of a diet omitting milk is often rewarding. In other children, in whom the recurrent cycle of infections continues unabated, a diet eliminating milk, wheat, corn, eggs, chocolate, soy, peanuts, and chicken should be tried. Up to 3–4 months may be required to see a difference, although subtle signs of improved mood and sleep are often noticeable in 2–3 weeks. If improvement is noted, rechallenge with each food introduced one at a time at 4-day intervals can often spot the offender(s). Sugar should be drastically reduced or eliminated. Even full strength fruit juice may be a problem.

A surprising number of children have poor intake of important micronutrients, many even below the Recommended Dietary Allowances.[48] Addition of extra vitamin C (250–500 mg daily), vitamin A (5–20,000 IU daily for brief periods), vitamin B$_6$, vitamin E, and formulations of Echinacea and Astragalus membranaceous have all been shown to improve immune responsiveness.

Homeopathic prescribing can also help in treatment. Single homeopathic remedies used in one study (Aconitum napellus, Apis mellifica, Belladonna, Capsicum, Chamomilla, Kalium bichromicum, Lachesis, Lycopodium, Mercurius solubilis, Okoubaka, Pulsatilla, Silicea) shortened the course of treatment and pain and resulted in fewer recurrences compared to antibiotic treatment.[49]

REFERENCES

1. Ogle KA et al. Children with allergic rhinitis and/or bronchial asthma with elimination diet. *Ann Allergy* 1977; 39(1):8–11.
2. Pelikan Z et al. Bronchial response to the food ingestion challenge. *Ann Allergy* 1987; 58(3):164–72.
3. Peat JK. University of Sydney. American Lung Association International Conference, New Orleans, 1996. *Medical Tribune* 1996; 37(11):7.
4. Britton J et al. Dietary magnesium, lung function, wheezing and airway hyperreactivity in a random adult population sample. *Lancet* 1994; 344(8919):357–62.
5. Rahman I et al. Systemic ocidative stress in asthma, COPD, and smokers. *Am J Respir Crit Care Med* 1996; 154(4 pt 1):1055–60.
6. Reynolds RD et al. Depressed plasma pyridoxal phosphate concentrations in adult asthmatics. *Am J Clin Nutr* 1985; 41(4): 684–8.
7. Kemp et al. Is infant immunization a risk factor for childhood asthma or allergy? *Epidemiology* 1997; 8(6):678–80.
8. Braun BG. Psychophysiologic phenomena in multiple personality and hypnosis. *Am J Clin Hyp* 1983; 26(2):124–37.
9. Strunk RC. Physiologic and psychological characteristics associated with deaths due to asthma in childhood. *JAMA* 1985; 254(9):1193–8.
10. Ben-Dov I et al. Effect of negative ionisation of inspired air on the response of asthmatic children to exercise and inhaled histamine. *Thorax* 1983; 38(8):584–8.
11. Rowe AH et al. Bronchial asthma due to food allergy alone in ninety-five patients. *JAMA* 1959; 169(11):1158–62.
12. Sanchez A et al. Role of sugars in human neutrophilic phagocytosis. *Am J Clin Nutr* 1973; 26(11):1180–4.
13. Okayama H et al. Treatment of status asthmaticus with intravenous magnesium sulfate. *J Asthma* 1991; 28(1):11–17.
14. Ciarello L et al. Intravenous magnesium therapy for moderate to severe pediatric asthma: results of a randomized, placebo-controlled trial. *J Pediatr* 1996; 129(6):809–14.
15. Carey OJ et al. Effect of alterations of dietary sodium on the severity of asthma in men. *Thorax* 1993; 48(7):714–18.
16. Middleton E Jr et al. Quercitin: an inhibitor of antigen-induced basophil histamine release. *J Immunol* 1981; 127(2):546–50.

17. Foreman JC. Mast cells and the actions of flavonoids. *J Allergy Clin Immunol* 1984; 73(6):769–74.
18. Maffei Facino R et al. Differential inhibition of superoxide, hydroxyl and peroxyl radicals by nimesulide and its main metabolite 4-hydroxynimesulide. *Arzneimittelforschung* 1995; 45(10):1102–9.
19. Okimasu E et al. Inhibition of phospholipase A2 and platelet aggregation by glycyrrhizin, and inti-inflammatory drug. *Acta Med Okayama* 1983; 37:385–91.
20. Gopalakrishnan C et al. Effect of tylophorine, a major alkaloid of Tylophorine indica, on immunopathological and inflammatory reactions. *Ind J Med Res* 1980; 71:940–8.
21. Gupta S et al. Tylophora indica in bronchial asthma—a double-blind study. *Ind J Med Res* 1979; 69:981–9.
22. Cohen HA et al. Blocking effect of vitamin C in exercise-induced asthma. *Arch Ped Adoles Med* 1997; 151(4):367–70.
23. Fung KP et al. Attenuation of exercise-induced asthma by acupuncture. *Lancet* 1986; 2(8521-22):1419–22.
24. Rider MS et al. Effect of immune system imagery on secretory IgA. *Biof Self Regul* 1990; 15(4):317–33.
25. Luparello T et al. Influence of suggestion on airway reactivity in asthmatic subjects. *Psychosom Med* 1968; 30(6):819–25.
26. Turner JA et al. The importance of placebo effects in pain treatment and research. *JAMA* 1994; 271(20):1609–14.
27. Collison DR. Which asthmatic patients should be treated with hypnotherapy? *Med J Aust* 1975; 1(25):776–81.
28. Smyth JM et al. Effects of writing about stressful experiences on symptom reduction in patients with asthma or rheumatoid arthritis: a randomized trial. *JAMA* 1999; 28(14):1304–9.
29. Lehrer PM. Relaxation decreases large-airway but not small airway asthma. *J Psychosom Res* 1986; 30(1):13–25.
30. Jain SC et al. Effect of yoga training on exercise tolerance in adolescents with childhood asthma. *J Asthma* 1991; 28(6):437–52.
31. Bowler SD et al. Buteyko breathing techniques in asthma: a blinded randomised controlled trial. *Med J Aust* 1998; 169(11–12):575–8.
32. Smith GR et al. Psychologic modulation of the human response to varicella zoster. *Arch Intern Med* 1985; 145(11):2110–12.
33. Koar WH. Meditation, T-cells, anxiety, depression and HIV infection. *Subtle Energies* 1995; 6(1):89–97.

34. Hemila H. Does vitamin C alleviate the symptoms of the common cold? A review of current evidence. *Scand J Infect Dis* 1994; 26(1)1–6.
35. Glasziou PP et al. Vitamin A supplementation in infectious diseases: a meta-analysis. *BMJ* 1993; 306(6874):366–70.
36. Mossad SB et al. Zinc gluconate losenges for treating the common cold: a randomized, double-blind, placebo-controlled study. *Ann Intern Med* 1996; 125(2):81–8.
37. Weber ND et al. In vitro virucidal effects of *Allium sativum* (garlic) extract and compounds. *Planta Med* 1992; 58(5):417–23.
38. Melchart D et al. Echinacea root extracts for the prevention of upper respiratory tract infections: a double-blind, placebo-controlled randomized trial. *Arch Fam Med* 1998; 7(6):541–5.
39. Gassinger CA et al. A controlled clinical trial for testing the efficacy of the homeopathic drug eupatorium perfoliatum D2 in the treatment of common cold. *Arzneimittelforschung* 1981; 31(4):732–6.
40. Maiwald VL et al. Therapy of common cold with a homeopathic combination preparation in comparison with acetylsalicylic acid. A controlled, randomized double-blind study. *Arzneimittelforschung* 1988; 38:578–82.
41. Suter PM et al. N-acetylcysteine enhances recovery from lung injury in man. A randomized, double-blind, placebo-controlled study. *Chest* 1994; 105(1):190–4.
42. Ferley JP et al. A controlled evaluation of a homeopathic preparation in the treatment of influenza-like syndromes. *Br J Clin Pharmacol* 1989; 27(3):329–35.
43. Etzel RA. Passive smoking and middle ear effusion among children in day care. *Pediatrics* 1992; 90(2 pt 1):228–32.
44. Sassen ML et al. Breast-feeding and acute otitis media. *Am J Otolaryngol* 1994; 15(5):351–7.
45. Hurst DS. Association of otitis media with effusion and allergy as demonstrated by intradermal skin testing and eosinophil cationic protein levels in both middle ear effusions and mucosal biopsies. *Laryngoscope* 1996; 106(9 pt 1):1128–37.
46. Nasouli TM et al. Role of food allergy in serous otitis media. *Ann Allergy* 1994; 73(3):215–19.

47. Kleinman LC et al. The medical appropriateness of tympanostomy tubes proposed for children younger than 16 years in the United States. *JAMA* 1994; 271(16):1250–5.

48. Food and Nutrient Intakes in the United States: *Nationwide Food Consumption Survey*, 1977–78. USDA Science and Education Administration, 1980 Sep.

49. Friese KH et al. The homeopathic treatment of otitis media in children—comparisons with conventional therapy. *Int J Clin Pharmacol Ther* 1997; 35(7):296–301.

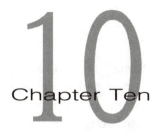

Chapter Ten

Musculoskeletal Diseases

Osteoarthritis

■ DESCRIPTION

Arthritis is an inflammation of the joints that deteriorates the integrity of the synovial cartilage of joints. Osteoarthritis (OA) is a degenerative articular process involving modest inflammation, but loss of articular cartilage, and hypertrophy of bone at the joint margins, which tends to be progressive with advancing age. It is also called degenerative or hypertrophic arthritis. It appears to occur when the regenerative ability of cartilage to repair and refurbish itself is outstripped by the degenerative processes. It is characterized by gradual onset of pain, stiffness, joint crepitation, limitation of motion, and swelling of the involved joints.

The commonest sites are the proximal and middle interphalangeal joints, knees, hips, cervical, and lumbar spine. Marked pain from spinal involvement is not common, and indeed, on X-raying the spine, it is not uncommon to inadvertently discover osteoarthritis which has been totally asymptomatic. There are no definitive laboratory tests. The diagnosis is based on findings of the history, physical examination, X-rays, and analysis of joint fluid. Osteoarthritis can be classified as primary, apparently resulting from normal wear and tear, or secondary, in which the changes can be attributed to chronic trauma from injury, obesity, postural problems, or occupational overuse.

■ PREVALENCE

Osteoarthritis is the most common form of arthritis, afflicting about 40 million Americans of all ages. It is uncommon before the age of 40, but the incidence in persons over 65 approaches 60 percent. Under the age of 45, it affects more men than women, with the reverse in those over 55. The majority of osteoarthritis patients do not seek medical treatment. In about one-third of those afflicted, the process is progressive, eventually causing significant disability.

■ ETIOLOGY AND RISK FACTORS

Hereditary patterns of incidence are commonly observed by primary-care physicians. Severe or recurrent joint injury from heavy physical activity is known to play a significant role. Congenital joint instability and skeletal postural defects are also contributory. Excess weight plays an extremely important role for the weight-bearing hip and knee joints. The risk for arthritis of the knee in men is 50–350 percent greater in men who are the heaviest compared to those of normal weight.[1]

Only the most taxing and violent joint-pounding activities (e.g., long-distance running, basketball) persisting over decades appear to predispose to the development of osteoarthritis. The mechanical knee strain incurred with the use of high-heeled shoes also significantly increases risk.[2] Cold climates and barometric pressure changes increase symptoms in some patients.

A diet high in animal products is associated with increased risk, and food sensitivity plays a definitive role in a significant number of patients; the most common food culprits are the Solanum (nightshade) foods (potatoes, tomatoes, peppers, eggplant, tobacco), wheat and cow's milk and derivatives.

Low-grade infections (e.g., gingivitis and prostatitis) play a contributory role, and it also appears that a marginally low pH increases the amounts of calcium, minerals, and acidic toxins deposited in the joint, leading to more inflammation. Other systemic disorders often associated with osteoarthritis include nutritional deficiencies, small-bowel assimilation disorders, constipation, fatigue, emotional stress, and endocrine disorders.

■ CONVENTIONAL MEDICAL TREATMENT

Conventional treatment of osteoarthritis includes reduction of stresses on joints through extra rest, weight loss, and the use of splints, braces, neck collars, crutches, or canes. Physical therapy is commonly utilized, consisting of: therapeutic exercise—swimming, water aerobics, walking, bicycling, and cross-country skiing; strengthening and stretching exercises; hot and cold packs; diathermy; and paraffin baths.

Relief of pain is sought with suggestions for using acetaminophen and progressing to non-steroidal anti-inflammatory drugs (NSAIDs), available either OTC or by prescription. The more commonly used are ibuprofen (Advil, Nuprin, Motrin), Alleve, Naprosyn, Orudis, Naprosyn, Tolectin, Indocin, and Feldene. Aspirin is not often recommended for osteoarthritis because the high doses required for relief may have adverse gastric effects. The NSAIDs *do not stop joint deterioration*, and long-term use increases risks for kidney and liver damage, as well as stomach and small-bowel irritation.[3] One half of all patients admitted to a hospital for gastrointestinal bleeding have been taking NSAIDs, leading to an excessive mortality in users. Even long-term use of acetominophen is attended with risk for renal failure.[4] New-generation non-steroidal anti-inflammatories (cyclooxygenase-2 inhibitors), which appear to have less risk for gastrointestinal erosions and bleeding, include Celebrex and Vioxx.

Corticosteroids are prescribed for their anti-inflammatory effects. The least harmful and most beneficial route is probably intra-articular injection. Hazards, especially with higher doses, include cushingoid changes, suppression of intrinsic corticosteroid synthesis, and acceleration of osteoporosis.

Surgery, as a late-stage intervention with onset of significant disability, includes reconstruction or replacement of knees, hips, knuckles, and other joints. Surgery for hip and knee replacement have the best results.

■ **HOLISTIC MEDICAL TREATMENT**

Osteoarthritis, like any other chronic condition, is a systemic disease targeted locally to specific joints. If joints have not yet deteriorated to the point that articular bone is denuded of the full thickness of its cartilaginous covering, it is often controllable or reversible.

Nutritional treatment. It is imperative to remove all contributing inflammatory causes, including food sensitivity. A food elimination trial is usually warranted, and must be continued for at least a month to be certain to fully assess its relationship to symptoms. Blind trials removing dairy products, wheat, and nightshade foods imposes less drastic restrictions and often bring noticeable changes. Each omitted food can be tested every 4–5 days during the rechallenge phase of the trial.

Generically reducing or eliminating animal foods other than fish is also important. The resulting diet will be wholly or marginally vegetarian. Vegetarians have less osteoarthritis. In addition, alcohol, coffee, sugar, and cranberries should be omitted, and spinach, plums, buckwheat, nuts, oil-rich seeds, and nut butters should be greatly reduced.

In severe cases, fasting, except for intake of fresh-juice vegetables and fruits also has a very high success rate in diagnosis and treatment. Fasting enhances the elimination and cleansing capacity of the lungs, skin, liver, and kidneys. Patients with advanced disease processes need to be carefully monitored.

The osteoarthritis diet should usually include green vegetables, carrots, avocado, seaweeds, spirulina, barley and wheat grass products, pecans, soy products, and whole grains (e.g., brown rice, millet, oats, and barley), and cold-water fish (e.g., salmon, sardines, herring, and tuna).

Supplements. Antioxidant supplements are essential to enhance healing and repair and restrain the destruction from oxidative stress. These include vitamin C 1–6 g daily, vitamin A 10,000 to 25,000 IU daily, and vitamin E 400–1,200 IU daily. Vitamin B-complex with 50 mg daily of each individual vitamin is recommended. Folic acid and B$_{12}$ supplementation reduces NSAID use and improves grip strength in patients with osteoarthritis of the fingers.[5] Vitamin D greatly decelerated cartilage loss and osteophyte formation.[6] Proanthocyanidin (grape seed extract or Pycnogenol), in doses of 100–300 mg daily has anti-inflammatory effects. Omega-3 oils 2 g daily from fish oil successfully treat rheumatoid arthritis and are moderately helpful in OA.

Niacinamide, a form of vitamin B_3, 250–500 mg q.i.d. has marked, occasionally striking benefits in osteoarthritis.[7] Liver damage is extremely rare. Zinc 30–50 mg, selenium 200 µg, copper aspirinate 2 mg, calcium 1 g, magnesium 400–800 mg, and manganese 10–20 mg should also be included daily.

Biomolecular options. Glucosamine sulfate is an endogenous amino-monosaccharide is an essential substrate for glycosaminoglycans and proteoglycans. These compounds comprise 50 percent of the makeup of hyaluronic acid, a major component in synovial fluid. These compounds function to oppose inflammation and enhance cartilage repair. Numerous controlled studies document reduction in pain, stiffness, and swelling in osteoarthritis, and there is good evidence for enhanced structural repair.[8] Gastrointestinal intolerance, the only reported side effect, is quite rare. A trial of 4–12 weeks is necessary to assess progress. The recommended dose is 500 mg t.i.d. It has become a popular seller in health food stores. Its effect may be enhanced in combination with boron 6–9 mg daily, and marginal added benefit may be seen in combination with chondroitin.

S-adenosylmethionine, an amino acid utilized in cartilage synthesis, has been shown in some studies to be more effective than ibuprofen in treating osteoarthritis. Essential fatty acids omega-3 oils from cold-water fish (salmon, sardines, and tuna) and flaxseed oil, have been effective in treating arthritis.[9] Flaxseed oil should be taken in a dosage of 2 tbsp daily, and is better absorbed if taken with a small amount of cottage cheese. Helpful fish oil doses of EPA and DHA combined range upward from 2 g daily.

Some evidence has been presented demonstrating therapeutic efficacy of hydrotherapy and hot mineral baths, resulting in greater range of movement and decreased use of analgesics. A traditional folk remedy, application of castor oil packs, has little research but fairly wide empirical evidence of benefit when used for several consecutive days. Flannel cloths saturated with castor oil are applied topically over painful areas and affected joints and left in place overnight, or covered with a heating pad for 30–60 minutes at a time once or twice daily.

Botanical options. Among effective herbs are included ginger, which exhibits anti-inflammatory effects, taken as fresh ginger powder 0.5–1 mg daily or as a tea—1 grated tsp of fresh ginger in a cup of hot water b.i.d.; curcumin (*Curcurma longa*), an extract of the common spice, tumeric, which also has anti-inflammatory effects, 400 mg t.i.d.; devil's claw (*Harpagphytum procumbens*) which manifests analgesic and anti-inflammatory properties, 1–2 g t.i.d.; licorice root (*Glycyrrhiza glabra*), exhibiting anti-inflammatory effects in doses of $\frac{1}{8}$ to $\frac{1}{4}$ tsp, of a 5 : 1 solid extract t.i.d. (long-term use may elevate blood pressure); cayenne (capsaicin), which blocks substance P in arthritic joints, available OTC for topical use t.i.d.; boswellin (*Boswellia serrata*) 400 mg t.i.d. for its anti-inflammatory properties; and hawthorn (*Crataegus oxycantha*) 100–200 mg of dried extract t.i.d. for its attribute of maintaining cartilage integrity.

Acupuncture. Traditional Chinese Medicine, using acupuncture and Chinese herbs, can be quite effective. A variety of herbs and oils used in Ayurvedic medicine, include camphor, used as a massage oil, or topical compress over the affected joints, eucalyptus, ginger, and rosemary.

Homeopathy. Remedies more commonly used in homeopathty in 12X to 30C potency, 3–5 pellets q 1–4 h, include *Arnica montana* for soreness and stiffness worse in cold, damp weather, Bryonia for pain aggravated by the slightest movement and cold, Pulsatilla for migratory symptoms relieved by continual movement, and *Rhus tox* for morning symptoms. A homeopathic gel (*Rhus tox, Symphytum officinale, Ledum palustre*) was recently shown to give equivalent benefits to an NSAID gel in knee osteoarthritis.

Manual medicine. Manipulative chiropractic and osteopathic treatment can sometimes be helpful with the soft-tissue component of the process, and body movement therapies such as Feldenkrais, Trager, and Pilates can help to improve mobility and increase range of motion.

Less documented, many practitioners observe benefit deriving from patient use of affirmations, imagery, relaxation, biofeedback, and meditation. The mechanisms involved are yet to be brought to light.

The energy medicine therapies (e.g., healing touch, Reiki, Jin shin jyutsu) may benefit, and a particularly good controlled study documenting very significant benefit of Therapeutic Touch in osteoarthritis of the knee has recently been published.[10]

Rheumatoid Arthritis

■ DESCRIPTION

Rheumatoid arthritis (RA) is a chronic systemic autoimmune disease. The deterioration caused by RA begins with a symmetrical synovitis and joint cartilage erosion. This progresses to a thickening of the membrane resulting from overgrowth of synovial cells and an accumulation of leucocytes. As the disease progresses, the production of excess fibrous tissue leads to pain, swelling, and limitation of joint motion. Fingers, wrists, ankles, and toes are often involved early; in the hands, the distal interphalangeal joints are usually spared. Rheumatoid nodules often develop over affected joints. Morning stiffness is a hallmark. In advanced disease, deformed and gnarled joints are common, especially severe in the hands.

Extra-articular manifestations of the disease can affect the eyes, lungs, heart, and blood vessels. Early in the course of the illness, even before the joints are involved, the patient may be aware of fatigue and weakness, a general malaise, low-grade fever, anorexia, and weight loss. The disease may worsen steadily, but often stabilizes over long periods with little progression.

The diagnosis is made with a typical history and physical examination. Splenomegaly and lymphadenopathy may be present. Rheumatoid factor is positive in about 80 percent of patients, and antinuclear antibodies in 25 percent. An elevated sed rate is common, and thrombocytosis and leukopenia are fairly common. X-rays are usually confirmatory, amd joint fluid usually manifests a high white blood cells (WBC) count and low glucose levels. The diagnostic criteria of the Arthritis Foundation requires 7 of 8 of the following to be present for at least 6 weeks: morning stiffness for > 1 hour; pain on motion in at least one joint; soft tissue swelling in at least one joint; swelling of at least one other joint; symmetrical joint swelling not including the terminal interphalangeal joint; subcutaneous nodules below the elbow; typical radiographic changes; positive rheumatoid factor.

■ PREVALENCE

Rheumatoid arthritis affects between 2 and 3 percent of the American population. Less common and often more disabling than osteoarthritis, the incidence is 3-fold higher in women than men. People in their 30s and 40s are most commonly affected, but RA can begin at any age. It afflicts about 70,000 children each year, with the female to male ratio about 6 to 1.

■ ETIOLOGY AND RISK FACTORS

The precise etiology remains obscure. There are multiple contributing factors for the development of RA. There is strong evidence of a genetic link involving histocompatibility complex class II antigens. Autoimunological factors play a major role, and some authorities think RA may be related to viral or bacterial infections, hormonal imbalances, or disordered permeability of the mucosa of the small bowel. Allergy plays a definitive role in some patients, and psychosocial factors are often cited. Personality traits which have been frequently cited as factors include tendencies to be more compulsive, perfectionistic, over-conscientious, inflexible, rigid, and moralistic. Psychosocial factors also loom large in the total picture. A study of 88 children with juvenile RA found that the odds for coming from a single parent home was $2\frac{1}{2}$ times greater, and the odds of having been adopted was 3 times greater than the incidence in health control children. The social disruptions (divorce, separation, death, or adoption) were associated with onset of the RA 51 percent of the time.[11] Any instance of separation, either real or imagined, may make patients of any age more vulnerable to RA.

■ CONVENTIONAL MEDICAL TREATMENT

Conventional treatment is directed at relief of the pain and stiffness. The severity of symptoms determines the potency of the anti-inflammatory drugs selected. Initial medications most often include aspirin, favoring enteric-coated forms; NSAIDs; and cyclooxygenase-2 inhibitors. Corticosteroids have anti-inflammatory and disease-modifying properties. Side effects include immune suppression, osteoporosis, adrenal suppression, mood changes, weight gain, and edema. Disease-modifying anti-rheumatoid drugs (DMARDS) include injectable and oral gold salts (Ridaura); antimalarials (Plaquenil, hydroxychloroquin); chelating agents (penicillamine); salicylate-sulfonamides (Azulfidine); and immune suppressants (azathioprine, methotrexate, cyclophosphamide). The latter group of drugs can slow the destructive progression of the disease, but can also cause serious and even life-threatening side effects, including nausea, vomiting, and diarrhea; myelosuppression; thrombocytopenia; proteinuria; and hepatotoxicity. Enbrel is a new tumor necrosis factor inhibitor for subcutaneous injection. Early experience with this drug has raised concern about increased susceptibility to infections which may be serious. Zileuton is a 5-lipoxygenase inhibitor for treatment of RA not yet released by the FDA.

Physical therapy is often a helpful option, and surgery may be recommended for the most disabling joint symptoms.

■ **HOLISTIC MEDICAL TREATMENT**

Most patients with RA initially undergo conventional treatment for their disease; consequently, practitioners of holistic medicine usually do not see RA patients in the early stages.

Nutritional treatment. A vegetarian diet eliminating all animal foods including eggs and dairy products is strongly recommended.[12] Omission of wheat, sugar, corn, chocolate, coffee, and artificial food coloring converts this to an elimination diet as well, for the identification of possible food allergens. When an RA patient identifies and eliminates a suspect food or foods, the result is often dramatic.[13] Some practitioners report complete or partial success in up to *50 percent* of patients.

Supplements. Specific nutrients in supplement form are all beneficial. The most important, with daily dosages in parentheses include copper (2–3 mg), omega-3 fatty acids (fish oil and flaxseed oil, 2 g and 2 tbsp, respectively),[14] all antioxidants (see previous), selenium (200 µg),[15] zinc (45 mg), manganese (20 mg).[16] Folic acid 5 mg weekly greatly reduced the toxic effects of Methotrexate (a folic acid inhibitor) without any reduction of the drug's effectiveness.[17]

Two supplements deserve special mention. Gamma linolenic acid from borage or black currant seed oils (500 mg) significantly reduced IL-6, TNF-α and IL-1β, all proinflammatory moities, as well as bringing clinical improvement in one study.[18] In another study which included objective measurements as well as subjective end points, 100 percent of 660 arthritis patients showed some improvement on niacinamide (250–1,000 mg t.i.d.) treatment for a year.[19]

Biomolecular treatment. Glucosamine sulfate, markedly helpful in OA is also moderately helpful in RA. Quercetin stabilizes mast cells (250–500 mg t.i.d.), and bromelain has anti-inflammatory activity when not mixed with food (2,000 mg b.i.d. between meals). Digestive enzymes such as pancreatin have been helpful in treating RA, possibly by mitigating the effects of food allergies (500–1000 mg with each meal).

Herbs. Curcumin (turmeric) is the botanical with the best documentation for treating RA. It is a potent anti-inflammatory (400–600 mg t.i.d.), usually given with bromelain, a pineapple extract. Others include ginger;[20] devil's claw; licorice root; *Panax ginseng* (Asian ginseng, 200–600 mg liquid extract daily), an adaptogen in long-term stress; *Bupleuri falcatum*, a Chinese herb that seems to be as effective an anti-inflammatory as steroids, but without the harmful side effects (2–4 g daily); *Eleuthrococcus senticosus* (Siberian ginseng), another adaptogen (500 mg b.i.d. of solid extract, 1 percent eleuthroside F); hawthorn berries, rich in flavonoids that promote the reconstruction of collagen ($\frac{1}{2}$ tsp or 2 capsules t.i.d.); and horsetail (*Equisitum arvense*) tea (see also osteoarthritis).

Homeopathy. Homeopathic symptomatic remedies commonly used in 12X to 30C preparations include *Rhus toxicodendron* for patients with pain worst in the morning, and in cold and stormy weather; *Bryonia alba* for symtoms that feel worse with any movement and respond to pressure; *Ruta graveolens* if pains are greatly aggravated by exertion and relieved by rest; and *Calcarea carbonica* for arthritis accompanied by great weakness. The optimal utilization of homeopathic remedies depends on constitutional prescribing.

Traditional Chinese medicine. TCM treatment with acupuncture and herbs includes the use of thunder vine (*Triptyrygium wilfordii*), shown to significantly improve stiffness, tenderness, and numbers of swollen joints compared to placebo.[21] Manual therapies including massage also have a place here as well as in OA.

Exercise. Physical movement and exercise are an important part of the global treatment approach. Gentle exercise which can usually be tolerated by most patients includes underwater exercise, stretching exercise, Tai Chi or Qi Gong, and dancing. A recent report documents significant improvement in those who regularly went to the dance floor.

Mental and emotional treatment. Psychotherapy may be very important to identify and release deep-seated emotional issues for RA patients. Those most commonly found include issues of trust, intimidation, self esteem, difficult decision making, and sensitivity to criticism. The benefits of relaxation exercises, affirmations, imagery, and writing about significant previous and present emotional traumas is supported by recently published research.[22] Social support is a factor in functionality and encouragement for maintaining personal contacts is important.

Low-Back Pain

■ DESCRIPTION

Backache is the term used to describe a persistent tenderness, stiffness, and pain in the lumbar spine ranging from mild discomfort to excruciating pain that limits motion. The stiffness generally worsens after prolonged sitting. X-rays usually reveal no abnormality. The diagnosis is made from the history and physical examination, which often reveals excessive muscle tightness and spasm, and significant limitation of flexion, extension and lateral flexion. The most common associations include strains and sprains secondary to overstretching or minor injury; muscle spasms; disc problems ("slipped" discs)—accounting for only 2–4 percent of backaches; and structural problems.

The symptoms of muscle strain and muscle spasm include persistent pain in the lower back, muscle spasms which often follow strenuous activity, stiffness, especially after sitting for extended periods without changes in posture, and limitation of mobility and activity. The normal healing process can take from 2 to 4 weeks in 90 percent of people with backache, but the pain usually starts to decrease after a few days or a week.

Other causes of back pain should be entertained in the differential diagnosis. Sudden severe back pain accompanied by abdominal pain suggests an aortic aneurysm, and unilateral back pain with subcostal referral suggests a renal stone. Persistent focalized pain requires malignancy to be ruled out, and sciatica with loss of motor power in the leg suggests a ruptured disc.

■ PREVALENCE

About 80 percent of all Americans will suffer from low-back pain at some point in their lives. Backache becomes more common between the ages of 30 and 50 as the intervertebral discs lose some of their ability to absorb shock, and backs become more unstable from inactivity. The United States National Center for Health Statistics says that back pain is the fourth most common chronic ailment, the sixth most common reason for visiting an emergency room, and accounts for 13 million visits to primary-care physicians' offices each year. Back pain is responsible for 60 million lost work days each year, which in turn costs the economy $5.2 billion.

■ ETIOLOGY AND RISK FACTORS

Physical causes include lifting heavy objects improperly, e.g., moving too quickly or awkwardly; poorly conditioned muscles (both back and abdominal) due to lack of exercise and flexibility;[23] excessive exercise; postural problems and leg length discrepancy; prolonged standing, insufficient arch support, and inappropriate footwear, such as high heels; obesity and pregnancy; inadequate support from a soft mattress; uncomfortable workstations, such as chairs with improper support or working under an automobile or with heavy equipment; nutritional deficiencies, especially low-protein and magnesium intake (diuretics used to treat hypertension lower magnesium); constipation; and congenital abnormalities predisposing to instability such as a transitional articulated sixth lumbar vertebra.

Mental and emotional factors loom large in the admixture of predisposing factors. Psychologists find the most common emotional issue contributing to backache is fear, involved with questionable ability to provide for life's necessities, inability to stand up for oneself, and discomfort in occupying one's home. Also related are issues around blame, guilt, money, sex, power, and control. The pain tolerance in those with intense emotional experience and depression is always significantly lower. Back pain is highly significantly related to unsatisfactory interpersonal relationships in social and work settings.[24] Those with less education are also at higher risk.[25]

■ CONVENTIONAL MEDICAL TREATMENT

X-rays and CT scans help to rule out destructive bone lesions, herniated discs and severe osteoarthritis. Once the diagnosis of chronic low-back pain has been made, bedrest and severe limitation of activity are usually prescribed for up to 48 hours. Other recommendations include sleeping on the back with a large pillow behind the knees or on the side with the pillow between the knees; ice to the affected area for the first 2 days, applied hourly for 20 minutes at a time to help decrease swelling and pain followed after 48 hours with moist heat (heating pad, hot bath, or shower) to help relax muscles and decrease spasm; gentle stretching to the point of tolerance (no pain). It is very important for patients to listen to their bodies and not over-stretch. The intensity of the stretches may be very gradually increased daily until a return to full motion (or even better motion than originally) is attained. If patients are impatient with this healing process, muscles may be re-injured. Physical therapy is commonly prescribed. The measures usually include strapping and taping to reduce motion, bracing, hot and cold packs, and therapeutic exercise.

Pain medications usually prescribed include: Tylenol, 1 or 2 extra strength 500 mg tablets, q.i.d. (maximum 8 per day); aspirin, 1 to 2 tablets q4h; ibuprofen (Advil, Nuprin, Motrin), 200 mg tablets, 2 tablets, t.i.d. to q.i.d.; or naproxen sodium (Aleve), 220 mg, 1 tablet, b.i.d. to t.i.d. The Tylenol has fewer potential side effects than the other medications but may not provide as much pain relief. For short periods of time, all of these medications are relatively safe. The exceptions are for persons with stomach ulcers, kidney, and liver problems. None of them should be taken with alcohol, including the Tylenol. Muscle relaxants offer some benefits, which are usually modest: Flexeril, Norflex, Parafon Forte, Robaxin and Soma. Drowsiness is a problem with some of these prescriptions.

Injections of local anesthetics and saline into muscle trigger points frequently give temporary and sometimes long-lasting relief.

It can be important to address, ergonomics of workstations, and proper instruction for lifting and carrying.

■ HOLISTIC MEDICAL TREATMENT

In *acute* back pain, a number of options are helpful. Vitamin C, L--carnitine, and coenzyme Q_{10} reduce the degree of subtle muscle injury and pain following overuse. Bromelain, a pineapple enzyme extract, 500 units t.i.d. reduces inflammation. Herbs with benefit are ginger, 100 mg b.i.d. (can also be used topically massaged into the back); white willow bark (a natural aspirin-like compound) $\frac{1}{2}$ to 1 tsp t.i.d.; and cramp bark (*Viburnum opulus*) relieves muscle tension and spasm, $\frac{1}{2}$ to 1 tsp t.i.d. or used topically as a massage vehicle. Feverfew and valerian, previously discussed, also offer relief. Herbs have practically no adverse gastrointestinal effects compared to standard analgesics. St. John's wort, taken orally or topically in appropriate preparations, helps with the commonly associated depression. Soft-tissue injections of Sarapin (North American pitcher plant, *Sarracenia purpurea*), 2–15 cc into multiple painful muscles and trigger points) has a local anesthetic effect which lasts up to 3 weeks and gives superb relief from acute and subacute pain of muscular origin.[26]

Homeopathic remedies having demonstrable benefits include Arnica as a topical preparation or for oral ingestion (markedly beneficial in sprains and strains and superficial trauma); rhus tox; and ruta graveolens. Aconite can be taken when the pain comes on suddenly or in cold or dry weather.

Osteopathic or chiropractic manipulation is frequently prescribed or chosen by the patient. Some studies show significant success with manipulation,[27] while others conclude the benefit is marginal.[28] Benefit from prolonged repeated or prophylactic manipulative treatment has not been documented. Research and experience with acupuncture as treatment is encouraging.[29,30]

In *chronic* low-back pain, additional approaches supplementing the acute care plan include addition of vitamins B_1 50 mg, B_6 50 mg and B_{12} 0.25 mg daily with NSAIDs was significantly better than NSAIDs alone, and NSAID dosages were reduced.[31] In patients with chronic pain, molybdenum 0.5 mg daily reduced pain and improved general perception of health far better than placebo.[32] Weight loss is important in overweight patients (see Chapter 13). Muscle spasm is much more common in patients with depleted levels of calcium and magnesium. This is particularly important for patients who have episodes of sudden onset of back spasms, or who commonly have muscle cramps when inactive or settling into bed for sleep.

Physical therapy performed by highly skilled personnel involves heat, ice, ultrasound, electrical stimulation, and other modalities. They appear to help symptomatically. Improving the structural alignment of bones and joints and the strength of muscles, ligaments, tendons, and fascia is an essential component of the holistic treatment for chronic back pain. A series of treatments by osteopathic physicians or chiropractors. Approaches which appear to be most helpful are myofascial release, craniosacral osteopathy, Feldenkrais training, Trager® psychophysical integration, the Alexander technique, Rolfing structural integration, and Pilates. These approaches usually combine hands-on treatment and instruction from the practitioner for exercises to be done by the patient at home.

Yoga has demonstrated remarkable success in both treating and preventing chronic low-back pain, and can safely be encouraged. Patients can begin with a class, a book, or a videotape. Stretching exercises also bring about improvement. Aerobic and resistance exercise to strengthen specific extensor back muscles shows great promise.[33] Brisk walking, swimming, or any other gentle form of aerobic exercise is routinely recommended.

A series of intravenous injections of colchicine injections for resistantly painful spinal and disc disorders appeared to achieve a high degree of success in a series of 6,000 patients. One to 2 mg, diluted to 10–15 cc with calcium gluconate, sodium salicylate, or saline, is administered 2–3 times weekly for 3–6 weeks. Good, sometimes dramatic, success was reported, apparently due to the anti-inflammatory activity of colchicine.[34] Acu- puncture appears to be helpful for both acute and chronic back pain. It may offer substantial and long-lasting relief, and often works well in combination with structural approaches.

Hot baths with mineral salts or therapeutic oils such as cha- momile, marjoram, lavender, or a combination of wintergreen, camphor, and eucalyptus have some tradition of helpfulness. If the patient with back pain does not sleep well, experimentation for the mattress giving the greatest comfort is to be encouraged. Soft mattresses and water beds are usually not helpful.

The relaxation afforded with consistent practice of progres- sive relaxation, autogenics, biofeedback, and meditation is always beneficial. Health practitioners will have greater success with patient motivation to practice these skills when working with people in groups. Affirmations and an optimistic attitude are associated with success. It is supremely important to address underlying unresolved psychological issues. Proactive treatment by practitioners who have an acute interest in these initiatives is always rewarding.

Energy medicine, using healing or therapeutic touch, Reiki, or more advanced techniques can be helpful in treating chronic low-back pain. Patients can make their own judgment of efficacy after a small number of treatments.

Osteoporosis

■ DESCRIPTION

Osteoporosis literally means "porous bones." In this process, bone loses density, becoming fragile and brittle due to progressive demineralization. Bone mass reaches its maximum in women at age 30–35, but by the age of 55–70, the average woman will have lost 30–40 percent of her bone mass. The most rapid rate of bone loss occurs in the first 5 years after menopause. The rate of loss then slows to about 1 percent each year. Men generally have bone loss beginning in the 70s.

Osteoclasts function to remove damaged or weak bone tissue, and osteoblasts function to build new bone. When the equilibrium of these two opposing functions tilts toward osteoclastosis, bone mass declines. Estrogen slows osteoclastosis, while progesterone stimulates osteoblastosis. Testosterone stimulates osteoblastosis in men. Calcitonin, produced by the thyroid gland, helps maintain levels of calcium, contributing to bone formation. Besides calcium, bone synthesis also requires adequate amounts of magnesium, phosphorus, manganese, zinc, copper, boron, strontium, and silicon, plus vitamins A, C, D, E, K, B_6, and folic acid. Physical stresses on bones, caused by gravitational pull and muscle contraction are also necessary. Integration of all these factors is required for maintenance of bone mass.

The most common clinical sign of osteoporosis is loss of height. In the extreme, the partial compression of vertebral bodies can lead to the so-called dowager's hump and compensatory posturing of the lumbar spine with pain. There may be no warning signs at all until relatively minor trauma causes a fracture, most often a Colles' fracture of the wrist, or an intertrochanteric fracture of the femur.

Comparative height measurements are the simplest clinical way to make the diagnosis, and patients can be encouraged to do this for themselves. A loss of $\frac{1}{2}$ in. from one's usual height is significant, and should trigger the ordering of bone densitometry. Dual photon absorptiometry is the most accurate measure of mineral density of bone. Standard X-rays detect osteoporosis only after a 25 percent loss of bone mass. Multiple sites may be screened; the lumbar vertebrae are the best single site for measurement.

■ PREVALENCE

Potentially a disabling disease, osteoporosis affects approximately 25 million Americans. It is 8 times more common in women than men. One half of women between the ages of 45 and

75 have some bone loss, and, nearly one-third of all post-menopausal women suffer from serious osteoporosis. Caucasians and Asians are more often affected. Osteoporosis affects more women than heart disease, stroke, diabetes, breast cancer, and arthritis. Incidence of osteoporotic fractures in the United States is the highest in the world. The incidence of hip fractures in women rises steeply after the age of 40, indicating significant bone loss before menopause.

■ ETIOLOGY AND RISK FACTORS

Risks increase with female gender; advancing age; being Caucasian or Asian; family history of osteoporosis; cigarette smoking (decreases both estrogen and progesterone); high dietary intake of sodium, fat, protein, processed food, sugar, alcohol (2 or more alcoholic drinks/day significantly increases risk); ingestion of soft drinks (high in phosphate) and caffeine; inadequate intake of any or many of the essential nutrients mentioned under description; hormonal deficiency (low progesterone is even more significant than low estrogen); exposure to heavy metals (lead, cadmium, tin from tin cans, aluminum), and acid rain (calcium from bone buffers the acidity; insufficient calcium absorption (vitamin D and adequate gastric HCl are necessary for adequate absorption); low body fat; being chronically underweight (reduces progesterone); hyperthyroidism or excessive thyroid medication (may cause excess bone catabolism); nulliparity; broad-spectrum antibiotics (destruction of intestinal flora necessary for vitamin K production); corticosteroid medications (impairs calcium absorption, and inhibits osteoblastosis); renal failure; hyperparathyroidism; Cushing's syndrome; chronic heparin treatment (induces relative vitamin K deficiency); low gastric acidity (leads to poor calcium and mineral absorption); and insufficient weight-bearing and resistance exercise. The latter is the *paramount reason* for the epidemic of osteoporosis in western society.

■ CONVENTIONAL MEDICAL TREATMENT

A calcium-rich diet and calcium supplements are usually recommended. Hormone replacement therapy (HRT) with estrogen (Premarin) or a combination of estrogen and a progestin (Premarin, Provera, Prempro) is standard treatment. Medication is usually continued until age 70 when the rate of bone loss slows. The longer estrogen is taken, the greater the risk of adverse side effects including water retention, increased fat synthesis, uterine fibroids, heart disease, gall bladder and liver disease, stroke, and breast cancer. Recent studies indicate that the benefit of HRT is limited to the first 10 years of treatment beyond menopause. The influence of HRT on reduction of fractures disappears by the age of 80, when the incidence reaches its peak.[35] The significant risk of endometrial cancer can be offset by taking progestins along with the estrogen, but the combination does not appear to reduce the debated risk of breast cancer.[36] Slightly over one-half of women prescribed hormone replacement hormones do not refill their prescription beyond a year. Bothersome side effects apparently explain most of the reticence to continue.

Newer agents include the biphosphonates (Fosamax, Didronel) which promote bone deposition given in 10 mg daily doses; they must be taken with a full glass of water on an empty stomach at least 30 minutes before a meal; side effects are mild and unusual. Another agent, Miacalcin, supplies salmon calcitonin in a nasal spray; lack of widespread use makes conclusive evaluation difficult. Selective estrogen receptor modulators (e.g., raloxifene 60 mg daily) have selective estrogen effects on bone maintenance, but do not target breast tissue and apparently do not increase breast cancer risk. Hot flashes are seen, and clotting abnormalities may occur.

A weight-bearing and resistance exercise program, including walking, jogging, dance, or weight training is commonly recommended.

■ HOLISTIC MEDICAL TREATMENT

Periodic monitoring in a patient whose bone density has been shown to be signficantly below normal for her age, can assess the benefit of any given treatment regimen.

Nutritional and environmental treatment. Highly beneficial is a vegan diet low in animal products (high in phosphorus) and rich in the high calcium foods: whole grain flours (amaranth, carob, cottonseed, garbanzo, quinoa, rice bran, soy); fresh vegetables (collard, kale, lambsquarters, mustard greens, okra, parsley, bok choy); legumes; nuts (brazil nuts, walnuts, almonds, pistachios); seeds (sesame, sunflower, flax); sprouted seeds and beans; soybeans; microalgae; lemon and orange peel; and seaweeds. Nuts and seeds have the highest values of calcium and many other critical minerals, besides supplying fat in its ideal, unsaturated, unoxidized form. For patients who cannot or will not incorporate the whole program, partial compliance is helpful. Alcohol, cigarettes, soft drinks, salt, coffee, and hot spices are all to be discouraged (see foregoing). Spinach, chard, beet greens, chocolate, cranberries, and plums contain not only calcium, but calcium oxalate as well, rendering the calcium nutritionally unavailable. It is also of note that countries with the highest consumption of milk products have the highest incidence of osteoporosis. While cow's milk is a good source of calcium it is often the cause of food sensitivity reactions and contributes to heart disease, diabetes, and other health problems.

Filters (charcoal or reverse filtration types) for water used for drinking and cooking eliminate the risk associated with lead and aluminum. High intake of foods packaged in tin cans increases exposure to tin and lead.

Supplements. The daily intake of β-carotene should be 15 mg; B complex 25–50 mg; folic acid 400 µg; C 1–3 g; D 200–600 IU (greater amount for postmenopausal women); E 400 IU; K 300 µg; calcium 500–1,200 mg (diets low in protein require less calcium); citrate, malate, fumarate, and aspartate forms of calcium are better absorbed than lactates and carbonates); magnesium 500–800 mg; zinc 30 mg; copper 2–3 mg; manganese 15 mg; silicon 1 mg; boron 2–3 mg; and hydrochloric acid (if needed and especially over 70).

Health food and nutrition stores often have combination products with many of these elements. Acidophilus supplements are important after antibiotics.

Biomolecular treatment. Because of side effects, many women dislike taking pharmaceutical hormones. Natural hormonal therapy offers estrogens and progesterone whose molecules are identical to the endogenous hormones, whereas Premarin and Provera are modified molecules. Natural progesterone, available from soybean and wild yam plant sources, appears to be safe and effective in treating and reversing osteoporosis, and better managing PMS and menopause[37] (see Chapter 7). Natural progesterone is available in topical forms (usual dose $\frac{1}{8}$ to $\frac{1}{2}$ level tsp applied to the skin daily. The cream is placed on 7 rotating sites of smooth skin each week. An oral micronized form (10–15 mg daily) is also available. Supplying progesterone to patients who must be on corticosteroids for a variety of reasons will also partially mitigate the degenerative effects of the steroids on bone metabolism.

Natural estrogens from the same vegetable sources, mixed in an 80 : 10 : 10 ratio of estriol : estrone : estradiol can be prescribed through compounding pharmacies. Appropriate doses result in relief from vasomotor menopausal symptoms and vaginal dryness equivalent to the effects from pharmaceutical estrogens. Effects on bone metabolism appear to be similar as well. This combination is informally called triple-estrogen, or tri-est. It can be prescribed in oral form and or can be prepared for topical use. Oral doses range from 2.5 to 5.0 mg daily. Occasional vaginal spotting may occur with the use of this estrogen, but is usually transient. The use of estriol has not been associated with cancer, and may actually reduce the risk of breast cancer.[38]

The ovaries produce small amounts of testosterone and DHEA. The majority of DHEA is synthesized in the adrenal cortex. Both of these hormones promote bone anabolism, and may be deficient in post-menopausal women, especially DHEA.

There is some evidence that replacing DHEA in modest doses after appropriate testing reveals deficiencies may improve bone density.[39]

Wild yam, from which natural progesterone is derived, has value in osteoporosis treatment. Herbs high in calcium and minerals include nettles, parsley, dandelion leaves, kelp, and horsetail. Both hops and sage contain estrogen-like substances which can protect against bone loss. Ipriflavone, a bioflavonoid with phytoestrogenic properties, given 200 mg t.i.d., has been shown to increase bone mineral density 5 percent in 2 years compared to a 3 percent loss in the placebo group.[40] Other phytoestrogens are discussed in Chapter 7.

With a serious approach to homeopathic treatment, an experienced homeopath should be consulted. For acute prescribing, 3–5 pellets of a 12X to 30C potency remedy containing *Calcarea carbonicum*, *Calcarea fluoricum* and silica taken every 1–4 hours would often be given.

Weight-bearing exercise is a quintessential component of treatment. Resistance exercise must involve all major body parts; walking does not prevent cervicothoracic spine bone mineral loss. Walking, jogging, stair-climbing, bicycling, skiing, and weight-training are all beneficial. Thirty to 45 minutes, 3 times a week, or more appears sufficient to make a difference. A recent report documents a highly significant reversal of falling bone densities in osteoporotic patients who danced 3 hours a week.[41] Yoga, also, achieves surprisingly good results.

Osteoporosis is an eminently preventable disease. It will tend to progress insidiously without exercise, regardless of other measures.

REFERENCES

1. Felson DT. The epidemiology of knee osteoarthritis: results from the Framingham osteoarthritis study. *Semin Arthritis Rheum* 1990; 20(3 Suppl 1):42–50.
2. Kerrigan DC et al. High-heeled shoes and knee osteoarthritis. *Lancet* 1998; 35(9113):1399–1401.

3. Redford MG et al. Reversible membranous nephropathy associated with the use of nonsteroidal anti-inflammatory drugs. *JAMA* 1996; 276(6):466–9.
4. Perneger TV et al. Risk of kidney failure associated with the use of acetominophen, aspirin and nonsteroidal anti-inflammatory drugs. *N Engl J Med* 1994; 331(25):1675–9.
5. Flynn MA et al. The effect of folate and cobalamin on osteoarthritis. *J Am Coll Nutr* 1994; 13(4):351–6.
6. McAlindon TE et al. Relation of dietary intake and serum levels of vitamin D to progression of osteoarthritis of the knee among participants in the Framingham study. *Ann Intern Med* 1998; 125(5): 353–9.
7. Kaufman W. *The Common Form of Joint Dysfunction, its Incidence and Treatment.* New York: Hildreth Press, 1949.
8. Drovati A. Therapeutic activity of oral glucosamine sulfate in osteoarthritis: a placebo-controlled, double-blind investigation. *Clin Ther* 1980; 3(4):260–72.
9. Stammers T et al. Fish oil in osteoarthritis. *Lancet* 1989; 2(8661): 503.
10. Gordon A et al. The effects of Therapeutic Touch on patients with osteoarthritis of the knee. *J Fam Pract* 1998; 47(4):271–7.
11. Henoch MJ et al. Psychosocial factors in juvenile rheumatoid arthritis. *Arthritis Rheum* 1978; 21(2):229–33.
12. Seignalet J et al. Diet, fasting and rheumatoid arthritis. *Lancet* 1992; 339(8784):68–9.
13. Darlington LG. Dietary therapy for arthritis. *Rheum Dis Clin North Am* 1991; 17(2):273–85.
14. Kremer JM et al. Fish oil supplements in active rheumatoid arthritis: a double-blind, controlled, crossover trial. *Ann Intern Med* 1987; 106(4):497–503.
15. Poretz A et al. Adjuvant treatment of recent onset rheumatoid arthritis by selenium supplementation: preliminary observations. *Br J Rheumatol* 1992; 31(4):281–6.
16. Simkin PA. Oral zinc in rheumatoid arthritis. *Lancet* 1976; 2(7985):539–42.
17. Morgan SL et al. Supplementation with folic acid during methotrexate treatment for rheumatoid arthritis: a double-blind, placebo-controlled trial. *Ann Intern Med* 1994; 121(11):833–41.

18. Watson J et al. Cytokine and prostaglandin production by mono-cytes of volunteers and rheumatoid arthritis patients treated with supplements of blackcurrant seed oil. *Br J Rheumatol* 1993; 32(2):1055–8.
19. Kaufman W. The use of vitamin therapy to reverse certain conco-mitants of aging. *J Am Geriatr Soc* 1955; 3(11):927–36.
20. Srivastava KC et al. Ginger (*Zingiber officinale*) and rheumatic dis-orders. *Med Hypotheses* 1989; 29(1):25–8.
21. Tao X et al. Effect of an extract of the Chinese herbal remedy *Triptorygium wilfordii* Hook F. on human immune responsiveness. *Arthritis Rheum* 1991; 34(10):1274–81.
22. Smyth JM et al. Effects of writing about stressful experiences on symptom reduction in patients with asthma or rheumatoid arthritis: a randomized trial. *JAMA* 1999; 281(14):1304–9.
23. Anderson B. *Stretching*. Bolinas, CA: Shelter Publications, 1980.
24. Spengler DM et al. Back injuries in industry: a retrospective study: III. Employee-related factors. *Spine* 1986; 11(3):252–6.
25. Deyo RA et al. Psychosocial predictors of disability in patients with low back pain. *J Rheumatol* 1988; 15(10):1557–64.
26. Rask MR. The omohyoideus myofascial pain syndrome: report of four patients. *J Craniomandibular Pract* 1984; 2(3):256–62.
27. Meade TW et al. Low back pain of mechanical origin: randomised comparison of chiropractic and hospital outpatient treatment. *BMJ* 1990; 300(6737):1431–7.
28. Cherkin DC et al. A comparison of physical therapy, chiropractic manipulation and provision of an educational booklet for the treatment of patients with low back pain. *N Engl J Med* 1998; 339(15):1021–9.
29. Gunn CC et al. Dry needling of muscle motor points for chronic low-back pain: a randomized clinical trial with long-term follow-up. *Spine* 1980; 5(3):279–91.
30. Coan RM et al. The acupuncture treatment of low back pain: a ran-domized control stury. *Am J Chin Med* 1980; 8(1–2):181–5.
31. Vetter G et al. Shortening diclofenac therapy by B vitamins. Results of a randomized double-blind study, diclofenac 50 mg versus diclofenac 50 mg plus B vitamins, in painful spinal diseases with degenerative changes. *Z Rheumatol* 1988; 47(5):351–62.
32. Moss M. Effects of molybdenum on pain and general health: a pilot study. *J Nutr Environ Med* 1995; 5(1):55–61.

33. Leggett S, Mooney V, Matheson LN et al. Restorative exercise for clinical low back pain. A prospective two-center study with 1-year follow-up. *Spine* 1999; 24(9):889–98.
34. Rask MR. Colchicine use in 6,000 patients with disk disease and other resistantly-painful spinal disorders. *J Neurol Orthop Med Surg* 1989; 10(4):291–8.
35. Felson DT et al. The effect of postmenopausal estrogen treatment on bone density in elderly women. *N Engl J Med* 1993; 329(16):1141–6.
36. Colditz GA et al. The use of estrogen and progestins and the risk of breast cancer in postmenopausal women. *N Engl J Med* 1995; 332(24):1589–93.
37. Lee JR. Osteoporosis reversal with transdermal progesterone. *Lancet* 1990; 336(8726):1327.
38. Lemon HM. Consideration in the treatment of menopausal patients with oestrogens: the role of estriol in the prevention of mammary carcinoma. *Acta Endocrinol Suppl* 1980; 94(Suppl 233):17–27.
39. Labrie F et al. Effect of 12-month dehydroepiandrosterone replacement treatment on bone, vagina, and endometrium in postmenopausal women. *J Clin Endocrinol Metab* 1997; 82(10):3498–3505.
40. Maugeri D et al. Ipriflavone treatment of senile osteoporosis: results of a multicenter, double-blind clinical trial for 2 years. *Arch Gerontol Geriatr* 1994; 19:253–63.
41. Kudlacek S, Pietschmann F, Bernecker P et al. The impact of a senior dancing program on spinal and peripheral bone mass. *Am J Phys Med Rehabil* 1997;76(6):477–81.

11

Chapter Eleven

Genitourinary and Men's Diseases

Benign Prostatic Hypertrophy

■ DESCRIPTION

Benign prostatic hypertrophy (BPH) is an enlargement of the prostate occurring with advancing age. The most common symptoms are increased daytime urinary frequency, nocturia, urgency and hesitancy with urination, a reduction in the force and caliber of urination, and a sensation of fullness in the bladder after urination due to incomplete emptying. The diagnosis is made by the suggestive history and confirmed by digital rectal examination.

Further information may be obtained by ultrasound examination and the prostate-specific antigen (PSA) blood test. Normal levels of PSA are less than 4 ng/mL, and elevated levels suggest prostate hypertrophy, prostatitis, or prostate cancer. Levels above 10 ng are suspect for cancer. Higher levels of the free PSA subfraction favor benign disease.

■ PREVALENCE

Benign prostatic hypertrophy is experienced by nearly 30 percent of men in the United States at age 50, 50 percent of men at 60, and almost 80 percent of men over 70.

■ ETIOLOGY AND RISK FACTORS

After the age of 50, free testosterone levels in the blood begin to decrease, while testosterone levels within the gland are increasing and conversion to the more potent compound dihydrotestosterone is accelerated. This leads to more rapid cell replication and eventual prostate enlargement.

The increased uptake of testosterone by the prostate also appears to result from action by prolactin, synthesized and secreted by the pituitary, and by estrogen, whose levels slowly increase with aging. Prolactin also increases the activity of the 5-α-reductase, the enzyme converting testosterone to dihydrotestosterone. Estrogen also appears to inhibit metabolic degradation of dihydrotestosterone, leading to higher levels.

Since alcohol, especially beer, and emotional stress increase prolactin levels, both may be significant contributors to causing BPH.

■ CONVENTIONAL MEDICAL TREATMENT

Depending upon the degree of symptomatology, primary-care physicians and urologists elect to treat men with BPH with pharmaceuticals, surgery, or "watchful waiting." In one recent study of 600 men with BPH who were treated with the latter approach, only 10 percent requested further treatment as the study was completed. Patients had learned to control many of their symptoms simply by limiting intake of liquids and bladder irritants (e.g., caffeine, alcohol) before bedtime. Regular ejaculations (cf. 3 times a week) also helped bring relief. The drug most often currently prescribed is Proscar, an inhibitor of 5-α-reductase. Some recent clinical studies have shown it to be only marginally effective. Proscar also causes impotence in about 4 percent of men who take it and decreases libido in 7 percent. Hytrin, Minipress, and Cardura are α_1-blockers which are also used. There is evidence that these drugs not only relieve symptoms, but also modestly slow the progression of the hypertrophy. They also may produce side effects such as dizziness and fatigue because of their tendency to lower blood pressure, and the manufacturers warn of the possibility of impotence. Flomax, an α_{1A}-blocker, may offer some advantages with greater specificity for prostatic action, and less effect on blood pressure. If symptoms progress in spite of drug treatment, transurethral resection (TUR) of the prostate may be suggested. Although the risk of incontinence is greater with surgery than it is with drug treatment, the relief from symptoms is greater. This surgical option, which results in a significant incidence of incontinence and impotence, should be reserved for men whose symptoms are not well managed medically. Nonetheless, 350,000 TURs are performed by urologists each year in the United States.

A relatively new procedure, transurethral microwave therapy, utilizes microwaves to accomplish destruction of periurethral tissue to enlarge the prostatic urethral channel. Another new therapy is transurethral hyperthermia which uses a series of heat treatments to shrink hyperplastic tissue. Longer term use will be needed to fully appreciate the place of these treatments in the armamentarium.

■ HOLISTIC MEDICAL TREATMENT

The dietary initiatives which have value in preventing and managing BPH emphasize avoidance of coffee, caffeine, refined carbohydrates, foods high in fat, alcohol, spicy foods, and avoiding smoking and nicotine as well. These nutrients and substances increase free-radical populations, requiring greater amounts of vitamins C and E, and zinc, which are all essential components of prostatic tissues and are essential in the formation of seminal fluid. Consumption of a whole foods, organic-sourced fruit, vegetable, and whole grain diet will supply more essential minerals since organic soils are not mineral depleted. Fresh, raw, pumpkin seeds (high in zinc and essential fatty acids, EFAs) are of benefit. Nuts, seeds, and whole grains are high in zinc, and all nuts and seeds, and their oils contain high amounts of mixtures of omega-3 and omega-6 oils. A high ratio of omega-3 to omega-6 oils is preferred for anti-inflammatory benefits; cold water fish (salmon, sardines, mackerel), flaxseed oil, and soybeans, are especially high in the omega-3 EFAs.

EFAs and zinc are particularly helpful in reducing the size of an enlarged prostate. Omega-6's can both increase inflammation of the prostate (prostatitis) by increasing pro-inflammatory prostaglandins. Six capsules daily of omega-3 fish oil or flax oil is a therapeutic level. Six 1,000 mg capsules of flax oil is equivalent to 1 tbs. Since the typical American diet is zinc-deficient, men usually need supplements in the form of zinc picolinate 15–60 mg per day. Zinc intake should not exceed 100 mg daily. Zinc deficiency can be assessed with a simple inexpensive liquid oral zinc sulfate/hydrate taste test. The test, called Zinc Tally, is available through Metagenics of Eugene, OR. Since zinc and copper compete for assimilation from the intestine, 2–4 mg of copper should be taken as a supplement as well at a different time of day. In addition to the above, the following daily intakes are also quite important: vitamin C 2 g t.i.d.; vitamin A 5–10,000 IU; β-carotene 10,000–15,000 IU; vitamin E 400 IU b.i.d. as natural D-α-tocopherol; vitamin B_6 100 mg b.i.d. (both B_6 and vitamin E can reduce prolactin levels); B-complex "50" (50 mg each element); magnesium 500 mg; copper 2–4 mg; selenium 200 µg; and amino acids (glutamine, alanine, and lysine) 500 mg each in divided dosages between meals.

Frequency, urgency, and dysuria may also be due to food sensitivities, even in the face of little to no anatomical obstruction. It is more common in those with other allergic symptoms (history of hay fever, asthma, eczema, urticaria). It should be considered in any patient whose symptoms seem to be in excess of physical findings, and who do not respond well to various therapies. In 900 patients refractory to conventional treatment, 73 percent of patients improved after elimination of suspect foods. When food elimination trials, detailed elsewhere, lead to elimination of offending foods and most symptoms, happy is the patient.[1]

Emptying the prostate through frequent ejaculation appears to reduce the incidence of prostate cancer (see Chapter 3) and may be important in preventing BPH. Prostatic massage has been often used by urologists as an effective therapy for relieving pressure and discomfort due to BPH. Patients undertaking frequent pubococcygeus muscle contractions accomplish some of the same effect.

Serenoa repens, an extract of saw palmetto berries, has been extensively researched; the liposterolic fraction inhibits the action of types 1 and 2 5-α-reductase in the conversion of testosterone to dihydrotestosterone, restraining the hyperplasia.[2] This action appears to be due to opposition to estrogen effects, and the reduction of dihydrotestosterone and epidermal growth factor is particularly marked in the periurethral tissues, the zone of the prostate most closely related to urethral obstruction. Its action is similar to that of Proscar but without reports of impotence or significant side effects. The clinical results are markedly positive and are usually realized after 2–3 months of treatment. The recommended dosage for a standardized liposterolic extract of saw palmetto berries containing 85–95% fatty acids and sterols is 320 mg daily in divided doses. 160 mg daily has some utility in preventing BPH.

Powdered bark of the tree *Pygeum africanum* has been shown to promote the regression of symptoms associated with BPH, with practically no reported side effects.[3] The most active principal is beta-sitosterol which, in addition to anti-inflammatory effects, appears to modulate age-related hypercontractility of the detrusor muscle. Objective measures of improvement exceed those for Serenoa. An extensive meta-analysis cites some studies reporting an effectiveness ratio of Pygeum to placebo of 91 to 4 percent. Recommended dose is 50–100 mg b.i.d. of an extract standardized to contain 14 percent triterpenes and 0.5 percent docosanol. Many health food stores currently have products that combine saw palmetto and *Pygeum africanum*. *Urticae radix* (stinging nettle) is useful in improving urinary flow in early stages of hypertrophy. The dosage is 4–6 g daily in divided doses.

Symptomatic homeopathic remedies that are often used include *Chimaphila umbellata* for bladder retention with BPH; Pareira for retention and painful urgency; *Thuja occidentalis* for BPH with an abnormal stream and Conium for BPH with a sensation of perineal heaviness and accompanied by premature ejaculation.

Again, comprehensive constitutional prescribing requires professional homeopathic expertise.

Physical activity and deliberate aerobic exercise are associated with a lower incidence of BPH and a decreased spectrum of symptoms. Excessive sympathetic tone contributes to increased prostatic smooth muscle tone and prostatic symptoms. Consistent aerobic exercise decreases sympathetic tone and one study has reported a 25 percent lower incidence of BPH, symptomatic BPH, and surgery for BPH in the top exercisers compared to the inactive sedentary patients.[4]

Prostatitis

■ DESCRIPTION

Prostatitis is an infection and/or inflammation of the prostate seen in three forms:

1. bacterial prostatitis—an infection of the gland that causes swelling;
2. non-bacterial prostatitis—swelling of the prostate without an infection;
3. prostadynia—an uncomfortable irritation of the prostate without infection or swelling

Symptoms of chronic prostatitis, which can be intermittent and can range from mild to severe, include pain or tenderness in the area of the prostate which might extend into the genitals; groin discomfort and lower back pain; difficult, frequent, and urgent urination; dysuria; a discharge from the penis after bowel movements; pain following ejaculation; and depression.

With chronic prostatitis, often undiagnosed and untreated because care is not sought, there is an increased risk of transmitting the infection to a sexual partner, as well as more severe complications such as nephritis, epididymitis, and orchitis. Other potential sequellae are bladder obstruction and prostate stones.

The prostate gland is also susceptible to acute infection or inflammation. An acute infection is noted by severe pain and tenderness in the area of the prostate, at times extending into the genitals, pelvis, and back. Fever, chills, and extreme fatigue are often present.

■ PREVALENCE

Abacterial prostatitis is usually seen in men between the ages of 20–50. Bacterial prostatitis is more common in men 70 and older.

■ ETIOLOGY AND RISK FACTORS

Bacterial prostatitis is due to bacterial invasion, resulting from a weakened immune system; depletion of prostatic glandular elements such as zinc, ascorbic acid (vitamin C), and proteolytic enzymes; increased amounts of sexual activity, particularly with multiple partners, which depletes the prostate of zinc and enzymes (both zinc and proteolytic enzymes function to sterilize the urethra and protect the gland from infection). Excesses of caffeine, alcohol, and spicy foods also contribute to a lack of glandular nutrition that ultimately adds to depletion of the prostate and reduced immune function. Bacteria in the urethra can invade the prostate, and retrograde urethral infection is thought to occur. Chlamydia, an intracellular parasite transmitted through sexual contact, is thought to be a common cause of prostatitis.

The cause of non-infectious or inflammatory prostatitis is unknown but may be an autoimmune disorder, resulting from a depleted glandular environment. Although it is a frequent but usually unconscious contributor to each of the men's health conditions discussed in this chapter, shame is an emotional factor contributing to prostatitis.

■ CONVENTIONAL MEDICAL TREATMENT

Medical treatment for both acute and chronic prostatitis consists almost exclusively of antibiotics. The most commonly prescribed drugs for chronic prostatitis are Bactrim and Septra, carbenicillin, Lorabid, and the quinolones (Cipro, Floxin, Noroxin). Four to 6 week regimens are often prescribed. For acute prostatitis, penicillins and occasionally parenteral aminoglycosides may be used. Mycoplasma and chlamydial organisms may be treated with macrolides (erythromycin, Biaxin, Zithromax). The acute condition usually responds well to the medication, but relapses in both acute and chronic situations are common. In a high percentage of cases, however, bacteria are not the primary cause of the symptoms, and may have only been an innocent bystander which is recovered on culture.

■ HOLISTIC MEDICAL TREATMENT

Dietary recommendations include creating a less acidic and therefore less irritating urine by avoiding spicy foods, caffeine, and acidic drinks like orange juice. Drinking copious amounts of water is also essential.

Zinc is an essential mineral for healthy prostate function, suggested doses 30–60 mg daily. One suggested regimen for zinc in treating chronic prostatitis is 150 mg daily for 2 weeks, followed by 30 mg daily. Doses above 100 mg daily should not be given long term. For reasons cited above, copper should also be supplemented.

Although it is commonly used for BPH, *Pygeum africanum* is also effective in treating chronic prostatitis. Recommended dose is 50–100 mg twice a day of a standardized extract. The standard course of treatment is 3 months; mild gastrointestinal discomfort is the only reported side effect. The evergreen plant, pipsissewa, is especially effective for chronic prostatitis. It helps provide the prostate and urinary tract with increased blood flow and nutrition. Horsetail (*Equisetum*) is a botanical used in the treatment of acute prostate infection. *Serenoa repens* (see foregoing) enhances blood flow and nutrition to the prostate: 160 mg of the standardized extract b.i.d. *Echinacea angustifolia*, an effective herbal anti-infective, can be a valuable part of the treatment program for both acute and chronic prostatitis: 2–4 mL of (1 : 5) tincture t.i.d., or

150–300 mg of powdered extract (3.5 percent echinacoside). Cernilton, a flower pollen extract has been moderately effective in resistant cases: 2 tablets t.i.d.[5]

Aerobic exercise, as detailed under prostate hypertrophy, reduces adrenergic nervous system activity. It is also helpful in preventing recurrent prostatitis by reducing obstructive symptoms, increasing blood flow and improving immunity. With acute prostatitis, jarring activity, and bicycle riding are discouraged. Swimming, walking, and yoga are reasonably gentle forms of exercise that are helpful.

As with BPH, emptying the prostate with ejaculation appears to be helpful in chronic prostatitis. Ejaculation should be avoided in early stages of acute prostatitis. Prostate massage in chronic infection is commonly done in urologic practices.

All previously discussed approaches to relaxation reduce sympathetic tone and improve prostate and urethral function. The tension and anxiety associated with stress in all its forms, and indeed the stress of serious urinary symptoms, is diminished in patients who practice meditation, biofeedback, progressive relaxation, yoga, and self-hypnosis. Persistent non-resolving symptoms may warrant locating an experienced therapist who can assist in dealing with past and present emotional issues, including those of unrecognized shame associated with past conditioning.

Impotence

■ DESCRIPTION

Impotence is defined as the inability to sustain a satisfactory erection to perform intercourse and ejaculation. Impotence may be the health problem that is most disturbing to men and for this reason might possibly be one of the most well-researched problems in medical science.

■ PREVALENCE

Impotence may well be the most common chronic condition afflicting men, with estimates of incidence as high as 30 million. Before Viagra, only about 200,000 men per year sought medical attention for this condition. Fifty-two percent of men 40–70 are thought to have some degree of impotence, and 85 percent of men over 70 have unsatisfactorily firm erections.

■ ETIOLOGY AND RISK FACTORS

The publicity surrounding Viagra uncovered a new epidemic. The majority of men believe impotence is a natural consequence of aging but, in fact, a man's physiological ability to have erections continues into his 80s and 90s. Masters and Johnson, authors of *Human Sexual Response,* found couples in their 80s who were still enjoying regular sexual intercourse. However, older men who had not been sexually active for a number of years, often due to the death of a spouse, were frequently impotent if they entered into a new relationship. As men age, the amount and force of ejaculation decreases, and the recovery time between ejaculations becomes longer, but the physiologic ability to have erections is still present.

Factors that contribute significantly to this epidemic in men of all ages are listed below.

Certain drugs, especially antidepressants, antihypertensives, anticholinergics, antihistamines and tranquilizers, tend to cause or intensify impotence. Alcohol and drug addiction amplifies chronic impotence even though many men who frequently drink or use drugs can be sexually active when they are under the influence, and become impotent when sober. Vascular disease, including diabetes and atherosclerosis reduce the blood supply to the penis, reducing the chance for normal function. High cholesterol is an issue; levels are positively correlated with impotence. Adequate testosterone levels not only contribute to normal libido but adequate erections as well. Since zinc appears to be important in synthesis and release of testosterone, low zinc intake can be problematic. Hypothyroidism and deficient anterior pituitary function also contribute to impotence. Neurological conditions, including multiple sclerosis, Parkinson's disease, and paraplegia also contribute.

Impotence most often results from a multitude of emotional causes, so-called psychogenic impotence. Self-esteem of many men is related to their ability to perform. Even one failure in sexual intercourse can be devastating and can lead to performance anxiety on the next occasion. Subsequent sexual encounters can create a downward spiral with more anxiety and less ability to perform, which eventually results in chronic impotence.

Although performance anxiety is often cited as the leading emotional cause of sexual dysfunction, other uncomfortable emotions can also cause a bout of impotence. Often ignored by men, these include fear of intimacy, guilt, shame, depression, and boredom. In *You Can Heal Your Life,* Louise Hay lists the probable emotional causes of impotence as "sexual pressure, tension, guilt; spite against a previous mate; and fear of mother."

In the first days of life, the majority of males were traumatized by circumcision. The resulting emotional wound is often much deeper than most men perceive. From childhood, most men were aware that their penis was the body part most associated with shame and had to be shielded from exposure. The unconscious awareness of the disparity of shamefully hiding the penis and yet having it as a major representation of power becomes a conflicted message which raises the psychological doubt which contributes to impotence. Impotence is truly a symptom of an imbalance or disease of mind, emotions and body that is not addressed by Viagra.

■ CONVENTIONAL MEDICAL TREATMENT

In 1998, Viagra (sildenafil) became one of the most publicized drugs in recent history. In its first year of availability, more than a million prescriptions for Viagra were written. It is the first pharmaceutical found truly effective in treating erectile dysfunction. It inhibits phosphodiesterase type 5, increasing levels of cyclic guanosine monophosphate, relaxing the smooth muscles which permit inflow of blood to the penis. The drug enhances the ability to achieve and maintain an erection with sexual stimulation.

The drug appears to offer substantial improvement in function in 60–90 percent of patients. It works best in men whose impotence is milder and whose basis is psychological or drug-effect-related. In men whose impotence is related more to physiological causes, it is not as successful. This would include men whose circulation is compromised with arteriosclerosis, men with diabetes, and men after prostate surgery.

Viagra is contraindicated in men taking nitroglycerin or nitrates for angina. The most common side effects are severe headache, skin flushing, indigestion, diarrhea, nasal congestion, urinary-tract infections, and abnormal vision (a bluish tint that can diminish sight by up to 50 percent and last up to 6 hours). Although no deaths have been conclusively shown to be related to the drug, enough doubt about complications has arisen that a number of foreign nations have banned its sale.

Prior to Viagra, drug treatment involved papaverine, or prostaglandin E-1 administered through self-injections into the penis. A urethral prostaglandin urethral suppository and an elastic device placed at the base of the penis to restrict blood outflow were also available.

Surgery for relief of erectile dysfunction has taken the form of penile revascularization, using a branch from an abdominal artery for a fresh blood supply. Some success in up to one-third of operations has been reported. Implantation of a penile prosthesis has also been offered to men with this diagnosis. Vacuum erection devices, available from urologists, are used to assist men who have trouble initiating or sustaining erections. Once the penis is erect, an elastic band at the base of the penis restricts blood outflow to maintain the erection.

■ HOLISTIC MEDICAL TREATMENT

Testosterone tends to be low in men with deficient zinc intake, and conversely, zinc supplements raise levels of testosterone.[6] It has also been shown that adequate zinc diminishes synthesis and release of prolactin from the pituitary, resulting in higher testosterone levels. The dosage of zinc is 30–60 mg a day along with copper 2 mg a day not taken together. Beta-carotene, 25,000 IU daily, vitamin C 3 g daily in divided doses, magnesium 500 mg daily, and omega-3 essential fatty acids are also important. Lycopene, another carotenoid found in red fruits and vegetables, such as tomatoes and watermelon; and arginine, an amino acid (found in nuts and animal meats) which improves circulation by enhancing nitric oxide, are also helpful.

The hormone DHEA has been successfully used in treating impotence. Blood levels should be first assessed to determine deficiency.

Yohimbine, from an African tree, heightens potency and maintains erections by increasing blood flow to the penis. Unlike Viagra, it does so by increasing the release of norepinephrine, which is also essential for erections.[7] A 1971 review of 10,000 men with impotence found 80 percent good to excellent results.[8] Yohimbine can potentially increase heart rate, raise blood pressure, and cause anxiety, hallucinations, headache, and skin flushing. The dose is 100 mg daily, although strength may vary with products of different concentrations.[9] Other herbs and supplements that can also contribute to enhanced sexual potency are: Damiana (*Turnera diffusa*), 2–4 mL or 60 drops daily, is an aphrodisiac long used by indigenous peoples which has not been researched; *Ginkgo biloba*—40 mg of a standardized extract 3x/day increases circulation; Ashwagandha, an Ayurvedic herb, 300 mg daily; *Panax ginseng*, endocrinological stimulant, 100 mg of a standardized extract b.i.d.; and Siberian ginseng, an adaptogen for stress, 400 mg of a standardized extract t.i.d. *Muira puama* (potency wood) from a Brazilian shrub, given in doses of one to 1 to $1\frac{1}{2}$ g daily, resulted in 50 percent significant improvement in erectile dysfunction after 2 weeks.

Physical exercise markedly enhances sexual performance and satisfaction, but systematic use of exercise for treatment of impotence has not been extensively studied. Homeopathic remedies and acupuncture have both been used to treat impotence.

After all physical causes for impotence have been ruled out, referral to competent therapists has moderate success in encountering and modifying beliefs, attitudes, and feelings adverse to full enjoyment of sexual activity, usually found to be rooted in past conditioning. Establishing greater intimacy, touching, and emotional closeness in non-sexual ways usually is helpful. Men are usually reluctant to acknowledge and discuss the problem; when they are willing to take some risk and discuss their impotence with their spouses or partners, the result is nearly always beneficial.

REFERENCES

1. Champault G et al. A double-blind trial of an extract of the plant *Serenoa repens* in benign prostatitis hyperplasia. *Br J Pharmacol* 1984; 18(3):461–2.
2. Powell NB et al. Allergy of the lower urinary tract. *J Urol* 1972; 107(4):631–4.
3. Berges RR et al. Randomised placebo-controlled, double-blind clinical trial of beta-sitosterol in patients with benign prostatic hyperplasia. *Lancet* 1995; 345(8964):1529–32.
4. Platz EA et al. Physical activity and benign prostatic hyperplasia. *Arch Intern Med* 1998; 158(21):2249–56.
5. Buck AC. Treatment of prostatitis and prostadynia with pollen extract. *Br J Urol* 1989; 64(5):496–9.
6. Prasad AS et al. Zinc status and serum testosterone levels of healthy adults. *Nutrition* 1996; 12(5):344–8.
7. Reid K et al. Double-blind trial of yohimbine in treatment of psychogenic impotence. *Lancet* 1987; 2(8556):421–3.
8. Margolis R et al. Statistical summary of 10,000 male cases using Afodex in treatment of impotence. *Curr Ther Res Clin Exp* 1971; 13(9):616–22.
9. Susset JG et al. Effect of yohimbine hydrochloride on erectile impotence: a double-blind study. *J Urol* 1989; 141(6):1360–3.

10. Waynberg J. Aphrodisiacs: contribution to the clinical validation of the traditional use of *Ptychopetalum guyana*. First International Congress on Ethnopharmacology, Strasbourg, FR, Jun 5–9, 1990.

11. White JR et al. Enhanced sexual behavior in exercising men. *Arch Sex Behav* 1990; 19(3):193–209.

12

Chapter Twelve

Vision Problems

Macular Degeneration

■ DESCRIPTION

The macula is the center of retinal vision for fine detail. Its yellow-ish hue arises from a high concentration of cells containing the yellow carotenoid pigments lutein and zeaxanthin. Degeneration of the macula results from free-radical damage, leading to the deposition of lipofucsin, in turn causing macular extrusions (drusen) which distort and dim the vision. The degenerative process is always well under way before any symptoms become apparent. The diagnosis is usually made by an ophthalmologist or optometrist at the time of an examination for a perceived need for lens correction. Earliest symptoms begin with the onset of subtle blurring in vision required for reading. Distortion of images or complaints of a dark spot in the central visual field are common.

■ PREVALENCE

Approximately 200,000 Americans suffer from blindness due to macular degeneration. It is the second most common reason for loss of vision in older people. A striking 30 percent of those over age 75 have some degree of macular degeneration. About 20,000 new cases of macular degenerative blindness are thought to occur yearly.

■ ETIOLOGY AND RISK FACTORS

Contributing factors include advanced age, atherosclerosis, excessive ultraviolet light exposure, smoking, and a high saturated fat diet. Deficient intake of carotenoids lutein and zeaxanthin are calculated to increase risk over 40 percent, and deficient intake of lycopene (another carotenoid) increases risk over 50 percent. There is a weak association with high alcohol intake.

■ CONVENTIONAL TREATMENT

There is no standard treatment for the atrophic form of macular degeneration which makes up 95 percent of all cases. Five percent of the problem presents as a "wet" neovascular form, treated very successfully by laser photocoagulation, especially when discovered in the earlier stages.

■ HOLISTIC TREATMENT

Nutrients

Nutrient sources of antioxidants are known to delay, halt, or reverse the degeneration. The most important vitamins are the carotenoids (lutein, zeaxanthin, lycopene, and beta carotene), riboflavin, C and E. Selenium, manganese, zinc, and copper are essential critical minerals. Of all these, lutein appears to be the most essential.[1]

The best food sources for the essential carotenoids are:

1. *Lutein and Zeaxanthin*: kale, collard greens, spinach, Swiss chard, mustard greens, red pepper, okra, romaine lettuce, parsley, dill, celery, fruits, carrots, tomatoes, corn, potatoes, egg yolks, paprika.
2. *Lycopene*: tomatoes, tomato juice, tomato catsup, watermelon, guava, pink grapefruit, dried apricots, green peppers, carrots.

3. *Beta carotene*: sweet potatoes, carrots, apricots, spinach, winter squash, collard greens, canned pumpkin, cantaloupe, Swiss chard, parsley.

The degree of macular degeneration is inversely correlated with the intake of fruits and vegetables. High on the list of desirable fruits are those with intense red, blue and purple colorings, containing high amounts of anthocyanidin bioflavonoids, including blackberries, raspberries, blueberries, huckleberries, and plums.

Supplements

In one study, daily intake of a combination of vitamins C 500 mg, E 400 mg, β-carotene 45,000 IU, and selenium 250 µg reversed or halted the visual decline in 60 percent of patients with macular degeneration.[2] Supplements of lutein (dosage 30 mg daily) derived from palm oil appear to be better absorbed than synthetic forms. Vitamin A intake is inversely correlated with the degree of macular degeneration.[3] Patients taking 80 mg of zinc for 1–2 years preserved their vision 42 percent better than those taking placebo. Zinc actually improved vision in a small percentage of subjects.[4]

Botanicals

Ginkgo biloba extract 80 mg b.i.d. for 6 months achieved significant improvement in distance vision scores.[5] Ginkgo improves circulation to the eye and brain.

Proanthocyanidins are potent bioflavonoids which have shown beneficial effects in macular degeneration.[6] Bilberry (*Vaccinium myrtillus*) 80 mg t.i.d. (25 percent anthocyanidin content) and grapeseed extract (*Vitis vinifera*) 150–300 mg/day (95 percent procyanidolin content) also restrain progression of the degeneration and have been clinically used with impressive success by holistic practitioners. Anthocyanidins, the key flavonoids, have potent antioxidant qualities.

Non-specific General Management Options

In addition to the specific biochemical, nutritional, and botanical options in preventing and delaying macular degeneration, all generic measures for neutralizing free-radical proliferation and slowing progression of or reversing atherosclerosis mentioned elsewhere are helpful, including exercise, avoidance of toxins from the environment, and adequate management of stress.

Active smoking and passive smoke exposure need to cease, and control of blood pressure is essential. Protection from excessively long hours of bright sunlight should be undertaken, particularly for those exposed to light reflection off snow and water, and those living in climates with long hours of bright sunlight for great portions of the year. In these situations, sunglasses which filter out 98 percent or more of the ultraviolet spectrum may be necessary.

Cataracts

■ DESCRIPTION

The cloudy, opaque degeneration that occurs in the crystalline lens of the eye in aging persons is called cataract. Ordinarily clear, the lens deteriorates as a result of dehydration and synthesis of polyols by the enzyme aldose reductase. Like macular degeneration, cataracts are moderately well under way before symptoms are noticed, and most diagnoses are made during routine eye examinations.

■ PREVALENCE

Cataracts are the leading cause of blindness in the US. Four million Americans experience visual impairment from cataracts and of these patients, 40,000 are legally blind. Medicare costs for surgical lens replacement total 3 billion dollars a year.

■ ETIOLOGY AND RISK FACTORS

The clouding of the lens of the eye is, in great part, the result of degeneration secondary to damage by free-radical proliferation.

Contributing factors are diabetes, toxic exposures such as cadmium (2- to 3-fold higher in cataracts compared to normal lenses; tobacco is a major source of cadmium), excessive ultraviolet and near-ultraviolet light exposure, smoking (2- to 3-fold excess risk), side effects of medications (long-term use of corticosteroids is hazardous), deficiency of antioxidants—vitamins A and E, carotenoids, and selenium (levels of selenium in the aqueous humor are 60 percent lower in people with cataracts), low superoxide dismutase levels (a major endogenous antioxidant enzyme), and depleted zinc (90 percent lower in cataracts compared to healthy lenses), copper (90 percent lower), and manganese (50 percent lower).[7]

■ CONVENTIONAL TREATMENT

Lens replacement surgery is highly successful, resulting in preservation of vision for millions of people. Surgery restores vision to its previous norm in over 98 percent of cases.

■ HOLISTIC TREATMENT

Nutrition

Higher intakes of fruits and vegetables with high antioxidant nutrient content are correlated with protection against cataracts. Foods which appear to be the most important are leafy greens (especially spinach), tomatoes, peppers, melons, cruciferous vegetables (broccoli), and citrus fruit.[8] Yams, carrots, and other highly colored yellow vegetables and fruits containing carotenoids are also important.

Supplements

Many studies document a 25 percent lower risk of cataracts in people who take multivitamins and minerals. The risk reduction from antioxidants is greatest in smokers. Validated case reports have documented partial regression of cataracts in 5 months of treatment with high supplemental doses of antioxidants.[9] Women taking supplements of vitamin C (250–1,000 mg/day) for 10 years or more reduced risk of cataract formation by 77 percent compared to non-supplementing women.[10] Epidemiological studies indicate that subjects with highest versus lowest intakes of: vitamin E reduced risk of cataract development 50 percent;[8] and mixed carotenoids 40 percent.[11] Beta carotene appears to act as a filter against light-induced damage to the fibrous part of the lens.[12]

Riboflavin up to 15 mg/day is beneficial.[13] Also extensively used with benefit are pyridoxine 50–80 mg; folic acid 400 µg; selenium 200–600 µg; calcium 500–1,000 mg; the bioflavonoid quercitin 400 mg t.i.d. a.c.; and amino acids methionine 500 mg b.i.d. and cysteine 500 mg t.i.d.

Biomolecular Options

Melatonin neutralizes hydroxyl radicals and inhibits cataract development in animals. The incidence of cataracts in humans increases with age, matching the decrease in melatonin levels with increasing age.

Botanicals

Reasonable doses for botanicals reported in research are bilberry 80 mg t.i.d. (25 percent anthocyanidin content) taken with vitamin E, grape seed extract 150–300 mg daily (95 percent procyanidin content), and Pycnogenol (pine bark extract) 30 mg q.i.d. or 85 mg b.i.d.

Glaucoma

■ DESCRIPTION

The cornea and lens of the eye have no blood supply. Nutrients are assimilated through the aqueous humor, a thick, clear liquid that is secreted into the central chamber of the eye. As it slowly circulates, the aqueous humor supplies nutrients and removes waste products, discharging them through the sponge-like connective tissue network of collagen around the margin of the eye, to then be absorbed into the blood stream. Damage to the collagen, the most abundant protein in the body, obstructs the egress of aqueous humor from the eye, increasing the pressure within the eye—the central problem in glaucoma. Glaucoma is usually diagnosed during a routine eye examination occasioned by the need for new prescription lenses. In early stages, glaucoma is usually totally asymptomatic. With the passage of time and increased pressures, chronic open-angle glaucoma manifests in gradually compromised peripheral vision, marked by blind spots, usually affecting both eyes.

Ocular pressure is measured by instrumentation or by digital palpation. Early diagnosis is important, since prompt treatment forestalls visual deterioration. Primary-care physicians can make testing for eye pressure a regular part of an interval examination, referring to ophthalmologists those whose pressure is borderline or elevated. People over 65 should have a screening examination every 2 years; African-Americans should be routinely screened after age 40.

A more rare condition, acute or closed-angle glaucoma, is heralded by severe pain of sudden onset, nausea, vomiting, one-sided presentation, blurring of vision, the impression of a halo effect around images, cloudiness of the cornea, redness of the eye and pressures over 40 mmHg. Acute glaucoma threatens sudden loss of vision and constitutes an emergency.

■ PREVALENCE

Two million Americans are thought to have glaucoma. The increased intraocular pressure of glaucoma in about a quarter of this group goes unrecognized, undiagnosed, and untreated. Glaucoma is the third leading cause for vision loss in aging people following cataracts and macular degeneration. The incidence in the elderly population is estimated to be about 3 percent.

■ ETIOLOGY AND RISK FACTORS

The immediate cause of increased intraocular pressure is free-radical-mediated deterioration of the sponge-like collagenous connective tissue which gradually obstructs the egress of aqueous humor from the eye. The obstruction results in a rise in pressure within the eye, leading to a subtle distortion of the eye globe itself, in which visual images fail to focus on the retina, causing blurred vision. The increased pressure also damages the functional parts of the visual apparatus. Normal intraocular pressures are 10–21 mmHg; with onset of chronic closed-angle glaucoma, pressures can be up to 40 mmHg.

The following contribute to risk for glaucoma:

1. Genetic factors.
2. Side effects of antihistaminic, anti-inflammatory steroid, and antihypertensive drugs.
3. Heritable diseases involving errors of collagen metabolism including Marfan's syndrome and osteogenesis imperfecta.
4. Diabetes and hyperglycemia.
5. Food sensitivities.
6. Being over 65.
7. Being African-American.
8. Severe myopia.
9. Sedentary deconditioning syndrome.
10. Stress. Increased stress and intense emotional experiences entrain increases in intraocular pressure. Conspicuous rises in pressures have been documented by initiating a discussion of a glaucoma patient's significant personal conflicts.[14]

■ CONVENTIONAL TREATMENT

Topical treatment includes α-agonists (lopidine), non-cardio-selective β-blockers (timolol, carteolol, metipranolol), cardioselective β-blockers (Betopic S), sympathomimetics, cholinesterase inhibitors (demecarium), carbonic anhydrase inhibitors, (brinzolamide), miotics (carbachol, pilocarpine), and prostaglandin agonists (latanoprost). Significant amounts of the topical agents are absorbed systemically, and the drug literature warns of possible respiratory and heart reactions, especially in those with asthma and arrhythmias, as well as local ophthalmic reactions. Bronchospasm, cardiac failure, hypotension, arrhythmias and other reactions are all reported. Beta blockers should be withdrawn slowly before any general anesthetic. Systemic agents for oral use include beta blockers, carbonic anhydrase inhibitors (diamox), and vasoconstrictors, the latter for use in acute closed-angle glaucoma. Occasionally, when medical management fails, conventional or laser surgery may be necessary.

■ HOLISTIC TREATMENT

Nutrition

Fruits and vegetables are indicated, supplying a variety of antioxidant, vitamin C, and bioflavonoid nutrients. Fish meals supply a high amount of salutary omega-3 fatty acids.

Supplements

1. A 1960s study documented an average fall of 16 mmHg in eye pressures after treatment with a daily dose of vitamin C of 200 mg per pound of body weight.[15] A recent study reaffirmed the same effect: addition of vitamin C to bowel tolerance levels (2–9 g daily) reduced pressures an average of 5.6 mmHg, or 28 percent.[16]
2. Addition of 240 mg of magnesium daily reduced intraocular pressures in glaucoma subjects 10 percent, while improving the visual field.[17]
3. Chromium deficiencies have been correlated with increased pressures. Addition of chromium (200–1,000 μg/day) often improves blood sugar control.
4. In animal studies, intraocular pressures are cut in half with the addition of fish oil to food intake and human studies likewise document substantial falls in pressures.[18] Omega 3 oils 2 g b.i.d. or flaxseed oil 1 tbs daily are reasonable doses.

Food Allergens

Elimination of food allergens accomplished through elimination and rechallenge trials has successfully lowered pressures in selected patients. In susceptible people, up to a 20 mmHg rise in pressure has been demonstrated following exposure to known allergenic foods.[19]

Exercise

Mean fall in pressures from 23 to 19 mmHg has been documented in sedentary glaucoma subjects following 12 weeks of regular aerobic exercise.[20]

Biomolecular Options

Two hundred to 500µg of melatonin in the evening decreases intraocular pressures about 10 percent through the rest of the night.[21] Intraocular pressures are 25 percent higher in people with hypothyroidism; they fall to normal when an appropriate dose of replacement thyroid or synthetic thyroxin (synthroid) is reached.[22]

Botanicals

Bioflavonoids from food and herbs containing anthocyanidins maintain capillary integrity, and stabilize the strength of collagen tissues by preventing free-radical damage and forming more cross-linked bonds within the protein matrix. Bilberry is outstanding in this regard.[23] Rutin, a citrus bioflavonoid, has been shown to lower pressures in patients unresponsive to medications alone.[24]

Stress Management

Regular relaxation practice and/or meditation, as well as regular aerobic exercise apply here as in most diseases. Both lower the toxic effects of stress and contribute to falls in free-radical populations. A degree of detachment from intense emotional and sympathetic nervous system responses to stressful situations insulates patients from the worst of the tension-related ocular pressure-raising mechanisms. Falls in intraocular pressures following disciplined practices of relaxation, biofeedback, and meditation are frequently great enough to be able to reduce medication or stop it altogether. Lower doses of topical and systemic medications reduce the risk for untoward side effects.

REFERENCES

1. Seddon JM et al. Dietary carotenoids, vitamins A, C, and E and advanced age-related macular degeneration. *JAMA* 1994; 272(18):1413–20.
2. Schalch W. *Free Radicals and Aging.* Boston: Birkhauser Verlag, 1992:1–10.
3. Goldberg J et al. Factors associated with age-related macular degeneration. An analysis of data from the first National Health and Nutrition Examination Survey. *Am J Epidemiol* 1988; 128(4):700–10.
4. Newsome DA et al. Oral zinc in macular degeneration. *Arch Ophthalmol.* 1988;106(2):192–8.
5. Lebuisson DA, Leroy L, Rigal G. Treatment of senile macular degeneration with *Ginkgo biloba* extract. A preliminary double blind drug vs. placebo study. *Presse Med* 1986; 15(31):1556–8.
6. Corbe C et al. Light vision and chorioretinal circulation: study of the effect of procyanidolic oligomers. *J Fr Ophthalmol* 1988; 11:453–60.
7. Swanson AA et al. Elemental analysis in normal and cataractous human lens tissue. *Biochem Biophys Res Commun* 1971; 45(6): 1488–96.
8. Tavani A et al. Food and nutrient intake and risk of cataract. *Ann Epidemiol* 1996; 6(1):41–6.
9. Ahlrot-Westerlund B. Remarkable success of antioxidant treatment [selenomethionine and vitamin E] to a 34-year old patient with posterior subcapsular cataract, keratoconus, severe atopic eczema and asthma. *Acta Ophthalmol (Copenh)* 1988; 66(2): 237–8.
10. Jacques PF et al. Long-term vitamin C supplement use and prevalence of early age-related lens opacities. *Am J Clin Nutr* 1997; 66:911–16.
11. Hankinson SE et al. Nutrient intake and cataract extraction in women: a prospective study. *BMJ* 1992; 305(6849):335–9.
12. Burton G. Beta carotene: an unusual type of lipid antioxidant. *Science* 1984; 224:569–73.
13. Prchal JT et al. Association of presenile cataracts with heterozygosity for galactosaemic states and with riboflavin deficiency. *Lancet* 1978; 1(8054):12–13.
14. Ripley HS. Life situations, emotions, and glaucoma. *Psychosom Med* 1950; 12(4):215–22.

15. Virno M. Oral treatment of glaucoma with vitamin C. *Eye Ear Nose Throat Mon* 1967; 46:1502–8.

16. Boyd HH. Eye pressure lowering effect of vitamin C. *J Orthomolec Med* 1995; 10(3–4):165–8.

17. Gaspar AZ. The influence of magnesium on visual field and peripheral vasospasm in glaucoma. *Ophthalmologica* 1995; 209(1)11–13.

18. Cellini M et al. Fatty acid use in glaucomatous optic neuropathy treatment. *Acta Ophthalmol Scand Suppl* 1998; (227):41–2.

19. Raymond LF. Allergy and chronic simple glaucoma. *Ann Allergy* 1964; 22:146–50.

20. Passo MS. Exercise training reduces intraocular pressure among subjects suspected of having glaucoma. *Arch Ophthalmologica* 1991;109(8):1096–8.

21. Samples JR et al. Effect of melatonin on intraocular pressure. *Curr Eye Res.* 1988; 7(7):649–53.

22. Centanni M et al. Reversible increase of intraocular pressure in subclinical hypothyroid patients. *Eur J Endocrinol* 1997; 136(6): 595–8.

23. Blumenthal M, ed. *The Complete German Commission E Monographs*. Boston. Integrative Medicine Communications, 1998.

24. Stocker FW. New ways of influencing the intraocular pressure. *NY St J Med* 1949; 49:58–63.

13

Chapter Thirteen

Systemic Diseases

Obesity

■ DESCRIPTION

In obesity, excess fat is distributed throughout the body, including increased deposition under the skin and in most of the internal organs. Two recognized patterns are seen: the android, "apple" pattern, with weight predominantly carried in the chest and waist, more commonly seen in men, and the gynecoid, "pear" pattern with fat distribution predominant in the low abdomen, buttocks and thighs, more common in women. Higher risks for a number of diseases are associated with the android pattern. Most often, an individual carrying the weight at age 60 comparable to that at age 20 has lost lean muscle mass and gained fat. In the United States, a mean of 4 percent of muscle mass is lost during each decade from age 25 to 50, and 10 percent each decade thereafter.

Obesity is diagnosed when patients are above the norms on weight/height tables, by above-normal measurements of abdominal girth, by the use of a body mass index chart, or by measures of excess content of body fat. The latter is and inexpensively done by measuring with a calipers the skin-fold fat layers, from which ideal weight can be determined from a standard chart. Body fat content can be determined, also, by weighing on a scale incorporating bioelectrical impedance

Excessive weight gradually leads to mild dyspnea, decreased stamina and increasing difficulty in managing the activities of daily living. Complications of obesity include higher incidence of some cancers (liver, gall bladder, colon, rectum, prostate, breast, uterus, urinary tract), hypertension, cardiovascular disease (myocardial infarction, strokes, sudden death events, poor leg circulation), type 2 diabetes, gout, gall bladder disease, hernias, intestinal obstruction, arthritis of weight-bearing joints, poor wound healing, excess risk of childbirth complications, sleep disorders, excess risk of injury and falls, respiratory disease susceptibility, and up to 20 percent shortening of lifespan.

■ PREVALENCE

Obesity is present in women whose body makeup is over 30 percent fat and men over 25 percent fat. Optimum body constitution is less than 24 percent body fat for women and less than 18 percent for men. Over one-half of American adults are thought to be obese. Since 1980, the incidence of obesity has increased 50 percent in children and 40 percent in teenagers.

■ ETIOLOGY AND RISK FACTORS

The roots of the increasing prevalence of obesity in "advanced" nations lie in a combination of physical, genetic, emotional, and social factors.

In spite of a mean decrease in caloric intake of 40 percent in the last 130 years, the decrease in physical exertion has been even greater, leaving more people overweight. The metabolism of stored body fat is considerably below that of lean tissue. Therefore, the metabolic rate of obese people is well below that of lean people, leading to a vicious cycle which is difficult to break without vigorous exertion.

Compared to the rest of the population, there is evidence that one-quarter of obese patients have to consume 25 percent fewer calories to maintain their weight in spite of adequate physical activity. The reasons for this marked difference in metabolism are thought to be predominantly genetic, including: decreased levels of serotonin, leading to increased hunger and craving for carbohydrate (aggravated by insufficient tryptophan intake); and insulin resistance, aggravated by lack of physical exercise and by increased caloric sources high in sugar, refined carbohydrates and saturated fat, which increase hunger, raise the "set point," and decrease the thermogenic effect of food. Impaired sympathetic nervous system activity also probably leads to decreased thermogenesis, and a lower percentage of brown fat leads to 25 percent higher efficiency in producing energy and heat, leaving a net saving of calories with more calories to go into fat storage. Coenzyme Q_{10} deficiency also appears to be present in up to 50 percent of obese subjects.

Obesity is also more common in hypothyroidism, hypertension, hyperlipidemias, and type 2 diabetes. For unknown reasons, both men and women whose birth weights were over 10 pounds are at significantly higher risk for adult obesity. Food allergies and sensitivities can evoke food craving and an addiction-like pattern. Overeating in these circumstances can often be traced to high intake of foods to which there is an addictive attraction. The most common of these offending foods are milk, wheat and corn—all commonly found in snacks.

Eating may be triggered by conditioning from admonitions in childhood associated with not wasting food, not depriving starving children of food, and cleaning one's plate. Juvenile and adult obesity are much more common in those whose parents used manipulative prompting to control their eating as young children. Emotional factors often associated with overeating include anger, self-hatred, anxiety, and boredom. Overeating is also commonplace as an easy source of pleasure when other sources of pleasure appear to be remote and unachievable.

Food is used everywhere in our society as a centerpiece of many social and business affairs of all kinds in which eating often carries a sense of obligation, and eating is often a reason for coming together. Excess eating is aggravated by intense advertising, and obesity is associated with television watching, contributing to our incredible habits of snacking in the United States, often associated with factors other than hunger.

■ CONVENTIONAL TREATMENT

Conventional management incorporates suggestions for consuming less and increasing exercise. Physicians are often discouraged by the poor success rate of most "diets," and referral to dietitians for nutritional help, or to commercial diet and weight-loss programs is common. About 70 percent of people on these programs initially lose weight, but 95 percent of the time regain it, sometimes becoming heavier than at baseline. Appetite-suppressant drugs are also used; in the 1960s and 1970s, amphetamines were prescribed, but all too often were abused. Amphetamine derivatives including fenfluramine, Bontril and Phentermine were used in the 1980s and early 1990s, but habituation problems were common, and side effects including heart valve abnormalities and pulmonary hypertension were encountered with the "Phen-fen" combination. Olestra—supplying non-assimilable fat—may be helpful in some patients, but may lead to bothersome diarrhea in some, and inhibit antioxidant nutrient absorption. Orlistat, a lipase inhibitor, prevents breakdown and intestinal assimilation of fat. Other drugs used include sympathomimetics, and Meridia, a new neurotransmitter reuptake inhibitor, contraindicated with use of other serotonergic drugs.

■ HOLISTIC TREATMENT

A high fiber intake, encouraging weight loss by accumulating a larger mass of food in the stomach, is commonly emphasized. High fiber, vegetarian, and near-vegetarian diets allow intake of larger quantities of food, and are nearly always helpful. Vegetarian obesity is uncommon. On the other hand, meals with an intake of high glycemic foods, refined carbohydrates, and sugars have been shown to lead to *50 percent greater snacking* in the hours afterward.[1] Guar gum, a derivative of the Indian cluster bean, is a fiber supplement which improves insulin sensitivity. In one study, initial doses of 2 g increased gradually to 10 g of guar gum b.i.d. a.c. achieved a weight loss of about one pound/week, while reducing insulin levels and cholesterol ratios.[2] Other effective individual and combination fiber sources include pectin, glucomannon (from konjac root), barley, and beets.

Medium-chain triglycerides, found in health food stores, have been found to be handled much less efficiently in the body than long-chain triglycerides, wasting 35–50 percent more calories. These triglycerides can be used as oils in salad dressings, or as a supplement taken in 1–2 tbsp amounts daily. This is best combined with a low-animal-fat diet containing small amounts of long-chain triglycerides[3] but should be used with caution in diabetics and those with chronic liver disease.

Overweight volunteers taking 200 µg of chromium picolinate, L-carnitine, and vitamin supplements not only lost about 15 pounds in 8 weeks but increased their metabolic rate.[4,5] Pantothenic acid (vitamin B_5) 2.5 g q.i.d. enabled a group of 100 obese subjects to comfortably tolerate a low calorie diet and lose 2.5 pounds a week over several months with no side effects.[6] 5-Hydroxytryptophan (5-HT), the direct metabolite of tryptophan, is in turn converted to serotonin; higher serotonin levels reduce carbohydrate craving and hunger. 5-HT is available in health food stores: doses of 300 mg t.i.d. in one study afforded a 12 pound weight loss in 12 weeks with marked elimination of excessive hunger, even in the face of caloric restrictions.[7] An appropriate starting dose is 100 mg before meals, increasing after 2 weeks if weight loss is under 1 pound per week. 5-HT should not be taken with SSRIs. Ten to 20 mg of DHEA daily in those who have low DHEA blood levels can contribute to weight loss. In coenzyme Q_{10}-deficient subjects, 100 mg of CoQ_{10} daily achieved a 30 pound weight loss in 9 weeks.[8]

Based on studies which show that excision of or interrupting the autonomic nerve fibers from the interscapular brown fat in animals leads to lowered metabolism and obesity in animals, one human study demonstrated that a daily combination of 30 mg of caffeine, 22 mg of ephedrine, and 50 mg of theophylline (calculated to increase metabolism) led to an 8 percent increase in metabolism and weight loss.[9] Hypertension, headache, and extrasystoles can occur if these minimal doses are exceeded.

Persistent patterns of food cravings, a tendency to consume large quantities of the same foods, or personal or family history of allergenicity, might prompt consideration of a food elimination trial. If elimination of the 8 most likely offenders (bovine milk, wheat, corn, sugar, eggs, chocolate, citrus fruits, and peanuts) for 5 days results in withdrawal symptoms (lethargy, irritability, headache, increased food cravings and other generalized symptoms of distress), each eliminated food should be reinstituted in a pure form, 1 every 3 days, to see if it provokes food cravings. If no withdrawal symptoms whatsoever occur after elimination, food sensitivity/addiction is less likely. If the thought of going a week without even a token amount of frequently consumed foods induces a sense of anxiety, then food sensitivities are more likely. If a food elimination and rechallenge trial gives significant results, proven offenders need to be eliminated or eaten on a limited rotation basis, once every 4–6 days.

Herbs which aid in managing obesity include yohimbine prescribed 15 mg daily in divided doses. Guggul derivatives (*Commiphora mukul*) 2.25 g b.i.d. have been shown to lead to 4 times the weight loss of those taking a placebo.[10] Hydroxycitrate 500 mg t.i.d. from the fruit of the Malabar tamarind (*Garcinia cambogia*) is helpful in reducing food cravings.

Exercise will not burn enough calories to lead to significant weight loss. For example, to lose 1 pound, a patient would have to jog 45 minutes daily. Exercise, however, does greatly increase thermogenesis not only during exercise, but also for up to 4–6 hours after finishing. Most people achieve about a 10 percent weight loss in 6 months with a well-designed aerobic exercise program alone. Aerobic exercise also increases insulin sensitivity and utilization, as well as lowering the "set point." The set point is an internally programmed, probably genetically determined threshold, below which it becomes increasingly difficult to adhere to a "diet" of lowered caloric intake. Therefore, *permanent weight loss almost always requires regular aerobic exercise.* Fidgeting, a manifestation of higher sympathetic nervous system energy, appears to burn an additional 5–700 calories daily.

Professional counseling help may be necessary for the obese, in order to commit to practicing a positive attitude of honoring and caring for the body; evoking motivation to be healthy and as attractive as possible; eating only when hungry; arranging to leisurely eat in pleasant circumstances; moving the body in ways which honor its need for physical activity; forging relationships with supportive people who esteem them no matter what; creating opportunities to experience pleasure without dependence on food; and becoming more aware of emotional eating patterns to gradually shift toward hunger as the major reason for eating. Biofeedback and relaxation procedures may be a helpful part of this process.

Chronic Fatigue Syndrome

■ DESCRIPTION

Chronic fatigue syndrome (CFS) involves severe, at times incapacitating, fatigue. CFS, at one time referred to as "yuppie flu," was first identified in the early 1980s. It was assumed for many years that patients complaining of this syndrome were either depressed or hypochondriacal. With the official adoption of the Oxford criteria in 1988, the Center for Disease Control officially recognized CFS as an actual disease and most physicians now accept CFS as a true illness. It appears that CFS is not a single specific condition, but rather a group of several related conditions, with multiple causes. The diagnosis is made on the basis of the typical symptoms and the exclusion of other ailments that might be causing these symptoms, including hypothyroidism, anemia, Lyme disease, or chronic hepatitis. Symptoms include debilitating fatigue, so severe that activities of daily living such as showering or brushing the teeth may be felt as too strenuous; fatigue unrelieved by rest and sleep; recurrent flu-like symptoms, including low-grade fever, sore throat, enlarged lymph glands, headache, muscle and joint aches; sleep disorder; depression, anxiety, and mood swings; weight loss; exercise intolerance; maladaptive immune response with increased allergenicity and chemical sensitivity; and cognitive dysfunction with poor memory, concentration and analytical thinking, "mental fog," and spatial disorientation.

■ PREVALENCE

CFS is common in America today. About 80 percent of the sufferers are women between the ages of 25 and 45; the majority of them had allergies prior to the onset of CFS. It is so often misdiagnosed that no estimates of its true prevalence can be accurately made.

■ ETIOLOGY AND RISK FACTORS

A definitive cause for CFS has never been determined. First thought to be caused by the Epstein-Barr virus, perhaps the best theory now explains CFS as an immune system disorder. Thus the reference in many cases to CFIDS (chronic fatigue and immunodeficiency syndrome).[11] Many who develop CFS have led overly busy, productive, and often stressful lives. Other common risk factors thought to possibly contribute to the syndrome include a history of a triggering viral infection;[12] recurrent courses of antibiotics, NSAIDs or other medications; chemical exposure or sensitivity to paints, refinishing oils, or other chemicals; inhalant and food allergies and sensitivities; adrenal exhaustion and low DHEA secondary to chronic stress or a serious illness; excessive emotional and work stress; insufficient sleep and relaxation; chronic candidiasis; hypoglycemia; chronic infection—sinusitis, prostatitis, or dental abscesses; subclinical hypothyroidism; sex steroid deficiencies; intestinal parasites; diets with excessive sugar, caffeine, alcohol, and/or chronic nutrient deficiency; toxicity from dental mercury amalgam fillings; and dysbiosis (leaky gut syndrome).

■ CONVENTIONAL MEDICAL TREATMENT

The role of conventional medicine in treating CFS is primarily to rule out treatable conditions, with a detailed medical history and laboratory tests. Once that evaluation is completed and the diagnosis of CFS is made, conventional medicine offers symptomatic relief with analgesics and antidepressants (SSRIs, tricyclics) and to improve sleep and decrease mood swings. Some practitioners prescribe a 6–8 week trial of Zovirax.

■ HOLISTIC MEDICAL TREATMENT

Investigation may include a standard chemistry blood profile, comprehensive digestive stool analysis (e.g., Great Smokies Laboratory, Asheville NC), cortrosyn-stimulated cortisol levels, testosterone, estrogen and progesterone levels, DHEA levels, complete thyroid profile, amino acid determinations, and oral mercury vapor testing. Sources of environmental toxicity need careful consideration.

A balanced, whole foods diet consists of high-nutrient, high-protein, complex carbohydrate foods including organic vegetables (parsley, cabbage, kale, carrots, beets, yams, leafy greens), whole grains, beans, fish, eggs, and poultry, avoiding mercury toxins in fish and antibiotics in poultry. Allergic and sensitizing foods need to be identified and eliminated if found. A rotation diet is recommended in order to minimize low-grade food sensitivities that may trigger symptoms. Sugar, caffeine, milk products, alcohol, aspartame, and refined carbohydrates (white flour, white rice) are discouraged.

Recommended daily supplements include mixed carotenoids, 15–25 mg; vitamin C 2–4 g; vitamin E 4–800 IU; vitamin B-complex (50–100 mg of each B-vitamin);[13] zinc picolinate 30 mg; magnesium glycinate or citrate 5–700 mg;[14,15] calcium citrate-malate 1,000 mg; vitamin D 400 IU; manganese 15 mg; omega-3 fatty acids (600 mg each of EPA and DHA);[16] pantothenic acid 500 mg; acetyl-L-carnitine 1,000 mg initially, later 500 mg;[17] coenzyme Q_{10} 1–200 mg; L-lysine 3,000 mg initially, later 1,000 mg; alpha lipoic acid 300 mg; L-glutathione 100 mg; and NADH (nicotinamide adenine dinucleotide) 10 mg.[18]

Supplements of amino acids found deficient on screening should be provided.[19] Acidophilus and bifidus probiotics are recommended, either empirically, or following stool analysis: $\frac{1}{2}$ tsp of mixed acidophilus/ bifidus in pure water on arising and at h.s. Vitamin B_{12} injections, 2 mg with folic acid, 5 mg, are often given 1–2 times weekly.[20] Gamma globulin injections weekly for several months may be included, and some complementary practitioners empirically use an intravenous "nutrient cocktail" consisting of 2 g of vitamin C, calcium 1 g, magnesium 1 g, and B-complex vitamins.[21]

Herbs used to treat CFS have antiviral and immunoenhancing properties. In the initial acute CFS phase, echinacea 3–325 mg, t.i.d. 3 weeks out of each month,[22] licorice 250 mg t.i.d. (20–28 percent glycyrrhizic acid, contraindicated in hypertension) for up to 2 months; and Lomatium 25–35 drops t.i.d. In the later chronic phase, helpful botanicals are Astragalus membranaceus 150 mg t.i.d.; licorice as above; Siberian ginseng 250 mg t.i.d.;[22] oats (Avena) 500 mg t.i.d.; Ashwagandha root 25 mg t.i.d. (with 1.7 percent anolides, 1.5 percent alkaloids); and Ginkgo biloba 60–100 mg t.i.d. (24 percent ginkgolides).

Hormone treatment may include DHEA, the dose dependent upon results of testing, hydrocortisone up to 20 mg daily if warranted by testing,[23,24] and estrogen, progesterone and testosterone replacement if deficient levels are found.[26]

Candidiasis is often present in CFS and should be treated if suspected or confirmed. If the diagnosis is in doubt, adhering to the anti-candida diet and taking probiotic supplements is still warranted. If parasites are identified, appropriate treatment is necessary.[26] Detoxification, herbal liver function enhancement with silymarin, and leaky gut repair have been well-documented and highly effective treatments for CFS.[27] Insomnia should be appropriately treated (see insomnia, Chapter 8, page 258).

Acupuncture alone or in combination with Chinese herbs has met with success in treating CFS. The treatment is directed towards strengthening the immune system and relieving soreness in the musculoskeletal system.

Walking and mild aerobic exercise is recommended, but exertion must be tailored to avoid any activity that increases fatigue for more than 2–3 hours after exercise. Stretching exercises, yoga, Qi Gong, Tai Chi are often more acceptable to the CFS patient, and breathing exercises are especially helpful since they stimulate lymph flow.

The depression which almost inevitably develops in CFS patients is responsive to a wide variety of cognitive and experiential approaches. Many CFS patients are so severely afflicted that they are forced to slow down, and re-assess their values and priorities, sometimes radically. Support groups are often helpful in chronic conditions. The CFS Association can be reached at (913) 321-2278, or the CFS Society at (503) 684-5261.

Fibromyalgia

■ DESCRIPTION

Fibromyalgia (FM) is a debilitating syndrome that often accompanies chronic fatigue syndrome. Health care costs for people afflicted with this condition average about $10,000 per year, and FM patients are almost 6 times more likely than the general public to apply for disability payments. More than a quarter of FM patients who remain employed report missing more than 120 days of work per year due to their disease.

Major symptoms of fibromyalgia include generalized muscle pain and tenderness, stiffness, and aching, accompanied by significant fatigue. Commonly experienced, also, are disruption of non-REM stage-4 sleep, tension, depression, poor memory and concentration, headache, dizziness, paresthesias, irritable bowel syndrome, irritable bladder, temporomandibular joint symptoms (TMJ), intolerance to cold, immune abnormalities, and allergic reactions to drugs, chemicals, and environmental toxins. Although most common test results are normal, altered levels of serotonin, norepinephrine, and substance P have been found. The American College of Rheumatology has established the qualifying criteria for making the diagnosis: history of generalized pain of ≥ 3 months' duration, present in all 4 quadrants of the body and in and around the spine; *and* pain, not just tenderness, on palpation with a force of 4 kg in at least 11 of 18 trigger points in the musculoskeletal tissues of the neck, shoulder, hip, knee and elbow.

■ PREVALENCE

Fibromyalgia afflicts 3–5 million people in the United States. The incidence ratio for women to men is 10 : 1. Typical age of onset is age 25–50. Fifteen to 20 percent of patients seen by rheumatologists are thought to have FM. Disability claims are 6-fold higher in FM patients compared to the general public. A quarter of FM patients who continue to work miss over 120 days of work each year.

■ ETIOLOGY AND RISK FACTORS

Although the cause of FM is unknown, most of the risk factors are similar to those for CFS. This is true of food allergy and sensitivity (dairy products, wheat, fermented foods, and nightshades—potatoes, tomatoes, eggplant, and peppers), stress, candidiasis, nutritional deficiencies, and adrenal exhaustion. Recent research suggests that damage to mitochondrial energy systems in the mitochondria from free radicals may be the primary cause. Compromised circulation to muscle cells and deficient levels of serotonin may also contribute to FM. The metabolic suppression in muscle cells might possibly be due to the accumulation of phosphate and uric acid. Some uricosuric agents used in gout (Zyloprim) and other drugs that raise excretion of uric acid and phosphate (Probenecid, Sulfinpyrazone, and Robinul) have significantly improved some FM patients. The expectorant Guaifenesin has recently been shown to help FM patients by increasing uric acid excretion. In FM patients, it is now known that the body metabolizes muscle protein excessively rapidly and converts it to glucose for energy. Some authorities believe that this accelerated muscle catabolism may be the cause of the pain, aching, and fatigue. It has been suggested that aluminum toxicity may also play a role.

Almost all FM patients have been overdoers and high achievers, but not balancing their overactive lives with rest and relaxation.

■ CONVENTIONAL MEDICAL TREATMENT

After many years of research, there is still no effective conventional treatment for fibromyalgia. Antidepressants have been used to provide short-term relief for sleep disorders and depression, while anti-inflammatory medications have been used for treating the pain with only fair results. Ruling out rheumatoid arthritis, lupus, and other autoimmune inflammatory conditions with similar symptoms including pain and fatigue is an important part of the diagnostic workup.

■ HOLISTIC MEDICAL TREATMENT

The holistic treatment for FM is similar to that for chronic fatigue syndrome. Additional issues include: magnesium malate 1.2–2.4 g daily,[28] vitamin B_1, and other synergistic nutritional factors are available in a product named Fibroplex, professionally supplied from Metagenics of San Clemente, CA. This supplement improves muscular energy production and accelerates aluminum detoxification. Quintessential nutrients for enhancing mitochondrial electron transport chain energy synthesis include daily acetyl-L-carnitine, L-glutathione, L-lysine, coenzyme Q_{10}, alpha lipoic acid, essential fatty acids, vitamins E and B-complex (especially thiamin), magnesium, manganese, and S-adenosyl-L-methionine 400 mg.[29] 5-hydroxytryptophane 50–100 mg b.i.d. tends to reduce muscle pain and insomnia. Intravenous vitamin and mineral injections described under chronic fatigue syndrome often produce significant improvement, but will usually require 3–4 injections weekly. Trigger point injections, massage therapy, hydrotherapy, biofeedback, electrostimulation, and acupuncture have all been reported to be effective in some patients. Soft-tissue injections of Sarapin, a derivative of the North American pitcher plant, give pain relief for up to 3 weeks at a time.[30] Topical Capsaicin 0.025 percent cream, from cayenne pepper, reduces pain and improves muscle strength.[31] Periodic use of UltraClear or UltraInflam (Metagenics) detoxification programs have been of great benefit to FM patients as a result of their reduction of free-radical activity, repair of leaky gut defects, and enhancement of liver function.[32]

Exercise is an essential part of the treatment program for FM, but impacting activities such as jogging, basketball, and other running sports are contraindicated. Gentler activities including walking, a stationary bicycling, treadmill walking, swimming, Qi Gong, Tai chi, and yoga breathing exercises can all be recommended. It is very helpful for patients to become observant and listen for signals and feedback from their bodies and act accordingly.

Patients receiving massage therapy report less depression, anxiety, pain, stiffness and fatigue, and better sleep. Electro-acupuncture has been reported beneficial, and the use of Rhus tox, a homeopathic remedy reduced the number of trigger points 25 percent in one study.

As with CFS, counseling is often advisable for FM patients. Dealing with depression, relearning the adoption of a healthy balance between activity and rest, and often the need to learn to play may require an insightful counselor who can guide patients to truly modify their worldview.

Fibromyalgia support groups can be located from the Fibromyalgia Network, (602) 290-5508.

Candidiasis (Yeast Overgrowth)

■ DESCRIPTION

Candida albicans infection is recognized conventionally as the offending microorganism in oral thrush, skin rashes, and vaginal infections. Its importance as an overgrowth of normal yeast populations in the intestine is largely rejected as clinically insignificant. Physicians practicing complementary medicine, however, have repeatedly observed significant infections, particularly in patients whose immune systems are overtly or subtly compromised. It is commonly overlooked or misdiagnosed, along with food sensitivity, with which it is not uncommonly inter-related.

Candida species are single-celled fungi that ordinarily exist innocuously in the body, inhabiting the mouth, intestine, vagina, and skin. The only postulated function of *Candida albicans* is to facilitate assimilation of B vitamins.

Widespread inflammation in the small bowel from the toxicity of candida may lead to gastrointestinal symptoms include bloating, diarrhea, constipation, alternating diarrhea and constipation, pruritis ani, flatulence, and cramps. Prolonged yeast overgrowth candida often leads to invasion of the tissues of the gastrointestinal tract, disrupting the normal control of assimilation, allowing incompletely digested food particles, pollens, pollutant molecules, antigenic yeast particles, and even the whole yeast organisms themselves to reach the bloodstream, as a manifestation of the "leaky gut syndrome."[33] Deliberate exposure to a large inoculum of candida organisms has been unequivocally shown to lead to invasion of the blood stream, even in healthy volunteers.[34] Candida organisms themselves are known to release 79 different allergenic proteins. These peptides inhibit suppressor T-cell function and increase antibody production, triggering autoimmune and allergic reactions. Antigenic particles and Candida organisms then tend to colonize sites in the body which are most favorable for growth—most often the moist mucous membranes of the sinuses, respiratory, and female genital tracts. Systemic symptoms from widespread bodily reactions include fatigue, irritability, emotionality, food cravings, headaches, vague malaise, insomnia, muscle and joint aches, recurrent sinusitis, chronic nasal congestion, vaginal itching, recurrent prostatitis, dermatitis, pruritis, and secondary depression.

Yeast organisms reduce the absorption of proteins and minerals, leading to suboptimal enzyme function. A yeast-impaired immune system also has less than the normal tolerance for ordinarily safe levels of common toxins including fumes from petro-chemicals, cleaning fluids, chlorine, and perfumes, in turn leading to increased synthesis of oxygen radicals. Candida organisms also synthesize acetaldehyde. Hepatic conversion into alcohol leads to reduced production of cellular energy, causing disorientation, dizziness, mental confusion, and spaciness often described by patients.

The diagnosis of candidiasis is made by a careful history, culturing of stool specimens done in specialized laboratories, and obtaining candida antibody titers from venous blood samples. Laboratory tests yield about 20 percent false negatives.

■ PREVALENCE

Candidiasis affects millions of Americans, most of whom are unaware that their symptoms, ranging from severe to subtle and vague, are related to the overgrowth of a yeast organism. Candida is kept under control by Lactobacilli and Bifidobacteria which also inhabit the gastrointestinal and genital tracts. These organisms synthesize enzymes and vitamins, fight pathogenic bacteria, and lower cholesterol levels. These organisms also compete with the yeast organisms, consuming them as a food source.

■ ETIOLOGY AND RISK FACTORS

Like most chronic disease, candidiasis usually results from a number of factors occurring simultaneously. In many respects, candidiasis is a 20th century disease, since many of the contributing causes include recent medical and societal factors such as antibiotics, oral contraceptives, environmental pollutants, today's typical high-sucrose, devitalized American diet, and the insidious but ubiquitous presence of unmanaged stress.

The most frequent cause of candidiasis is recurrent or extended use of antibiotics, which kill not only the pathogenic bacteria implicated in the condition for which the antibiotic is prescribed, but also the good bacteria needed to keep candida in check. Broad-spectrum antibiotics are particularly suspect, because their wide bactericidal effects are more likely to deplete the pool of lactobacilli and bifidus. Vaginal candidiasis often occurs soon after women are given antibiotics, for example. The majority of those with chronic sinusitis, who have taken 3 or more courses of antibiotics within a span of 6 months, also tend to harbor an increased population of yeast. Since most antibiotics are administered orally, the friendly bacteria in the intestines are particularly susceptible. Antibiotics are also commonly found in commercially grown meats and poultry, making these foods potential contributors to yeast overgrowth as well.

The prevalence of candidiasis is higher in menstruating women compared to men, children, or non-menstruating women. Progestins, found in most birth control pills and also intrinsically secreted at high levels prior to menstruation, have been shown to stimulate the growth of candida. The combination of high progesterone levels just prior to menstruation and a preexisting excess of candida contributes to particularly severe symptoms of premenstrual syndrome (PMS). The continuous high levels of progesterone in pregnancy also create favorable conditions for candida overgrowth in both the vagina and intestine.

Anything that weakens the immune system can contribute to yeast overgrowth. Cortisone derivatives, often used to treat chronic inflammatory conditions such as asthma, arthritis, lupus, and colitis, are well-known immune suppressants, and have the potential for stimulating yeast overgrowth, actually aggravating the disease for which the cortisone was prescribed. Direct immune suppressants such as methotrexate are also problematic. Chemotherapy and radiation treatments for malignancies also compromise immunity and open the door to candida.

Any medications, such as non-steroidal anti-inflammatories, that potentially cause gastrointestinal ulcerations or inflammation and weaken the lining of the gut can allow candida to displace normal friendly intestinal bacteria. Candida organisms thrive in a pH of 4 to 5. H_2 antagonists, such as Tagamet and Zantac, reduce acidity and increase gastric pH, creating a more optimal environment for candida proliferation.

Environmental toxins and chemicals such as pesticides, herbicides, solvents, paints, formaldehyde, fossil fuel combustion products (sulfur and nitrous oxides), and heavy metals such as lead, cadmium, arsenic, mercury, aluminum, and nickel can also weaken the immune system. People with occupational exposure to these substances are at higher risk for candidiasis. Most urban Americans are living in the polluted environment in which they experience exposure to these toxins.

A diet high in sugar and high glycemic foods is a major contributor to candidiasis. Candida organisms flourish on the high sugar content of the typical American diet. While candida thrive on it, sugar compromises phagocytosis.[35] It is therefore not surprising that diabetes is also a predisposing factor to candidiasis. Other risk factors for candidiasis include alcohol, food and inhalant allergies, chronic viral infections, amebiasis and giardiasis, physical trauma, adrenal dysfunction, hypothyroidism, and intrinsic deficiencies in gastric hydrochloric acid, pancreatic enzymes, and bile.

Unmitigated effects of excessive stress compromise immunity directly[36] as well as indirectly through the downstream effects of increased levels of corticosteroid production.[37]

■ CONVENTIONAL MEDICAL TREATMENT

Due to the unreliability of the currently available diagnostic tests, the majority of physicians do not believe candidiasis is a widespread problem. Notwithstanding, a number of powerful systemic antifungal drugs have reached the market in the last decade, facilitating the treatment of candidiasis. The systemically acting antifungal medications, such as Nizoral, Diflucan, and Sporanox, are usually required in moderately and severely afflicted individuals. Periodic liver function tests should be done to monitor the low risk of liver toxicity. Nystatin, long available for limited treatment of vaginal and intestinal candidiasis, is still widely used, though less effective on systemic disease.

■ HOLISTIC MEDICAL TREATMENT

The foregoing broad spectrum of risk factors requires a multi-faceted approach in treatment. For a successful outcome, patient commitment to dietary and lifestyle changes is required. When yeast overgrowth is confined only to the gastrointestinal tract or vagina, the treatment can be shorter and less complicated. In systemic cases, however, where yeast toxins or organisms have spread throughout the body, treatment protocols lasting up to a year may be required. The comprehensive holistic approach consists of four components: depopulating the candida overgrowth; eliminating the principal substrate for the growth of candida with appropriate diet; restoration of normal bacterial flora in the bowel; and restrengthening of the immune system.

During systemic treatment, the addition of 420 mg daily of milk thistle (silymarin), a hepatoprotective herb, will also mitigate risk.[38] A far more common side effect of the systemic drugs is a Herxheimer reaction, or "die-off" effect, in which a flood of candida toxins and allergens is released as the organisms are destroyed. Patients should be warned about the possible increase in candida-related symptoms, including fatigue, headaches, nausea, loose stools, or flu-like aches and pains. Using smaller initial doses of systemic drugs, increasing intake of distilled or filtered water, using water enemas, and taking vitamin C and ibuprofen all help to relieve this cataract of increased symptoms. This exacerbation of symptoms with treatment is actually confirmatory for the diagnosis. Systemic drug treatment should be continued for 4–6 weeks, in doses of 200 mg daily. Tapering doses at the end of the course of treatment also seems to be helpful. Nystatin may be adequate for limited infections, and should also be started with minimal doses and tapered at the close of treatment.

For patients who are unable to afford these drugs or who cannot take them due to potential side effects, a number of other options are available, although none works as quickly or effectively. Commonly available in health food stores are OTC homeopathic remedies and other products, including Yeast Fighters, Candida Cleanse, Cand-Ex, Caprystatin Yeast Defense, Cantrol,

Caprylic acid, garlic, and pau d'arco, acting either directly on candida or indirectly by strengthening the immune system. Also available are products which combine yeast suppressants with the probiotics acidophillus and bifidus. The herbal formula Intestinalis (available for physicians from BioNutritional Formulas at 800-950-8484) can treat both candida and some parasites. Two other effective products available through physicians are Candicin (from Metagenics) and SF 722 (from Thorne).

In addition to killing off candida, dietary changes are essential for most patients. The important principles include: consuming primarily protein and fresh vegetables, with a limited amount of complex carbohydrates and foods rich in healthy fats, along with a small amount of fresh fruit, avoiding fruit and juices for the first 2–3 weeks. Acceptable foods include raw or lightly steamed, fresh, organic vegetables high in water content and low in starch. These include all green, leafy vegetables (lettuce, spinach, cabbage, kale, sprouts, greens, and parsley), and low-starch vegetables (celery, zucchini, squash, green beans, broccoli, cauliflower, bell peppers, asparagus, tomato, onion, cucumber, garlic, radish, and Brussel's sprouts). Proteins can be eaten freely, but free-range and organic meats that are free of antibiotics and hormones are far more preferable. Nuts and seeds, preferably organic, are also acceptable. Carrots, beets, turnips, eggplant, artichokes, avocados, and peas, containing more starch, can be added after 1–2 months. Complex carbohydrates should be limited to one serving daily, including, sweet potatoes, yams, legumes, brown rice, millet, amaranth, quinoa, and buckwheat, also added after the first month. Flaxseed oil, 1–2 tablespoons daily, used on grains or vegetables, or as a salad dressing, should be used without heating. Other acceptable oils are cold pressed olive, linseed, walnut, and soy. Fruits which are acceptable after the first 2 weeks include melons and berries. With detectable progress, grapefruit, apples, pears, peaches, oranges, nectarines, apricots, cherries, and pineapple can then be added. Fruit juices are best avoided for several weeks; then, fresh squeezed juices are preferred, and they should be diluted 1 : 1 with water. Candida cookbooks are available in bookshops and health food stores. Acceptable foods should be rotated every 3–4 days. Strictly maintaining the restrictive diet for 3–6 months is usually required before broadening the foods ingested. The prohibition against sucrose and concentrated sweets, however, needs to be lifelong.

Foods to avoid include all those containing sugar (e.g., cakes, cookies, donuts, ice cream, soft drinks, most dry breakfast cereals, catsup, jello), sucrose, fructose, maltose, lactose, glucose, dextrose, corn sweetener, corn syrup, sorbitol, mannitol, honey, molasses, maple syrup, fruit sugars, barley malt, rice syrup. Milk, cheese, and dairy products should also be avoided, although butter is acceptable in limited amounts, as is non-fat, unsweetened yogurt if you are milk-tolerant. Unsweetened soy milk is a good substitute. Breads and baked goods made with yeast should be avoided. Other prohibited foods include all white and refined flour products, most packaged and processed foods, olives, pickles, sauerkraut, vinegar, mustard, mushrooms, margarines, refined and hydrogenated oils, soy sauce, tamari, alcohol, and caffeine.

The next phase of treatment emphasizes the restoration of normal concentrations of friendly bacteria in the bowel, adding *Lactobacillus acidophilus* and *bifidus* supplements which are commonly available at most health food stores. Until bowel yeast overgrowth is corrected, attempts to re-establish normal levels of friendly bacteria are frequently unsuccessful. To ensure potency of probiotic supplements, patients should buy refrigerated brands with an expiration date between 1 and 10 months from the date of purchase, and supplying between 1 and 10 billion organisms in divided doses daily. Liquid cultures and powdered forms containing whey, or non-dairy varieties, provide the best supply of organisms. Take two servings per day, morning and evening. Yogurt sources of probiotics are usually insufficient, and are often problematic for the many people sensitive to cows milk derivatives. Yogurts are also often sweetened.

Strengthening the immune system can be accomplished through avoiding toxins (petrochemicals and heavy metals), radiation, and excess ultraviolet exposure. Assuring an adequate intake of vital micronutrients, often through supplements, is essential. The most important micronutrients, many of which can be found in high-dose multivitamin–mineral products, include antioxidants, zinc, manganese, copper, calcium, magnesium, B-complex, and biotin. Essential fatty acids (omega 3 oils, black current seed oil) are helpful. Pancreatic enzymes (1–2 capsules t.i.d. a.c.) and hydrochloric acid (1 capsule with pepsin t.i.d. a.c.) may be necessary to restore normal digestive function. Incorporating adequate aerobic exercise, practicing meditation or regular deep relaxation, adequate sleep, utilizing measures to manage stress, and periodically supplementing with goldenseal and echinacea as indicated all enhance immune function.

Significant attenuation of symptoms should be seen within 1 month of instituting anti-fungal treatment and instituting the diet. If little or no change is noticed, additional complicating factors should be considered, including specific food reactions, the possibility of parasite infestation, hypothyroidism, adrenal exhaustion, chronic viral infection, chronic fatigue syndrome, chemical hypersensitivity, and heavy metal toxicity. People with full-fledged leaky gut syndrome symptoms can expect to progress quite slowly, among other possible causes. Candidiasis can also be sexually transmitted from regular sex partners.

Because symptoms are often variable and vague, and because laboratory tests have high degrees of false negatives, candidiasis remains one of the most elusive conditions to diagnose. Management remains to a great extent at the clinical and not the laboratory level. Often, however, the improving patient will experience a markedly improved physical, emotional, and mental sense of well being.

REFERENCES

1. Ludwig DS et al. High glycemic index foods, overeating, and obesity. *Pediatrics*, 1999; 103(3):E26.
2. Krotkiewski M. Effect of guar gum on body-weight, hunger ratings and metabolism in obese subjects. *Br J Nutr* 1984; 52(1):97–105.
3. Hill JO et al. Thermogenesis in humans during overfeeding with medium-chain triglycerides. *Metabolism* 1989; 38(7): 641–8.

4. Evans GW. Chromium picolinate is an efficacious and safe supplement. *Int J Sport Nutr* 1993; 3(1):117–22.
5. Anderson RA et al. Chromium and its role in lean body mass and weight reduction. *The Nutrition Report* 1993; 11(6):41–6.
6. Leung LH. Pantothenic acid as a weight-reducing agent: fasting without hunger, weakness and ketosis. *Med Hypotheses* 1995; 44(5):403–5.
7. Cangiano C et al. Eating behavior and adherence to dietary prescriptions in obese adult subjects treated with 5-hydroxytryptophan. *Am J Clin Nutr* 1992; 56(5):863–7.
8. Van Gaal L et al. Exploratory study of coenzyme Q_{10} in obesity. In: Folkers K, Yamamura Y, eds. *Biomedical and Clinical Aspects of Coenzyme* Q10, vol. 4. Amsterdam: Elsevier Science, 1984.
9. Dulloo AG et al. The thermogenic properties of ephedrine/methylxanthine mixtures: human studies. *Int J Obes* 1986; 10(6):467–81.
10. Paranjpe P et al. Ayurvedic treatment of obesity: a randomised, double-blind, placebo-controlled trial. *J Ethnopharmacol* 1990; 29(2):1–11.
11. Gupta S et al. A comprehensive immunological analysis in chronic fatigue syndrome. *Scand J Immunol* 1991; 33(3):319–27.
12. Lavy JA. Univ. California School of Medicine, San Fran. 1997 American College of Physicians Annual Meeting, *Fam Pract News* 1997; 27(12):20.
13. Lonsdale D. Red cell transketolase as an indicator of nutritional deficiency. *Am J Clin Nutr* 1980; 33(2):205–11.
14. Cox IM et al. Red blood cell magnesium and chronic fatigue syndrome. *Lancet* 1991; 337(8744):757–60.
15. Russell IJ et al. Treatment of fibromyalgia with supermalic: a randomized, double blind, placebo controlled crossover pilot study. *J Rheumatol* 1995; 22(5):953–8.
16. Gray JB et al. Eicosanoids and essential fatty acid modulation in the chronic fatigue syndrome. *Med Hypotheses* 1994; 43(1):31–42.
17. Plioplys AV et al. Amantidine and L-carnitine treatment of chronic fatigue syndrome. *Neuropsychobiology* 1997; 35(1):16–23.
18. Forsyth LM et al. Therapeutic effects of oral NADH on the symptoms of patients with chronic fatigue syndrome. *Ann Allergy Asthma Immunol* 1999; 82(2):185–91.

19. Bralley JA et al. Treatment of chronic fatigue syndrome with specific amino acid supplementation. *J Appl Nutr* 1994; 46(3):74–8.

20. Ellis FR et al. A pilot study of vitamin B_{12} in the treatment of tiredness. *Br J Nutr* 1973; 30(2):277–83.

21. Reed JC. Magnesium therapy in musculoskeletal pain syndromes—retrospective review of clinical results. *Magnesium Trace Elem* 1990; 9(6):330.

22. Bauer VR et al. Immunologic in vivo and in vitro studies on Echinacea extracts. *Arzneimittelforschung* 1988; 38(2):276–81.

23. Demitrack MA et al. Evidence for impaired activation of the hypothalamic-pituitary-adrenal axis in patients with chronic fatigue syndrome. *J Clin Endocrinol Metab* 1991; 73(6):1224–34.

24. Jeffries, W McK. *Safe uses of Cortisone.* Springfield, IL: C C Thomas, 1981:54–60.

25. Teitlebaum J. Effective treatment of severe chronic fatigue: a report on a series of 64 patients. *J Musculoskel Pain* 1995; 91–110.

26. Galland L. *Giardia lamblia* infection as a cause of chronic fatigue. *J Nutr Med* 1990; 1(1):27–31.

27. Bland J et al. A medical food-supplemented detoxification program in the management of chronic health problems. *Alt Ther Health Med* 1995; 1(5):62–71.

28. Russell IJ et al. Treatment of fibromyalgia with supermalic: a randomized, double blind, placebo controlled crossover pilot study. *J Rheumatol* 1995; 22(5):953–8.

29. Grassetto M et al. Primary fibromyalgia is responsive to S-adenosyl methionine. *Curr Ther Res* 1994; 55(7):797–806.

30. Rask MR. The omohyoideus myofascial pain syndrome: report of four patients. *J Craniomandibular Pract* 1984; 2(3):256–62.

31. McCarty DJ et al. Treatment of pain due to fibromyalgia with topical capsaisacin: a pilot study. *Semin Arthritis Rheum* 1994; 23(6 suppl 3):41–7.

32. Bland J et al. A medical food-supplemented detoxification program in the management of chronic health problems. *Alt Ther Health Med* 1995; 1(5):62–71.

33. Kennedy MJ et al. Ecology of candida adhesion, colonization, and dissemination from the gastrointestinal tract by bacterial antagonism. *Infect Immun* 1985; 45(3):654–63.

34. Krause W et al. Fungaemia and funguria after oral administration of *Candida albicans. Lancet* 1969; 1(7595):598–99.

35. Sanchez A et al. Role of sugars in human neutrophilic phagocytosis. *Am J Clin Nutr* 1973; 26(11):1180–4.
36. McEwen BS et al. Stress and the individual. Mechanisms leading to disease. *Arch Intern Med* 1993; 153(18):2093–2101.
37. Cupps TR et al. Corticosteroid-mediated immunoregulation in man. *Immunol Rev* 1982; 65:133–55.
38. Salmi HA et al. Effect of silymarin on chemical, functional, and morphological alterations of the liver. A double-blind controlled study. *Scand J Gastroenterol* 1982; 17(4):517–21.

14

Chapter Fourteen

The Future of Holistic Medicine

It is very clear that changes in American medicine are occurring rapidly in many aspects. The amazing technology of submolecular chemistry, outstanding feats of surgical complexity, and clear advances in emergency care generate headlines in newspapers and periodicals each week. All of these approaches have great potential to prolong life by bringing to bear exogenous options to modify our chemistry, reattach severed limbs, and resuscitate individuals who were presumed clinically dead.

Underlying this headline type of medicine, there is an awareness at both the consumer and professional level that we are doing considerably less well at managing the more common aspects of health failures involving chronic disease. Many of the strikingly successful techniques which facilitate pulling victims back from the brink of death from trauma or acute illness have considerably less utility in dealing with chronic illness. In fact, chronic rather than acute health problems comprise over 80 percent of the reasons for which patients seek medical help from primary care doctors.

The chronic issues with which most of our US population deals are closely associated with lifestyles and living habits. Physicians principally intervene in the course of a chronic illness by prescribing medications to alter bodily function. The problem with this one-modality response is the significant incidence of side effects. At a minimum, the appropriate use of medications in hospital settings is estimated to be the fifth leading cause of death each year in the United States.[1] Effect of medications, however, pales by comparison with the potential effects of shifts in lifestyle. Moreover, limitation of management of chronic disease to intervention with drugs is much less effective than giving attention to issues of prevention and health promotion.

Why is there so little emphasis on prevention and health promotion?

First, nobody is pushing these approaches. Pharmaceuticals are promoted heavily to practicing and teaching physicians through a variety of ways. The drug industry employs one pharmaceutical representative for every twelve physicians in the country. Most continuing medical education programs and medical journals are heavily supported by pharmaceutical support and advertising. And drugs certainly have their place, are extremely important, and may be life-saving in acute care.

Second, in terms of quality and longevity of life, the benefits of drug treatments in chronic illness pale by comparison to those accruing from positive lifestyle changes. Numerous examples in foregoing chapters have chronicled the benefits of exercise, relaxation practice, and consuming 5–9 servings of fruits and vegetables each day. And it doesn't end here. A recent 25-year study from the Mayo Clinic concluded that optimists live 19 percent longer than pessimists.[2] If this be true, the average lifespan would be increased by about 17 years. Contrast this to a statistician's calculation that if cancer were totally eliminated, the total longevity gain would be about 3.5 years. Modifying aspects of lifestyle has such potential benefit in store that we in 2001 can scarcely grasp its magnitude.

It is essential to re-emphasize that concepts of complementary or holistic medicine are not distinguished by a reliance on either–or thinking in regard to conventional and alternative concepts. As Astin and Eisenberg found in their research, few consumers rely on alternatives to the exclusion of conventional resources. Likewise, few practicing holistic medical and osteopathic physicians do so either. In many situations, it is a matter of choice about responding to a given question with a conventional response or an alternative one. The discovery of hypertension serves as a typical example. Upon the establishment of the presence of essential hypertension, the treating physician has a choice about simply prescribing a single pharmacological antihypertensive (monotherapy), or more likely in today's thinking, a combination of drugs. Repeat blood pressure readings and adjustments in dosage levels are then equilibrated until the blood pressure is observed to respond by falling to normal levels. The alternative choice begins with an elicitation, if possible, of the reason why the blood pressure has become elevated at this particular time in the life of the patient. Addressing that issue is often fruitful. *Drug treatment alone never halts the progression of whatever underlying process is elevating the blood pressure.* Once causation is addressed as completely as possible, then lifestyle modifications can be offered as the first line of treatment. These might include changes in the areas of nutrition, exercise, relaxation, herbology, psychology, energy medicine, spirituality, social health, or manual medicine. The choice of a pharmacological approach or a holistic approach is often dependent on the desires and willingness of the patient, and the degree of responsibility that they wish to assume. If the choice of lifestyle modification is not viable, then drug treatment is always an option. And again, if lifestyle modifications do not result in normalization of blood pressure, the pharmaceutical approach is always available as a secondary option.

In other words, the approaches depend on the choice of which options are elected as the primary approach, and which as the secondary. Many holistic physicians find that many patients, given an explanation of the options, including the discussion of the array of the potential side effects of pharmaceuticals, choose to make the effort to alter and change aspects of their thinking, emotions, and behavior. Holistic physicians consider this a more desirable option, since it more closely approaches the ideal of healing an underlying life issue rather than merely controlling the symptoms manifesting from that issue.

With the rise in public interest through the late 1980s and 1990s, professional awareness spawned greater attention in "alternative" and "complementary" approaches. Although many conventional authorities continue to resist the trend, saying "There is no proof [of efficacy]," the significant benefit experienced by enough consumers continues to fuel the growth of interest in alternative/complementary medicine. The trend toward the new paradigm is emboldened by the sheer numbers of those seeking more of the alternatives. Bias against this progress has been documented in numerous studies published in conventional journals themselves.[3,4]

The conclusions of the Astin report (see Preface) appear to identify a deeply experienced shift in values propelling public interest toward a new definition of healthcare for themselves. The fact that 97 percent of the users of alternatives utilized conventional care as well marks the trend as an interest in complementary care rather than alternative care. The generally more educated users of alternative services appeared to have concerns for earth ecology, women's issues, their own personal, psychological, and spiritual growth, and a commitment to spirituality. These qualities of users of alternatives, it would appear, mark the interest in complementary care as a serious, long-term, paradigmatic shift in a holistic direction, not only for medical care, but probably for society as a whole, as well. The fact that the great portion of the billions of dollars spent on alternatives was spent out-of-pocket and unreimbursed by insurance gives testimony to the assertive determination of consumers to make their own decisions about how to combine available treatment options.

The future appears to hold the elements of a new model of heath and sickness care, in which:

- The hierarchical model of patients being told what to do will gradually fade.
- The model of more collegial decision-making regarding a wide variety of choices of conventional and complementary options will become more commonly used.
- Elements of preventive medicine and health promotion will be increasingly emphasized.
- The conventional model of superb management of emergencies, acute illness, congenital disease, and genetic

problems will be supplemented with a model of superb complementary prevention and management of chronic disease.

- Practitioners of various disciplines will work together as members of a team, pooling their aggregate abilities and strengths.
- Increased use of alternative services and products will be a continuing trend, the conclusion of which is not yet clear.
- Medical practitioners will build strong, compassionate, and caring relationships with patients to foster optimal health and satisfying life experiences.

The last element deserves great emphasis. The boundaries of holistic medicine are significantly larger than those of complementary medicine. Holistic medicine extends beyond the incorporation of the best of the methods of conventional and alternative care. Holistic medicine is based on the core belief that unconditional love is life's most powerful healer. At its essence, the practice of holistic medicine embraces a spirit of interdisciplinary and physician–patient cooperation; balances the mitigation of causes with relief of symptoms; integrates conventional and complementary therapies; and facilitates the experience of being fully alive.

How will this manifest itself in coming decades? The most significant advances will come in the areas of what are known as energy medicine and psychoneuroimmunology. In contrast to the conventional offerings of drugs and surgery, i.e., potential for healing derived from exogenous sources, holistic medicine will increasingly research and utilize endogenous sources for healing. Recent research has begun to accumulate powerful evidence of effective contributions to health promotion and healing from meditation, contiguous and remote healing, prayer, positive beliefs and attitudes, hope, humor, and unconditional love. This published research points the way to the mobilization of these intrinsic attributes to enhance our health and the experience of being fully alive.

Many physicians who now define themselves as holistic doctors have found their way to this philosophy as a result of their own transformative experiences. In many situations it has reinjected a sense of vitality, conviction, and purpose into their practice of medicine. Some physicians have always had these leanings and predilections, and the philosophical aspect of this shift will not be new. It is my hope that *Clinician's Guide to Holistic Medicine* can make a contribution to the further espousal of these principles.

REFERENCES

1. Lazarou J et al. Incidence of adverse drug reactions in hospitalized patients. *JAMA* 1998; 279(15):1200–5.
2. Maruta T et al. Optimists vs. pessimists: survival rate among medical patients. *Mayo Clin Proc* 2000; 75(2):140–3.
3. Resch KI et al. A randomized controlled study of reviewer bias against unconventional therapy. *J Roy Soc Med* 2000; 93(4): 164–7.
4. Goodwin JS, Tangum MR. Battling quackery: attitudes about micronutrient supplements in American academic medicine. *Arch Intern Med* 1998; 158(20):2187–91.

I

Glossary of Terms and Commonly Used Abbreviations

ADD, ADHD. Attention-deficit disorder and attention-deficit hyperactivity disorder. A condition of children and adults in which heredity is thought to play a role, characterized by pathological distractibility or impulsiveness, or both.

Alternative medicine. Dealing with techniques or approaches not taught in medical schools and not generally available in United States hospitals. May involve practitioner-centered as well as client-centered approaches.

Antioxidants. In general, any substances exerting a neutralizing effect in circumstances of oxidative stress. These include nutrients, and intrinsic body enzymes, the best known of which are glutathione peroxidase, catalase, and superoxide dismutase.

Autoimmune. Referring to a tendency for the immune system to generate antibodies and immune complexes toward elements of host tissues. Examples of disease entities involving this process are thought to include rheumatoid arthritis, lupus erythematosus, Grave's disease, inflammatory bowel disease, and perhaps multiple sclerosis. Careful investigation of these processes must be carried out to establish whether the etiology is due to an allergic response to an exogenous inhalant or ingestant, or to a wholly endogenous process.

Ayurvedic medicine. The ancient traditional Indian medicine dating from at least 3000 B.C.E., utilizing a variety of modalities used according to their qualities and combined as necessary to restore the health or life force (*prana*) of the individual in terms of being in balance with nature. Some of those used include sound, color, herbs, diets, and aromas. Human diagnosis and treatment is accomplished through an understanding of biological energies, tissues, channels, and elements.

Biomolecular medicine. That holistic area of medical interest encompassing exogenous nonnutritional agents; endogenous biosynthetic agents (hormones, enzymes, chemical moieties); chelation and bio-oxidation; apitherapy; neural therapy; prolotherapy; intestinal dysbiosis; and innovative uses of existing drugs and protocols.

Botanical medicine/herbology. A mainstay of the practice of naturopathic medicine, the use of herbs has become widespread in the last five years in the US. Therapeutic formulations may consist of whole-substance derivatives or standardized extracts. A considerable database of information is available. The potency of herbs is such that they may interfere with certain drugs taken concomitantly, and a small number of herbs have serious toxicity potential.

CAD. Coronary artery disease, used synonymously with ischemic heart disease.

Chiropractic. Chiropractors utilize manipulation of the spine in a variety of ways, believing that spinal misalignments are responsible for an interrupted flow of bodily energy and the production of a variety of diseases.

Clinical ecology. A term referring to the study of the effects of allergy and sensitivity reactions to inhalants, contactants, and ingestants. Clinical ecologists disagree with classical allergists in suggesting that food reactions in adults are common rather than rare, and that inhalant and food reactions can affect any organ system of the body rather than just the nose, lungs, and skin.

Coenzyme Q_{10}. A quinone with an isoprenoid unit in a side chain occurring in the lipid fraction of the mitochondrial membrane and acting as an intermediate compound in electron transport.

Complementary medicine. Dealing with alternative techniques and approaches in combination with accepted conventional approaches in complementary fashion.

DHEA. Dehydroepiandrosterone. An adrenal cortex hormone, produced in amounts greater than cortisol and other compounds, acting as a substrate for conversion to testosterone and estrogen, and possessing intrinsic activity of its own.

Energy medicine involves consideration and use of conventional and subtle (quantum) energies in healing. Examples include prayer, distance healing, meditation, reiki, jin shin jyutsu, Therapeutic Touch, healing touch, and hands-on healing.

Environmental medicine. This area of holistic interest relates to the toxic nature of much of our human environments including noise, chemicals, radiation, pollution, and communicable diseases. It also includes the multiple allergies and sensitivities from inhalants and ingestants in our environment which can effect every organ system in the body.

Essential fatty acids. The two families of fatty acids not synthesized in the body, linolenic and linoleic acid, with their essential derivatives, eicosapentaenoic/docosapentaenoic acids and gamma-linolenic acids, respectively.

Feldenkrais. A bodywork discipline founded by Moshe Feldenkrais, D.Sc., directed at the healing of injuries and the enhancement of musculoskeletal function through twin principles of awareness through movement and functional integration. Many case studies give testimony to effectiveness in pain control and enhancement of motor function and control.

Free radical. An evanescent, extremely reactive and potentially destructive chemical form of oxygen with an unpaired electron in its outer orbit; an oxidative radical. The condition of excess free radical generation is known as oxidative or oxidant stress.

HDL. High-density lipoprotein.

HDL-C. High-density lipoprotein cholesterol.

HLA. Histocompatibility leucocyte antigens. Human glycoprotein antigens on the surfaces of nucleated cells determined by a region of chromosome 6 bearing genetic loci made up of multiple alleles and playing critical roles in tissue matching procedures.

HMG-CoA-reductase inhibitors. 3-Hydroxy-3-methylglutaryl coenzyme A-reductase inhibitors. Refers to a relatively new class of cholesterol-reducing agents which affect the liver's handling of lipids.

Holistic medicine. Dealing with the whole of an entity. In this context, dealing with the whole spectrum of experiences of the patient, or the whole spectrum of a series of potential healing options. Greater emphasis on client participation in decision-making and involvement with self-care measures, on improving the quality and healing nature of the practitioner-client relationship, and on the whole spectrum of changes required for movement in the direction of creating optimal health – physical, mental, emotional, spiritual, environmental, and social.

Homeopathy. Utilizing two primary principles, Dr. Samuel Hahnemann developed homeopathy in the late 1700s. First, "like cures like": repeated exposure to minute quantities, or even the residual energies of minute quantities of a substance which in large amount produces the symptoms of a given condition, can be curative for that condition. Second, "healing occurs from within outwardly." Homeopathic remedies reestablish the inner constitutional balance, healing from which proceeds layer by layer to the outside.

HRT. Hormone replacement therapy. The prescribing of estrogen and progesterone derivatives to women after menopause, singly or in combination.

Integrative medicine. A style of medical practice forged to utilize alternatives and conventional approaches not as side-by-side options, but attempting to form a whole from the sum of both parts. Includes emphasis on health maintenance and mind–body medicine.

LDL. Low-density lipoprotein.

LDL-C. Low-density lipoprotein cholesterol.

LVEF. Left ventricular ejection fraction. The percentage of the left ventricular blood content ejected by a single stroke of the heart; normal is 60% or more.

Macronutrients. Nutrients used in large amounts daily by the body for fuel, fiber value, and anabolic metabolism.

Micronutrients. Essential nutrients required in small amounts for minimal to optimal molecular function and organ function, including vitamins, minerals, and more broadly also including two essential fatty acids and eight essential amino acids. Intense recycling makes only small amounts necessary for normal function.

Mitogen. Any substance stimulating lymphocyte transformation and immune responsiveness.

NSAIDs. Nonsteroidal anti-inflammatory drugs. The class of drugs, some of which are available over the counter (e.g., ibuprofen), commonly used for relief of pain and treatment of inflammatory conditions. Users should be aware of gastric, hepatic, and renal side effects.

NYHA. New York Heart Association functional classification of heart function. Demonstrable but minimal deficiencies in function are described as class I, and severe debilitating cardiac function is described as class IV.

OR, ORs. Odds ratio(s). The likelihood that a given result will occur, compared to a control result. An OR of 2.0 means that the result with a given variable is twice as likely to occur when compared to the control whose likelihood is expressed as 1.0.

Osteopathy. This school of medicine includes much of allopathic medicine, and includes also training in the utilization of manipulative spinal and soft tissue techniques to relieve energy imbalances and re-establish homeostasis. Preventive practices receive strong emphasis.

PMS. Premenstrual syndrome. A complex of premenstrual symptoms affecting substantial numbers of women during their menstrual years of life. They include mood disturbances, fatigue, metabolic disturbances, retention of tissue fluid, and pain.

Psychoneuroimmunology. Used synonymously with mind–body medicine, this technique recognizes the powerful effects of the energies of mind (concepts, images, ideas) on the central nervous system, which in turn has power effects on and feedback loops from the endocrine, musculoskeletal, and immune systems.

Qi gong. An ancient healing art in traditional Chinese medicine involving meditation, movement exercises, self-massage, and special healing techniques. A core belief is that the integration of breathing, mental, and physical function restores, preserves, and promotes the store of *qi* (vital force) in one's being. Numerous studies document demonstrable success in treating specific conditions. The most sophisticated understanding of the mechanisms involved requires the invoking of quantum and chaos theory.

RR, RRs. Risk ratio(s). The risk that a given result will occur, similar to odds ratios.

Social medicine. In this area of holistic interest, recent research has shown the significant potential for the incidence of many diseases and the outcomes of treatment to be significantly influenced by the quality of human relationships. This has been referred to as social environmental medicine.

Stress. Any psychological or physiological stimulus demanding adaptation.

Syndrome X. A syndrome centered on insulin resistance and hyperinsulinism, spawning elevated lipids, diabetes, coronary artery disease, myocardial infarctions, gout, and hypertension.

Traditional Chinese medicine. The ancient practice of Chinese medicine dating back 3000 years and consisting of principally four elements: acupuncture, botanical medicine, massage, and Qi gong. All deal with enhancement or restoration of the balance of *qi* (*chi*) or vital energy.

Type A behavior. A combination of attitudes manifesting as "hurry sickness," impatience, hostility, and driven behaviors.

Type B behavior. A personality type manifesting much lower need to control, acceptance of the rate at which things happen, and greater comfort with periods of nonproductive relaxation.

Type D behavior. The defining characteristic of this type is the combination of experiencing intense emotions in the face of an inability to express them.

VLDL. Very low-density lipoprotein.

VLDL-C. Very low-density lipoprotein cholesterol.

Appendix II

Tables of Essential Information

RECOMMENDED AMOUNTS OF NUTRITIONAL SUPPLEMENTS

Vitamin	Daily Allowance (1995)	Suggested Maintenance Amounts
A (β-Carotene)	750 (3750 i.u.)	2–5000 µg (10–25,000 i.u.)
B$_1$ (Thiamine)	0.7–1.1 mg	50–100 mg
B$_2$ (Riboflavin)	1.0–1.5 mg	25–50 mg
B$_3$ (Niacin)	12–20 mg	100 mg
B$_5$ (Pantothenic acid)		500 mg
B$_6$ (Pyridoxine)	1.1–2.0 mg	75–100 mg
B$_{12}$ (Cobalamin)	3 µg	400 µg
Folic acid	200 µg	800 µg
Biotin		400 µg
Inositol		100–1000 mg
PABA		100–500 mg
Choline		100 mg
C	40–50 mg	1000 mg
D	5–10 µg (200–400 i.u.)	2.0–10.0 µg (100–400 i.u.)
E	7–10 mg (10–15 i.u.)	267 mg (400 i.u.)

Mineral	Daily Allowance (1995)	Suggested Maintenance Amounts
Boron		3 mg
Calcium	800–1000 mg	200–1500 mg
Chromium		200 µg
Copper		0–2 mg
Iodine	120–150 µg	200 µg
Iron	5.7–12.6 mg	0–15 mg
Magnesium	270–320 mg	400 mg
Manganese		15 mg
Molybdenum		100 µg
Phosphorus	800–1000 mg	0 mg
Potassium		100 mg
Selenium	45–70 g	200 µg
Vanadium		100 mg
Zinc	12 mg	15 mg

CONVERSION TABLES

Vitamin A (Retinol)
1 mg = 5000 IU; 1000 IU = 0.2 mg

β-Carotene (pro-vitamin A)
1 mg = 167 IU; 1000 IU = 6 mg

Other carotenoids
1 mg = 83.33 IU; 1000 IU = 12 mg

Vitamin E (tocopherol)
1 mg = 1.5 IU; 1000 IU = 667 mg

Vitamin D (calciferol)
1 μg = 40 IU; 1000 IU = 25 μg

IU = international units
1 μg = 1/1000 mg = 1/1,000,000 g
1 g = 1000 mg = 1,000,000 μg

THE SEVEN TRAITS OF HEALTHY PERSONS

Healthy people:

1. Tend to be attuned to their own mind–body signals of pleasure and pain, including such things as fatigue, anger, and sadness.
2. Have the capacity to confide their secrets, traumas, and feelings to others instead of keeping them locked up inside.
3. Exhibit the three Cs: a sense of control over their health and quality of life; a strong commitment to work, creative activities, or relationships; and an ability to see stress as a challenge rather than a threat.
4. Are appropriately assertive about their needs and feelings.
5. Tend to form relationships based on unconditional love rather than frustrated power.
6. Are altruistically committed to helping others.
7. Demonstrate willingness to explore many different facets of their personalities, which gives them strengths to fall back on if one fails.

Source: Dreher, H., *The Immune Power Personality*. New York: Dutton, 1995.

THE RELAXATION RESPONSE

Increase in:
immune response; water and sodium excretion; circulation to nose, skin, kidneys, and gastrointestinal tract; gastrointestinal peristalsis; resistance to digestive juices; reaction time; auditory perception; and pain tolerance.

Decrease in:
muscle tension; brainwave frequency; heart rate; BP; respiration rate; circulation to heart, brain, muscles, and lungs; perspiration; metabolism; glycogen consumption; potassium and magnesium excretion; epinephrine; cortisone; cholesterol; triglycerides; clotting factors; and oxidative stress.

Disease states benefiting:
heart rhythm disturbances; hypertension; tension headaches; migraine; seizures; Raynaud's; neck and back pain; IBS and ulcer; allergic responses; premenstrual syndrome; dysmenorrhea; insomnia; anxiety and panic disorder; ADHD; and all free-radical mediated disease.

Relaxation is a skill for which many persons require training similar to most learned behaviors. The *conditions* which facilitate the acquisition of the skill of relaxation are:

- A quiet environment with decreased environmental stimuli.
- A comfortable position with decreased muscle tone.
- Adoption of a passive attitude returning the focus of concentration gently from distractions as they occur.
- A mental device such as a repeated word, phrase, thought, or image; a repeated sound; or gazing at an object.

The *stages* of skill development are:

- Identification of the relaxed state.
- Recognition of the achievement path.
- Ongoing practice.
- Habit development.

The *techniques* which achieve the alpha brain-wave state of relaxation are:

- Biofeedback.
- Autogenics.
- Progressive relaxation.
- Self-suggestion and hypnosis.
- Meditation.

Sources: Benson, H., *The Relaxation Response*. New York: Avon, 1975; Anderson, R., *Stress Power!* New York: Human Sciences Press; 1978; Anderson, R., *Wellness Medicine*. New Canaan, CT: Keats, 1990.

III

Appendix III

Resource Guide

HOLISTIC/COMPLEMENTARY MEDICINE

American Holistic Medical Association (AHMA)
6728 Old McLean Village Drive
McLean, VA 22101-3906
(703) 556-9728
Fax (703) 556-8729
www.holisticmed.org

American Board of Holistic Medicine (ABHM)
P.O. Box 5388
Lynnwood, WA 98043-5388
(425) 741-2996
blh@halcyon.com

American Preventive Medical Association
459 Walker Road
Great Falls, VA 22066
(703) 759-0662
Fax (703) 759-6711

American Holistic Nurses Association
P.O. Box 2130
Flagstaff, AZ 86003
(800) 278-AHNA
http://www.ahna.org

The British Holistic Medical Association
179 Gloucester Place

London NW1 6DX
England
020 7272 5299
www.users.dircon.co.uk/
bhma/sec

Center for Science in the Public
Interest
1875 Connecticut Avenue NW,
Suite 300
Washington, DC 20009
(202) 332-9110
Fax (202) 265-4954

Holistic Dental Association
P.O. Box 5007
Durango, CO 81301
www.holisticdental.org

Institute of Noetic Sciences
475 Gate Five Road, Suite 300
Sausalito, CA 94965
(415) 331-5650
webmaster@noetic.org

Naturopathic Medicine

American Association of
Naturopathic Physicians
2366 Eastlake Avenue East,
Suite 322
Seattle, WA 98102
(206) 323-7610

Institute for Naturopathic
Medicine
66 1/2 North State Street

Concord, NH 03301
(603) 255-8844

ENVIRONMENTAL MEDICINE

American Academy of
Environmental Medicine
10 E. Randolph
New Hope, PA 18938
(215) 862-4544

NUTRITIONAL MEDICINE

American College of Nutrition
722 Robert E. Lee Drive
Wilmington, NC 28480
(919) 452-1222

American Natural Hygiene
Society
11816 Racetrack Road
Tampa, FL 33626
(813) 855-6607

American Dietetic Association
216 West Jackson, Suite 800
Chicago, IL 60606
(313) 899-0040

International Association of
Professional Natural Hygienists
Regency Health Resort and Spa
2000 South Ocean Drive
Hallandale, FL 33009
(305) 454-2220

BIOMOLECULAR MEDICINE

Chelation Therapy
American College of
Advancement in Medicine
(ACAM)
23121 Verdugo Drive, Suite
204
Laguna Hills, CA 92653
(800) 532-3688

American Board of Chelation
Therapy
1407-B North Wells Street
Chicago, IL 60610
(800) 286-6013
www.glccm.org

International Society for
Orthomolecular Medicine
16 Florence Avenue
Toronto, Ontario,
Canada M2N 1E9
(416) 733-2117
www.orthomed.org

The Institute for Functional
Medicine
5800 Soundview Drive # b
Gig Harbor, WA 98335-2057
(253) 851-3943
www.fxmed.com

EXERCISE MEDICINE

American Dance Therapy
Association
200 Century Plaza, Suite 108
10632 Little Patuxent Parkway
Columbia, MD 21044
(410) 997-4040
info@adta.org

ETHNOMEDICINE

*Acupuncture/Traditional
Chinese Medicine (TCM)*
American Association for
Oriental Medicine
433 Front Street
Catasaqua, PA 18032
(610) 266-1433
Fax (610) 264-2768

American Academy of Medical
Acupuncture
5820 Wilshire Blvd., Suite 500
Los Angeles, CA 90036
(213) 937-5514

Qigong Institute/East-West
Academy of Healing Arts
450 Sutter, Suite 916
San Francisco, CA 94108
(415) 788-2227

Qigong Institute
561 Berkeley Avenue
Menlo Park, CA 94025

www.healthy.net/
QiGonginstitute

Ayurvedic Medicine

Ayurvedic Institute
P.O. Box 23445
Albuquerque, NM 87192
(505) 291-9698
Fax (505) 294-7572

BEHAVIORAL MEDICINE/ PSYCHONEURO- IMMUNOLOGY/ MIND–BODY MEDICINE

National Institute for the
Clinical Application of
Behavioral Medicine
P.O. Box 523
Mansfield Center, CT 06250
(860) 456-1153
Fax (860) 423-4512

Association for Humanistic
Psychology
45 Franklin Street, Suite 315
San Francisco, CA 94102
(415) 864-8850

Center for Mind–Body Medicine
5225 Connecticut Avenue NW,
Suite 414
Washington, DC 20015
(202) 966-7338

Mind/Body Medical Institute
New Deaconess Hospital

185 Pilgrim Road
Boston, MA 02215
(617) 632-9530

Biofeedback

Association for Applied
Psychophysiology and
Biofeedback
10200 West 44th Avenue
#304
Wheat Ridge, CO 80033
(303) 422-8894

Guided Imagery

Academy for Guided Imagery
P.O. Box 2070
Mill Valley, CA 94942
(800) 726-2070/Fax (415)
389-9342
www.interactiveimagery.com

Hypnotherapy

American Association of
Professional Hypnotherapists
P.O. Box 29
Boones Mill, VA 24065
(540) 334-3035

Neurolinguistic Programming

American Board of NLP
16842 Von Karman Avenue,
Suite 475
Irvine, CA 92714
(949) 261-6400

MANUAL MEDICINE

Chiropractic

American Chiropractic
Association
1701 Clarendon Blvd.
Arlington, VA 22209
(703) 276-8800

International Chiropractors
Association
1110 North Glebe Road, Suite
1000
Arlington, VA 22201
(800) 423-4690
(703) 528-5000

Craniosacral Therapy

Cranial Academy
8606 Allisonville Road, Suite
130
Indianapolis, IN 46268
(317) 594-0411
Fax (317) 594-9299

Alexander Technique

North American Society of
Teachers of the Alexander
Technique
P.O. Box 5536
Playa del Rey, CA 90296
(800) 473-0620

Feldenkrais Method

Feldenkrais Guild of North
America
524 Ellsworth Street SW,
Box 489
Albany, OR 97321
(541) 926-0981
www.feldenkrais.com

Hellerwork

Hellerwork International
406 Berry Street
Mount Shasta, CA 96067
(916) 392-3900
www.hellerwork.com

Massage

American Massage Therapy
Association
820 Davis Street, Suite 100
Evanston, IL 60201
(847) 864-0123

Osteopathic Medicine

American Academy of
Osteopathy
3500 DePauw Blvd., Suite
1080
Indianapolis, IN 46268
(317) 879-1881

American Osteopathic
Association
142 East Ontario Street

Chicago, IL 60611
(312) 202-8000

Reflexology

International Institute of
Reflexology
P.O. Box 12462
St. Petersburg, FL 33733
(813) 343-4811

Rolfing

International Rolf Institute
205 Canyon Blvd.
Boulder, CO 80302
(303) 449-5903
www.rolf.org

Trager

The Trager Institute
21 Locust Avenue
Mill Valley, CA 94941
(415) 388-2688
admin@trager.com

ENERGY MEDICINE

International Society for the
Study of Subtle Energies and
Energy Medicine (ISSSEEM)
356 Goldco Circle
Golden, CO 80401
(303) 278-2228
Fax (303) 279-3539

Healing Touch

Colorado Center for Healing
Touch, Inc.
198 Union Blvd., Suite 204
Lakewood, CO 80228

Polarity Therapy

American Polarity Therapy
Association
2888 Bluff Street # 149
Boulder, CO 80301
(303) 545-2080
www.polaritytherapy.org

Reiki

Reiki Alliance
P.O. Box 41
Cataldo, ID 83810
(208) 682-3535

Therapeutic Touch

Nurse Healers Professional
Associates, Inc.
1211 Locust Street
Philadelphia, PA 19107
(215) 545-8079

Yoga

The American Yoga
Association
513 South Orange Avenue
Sarasota, FL 34236
(941) 953-5859
AmYogaAssn@aol.com

BOTANICAL/HERBAL MEDICINE

American Botanical Council
P.O. Box 201660
Austin, TX 78720
(512) 331-8868

Herb Research Foundation
1007 Pearl Street
Boulder, CO 80302
(303) 449-2265

HOMEOPATHY

International Foundation for
Homeopathy
2366 Eastlake Avenue East,
Suite 301
Seattle, WA 98102
(206) 324-8230

National Center for
Homeopathy
801 North Fairfax, Suite 306
Alexandria, VA 22314
(703) 548-7790

ART, SOUND, LIGHT, AROMA THERAPIES

Aromatherapy

National Association for
Holistic Aromatherapy
P.O. Box 17622
Boulder, CO 80308
(888) ASK-NAHA
info@naha.org

Art Therapy

American Art Therapy
Association (AATA)
1202 Allanson Road
Mundelein, IL 60060
(847) 949-6064
(888) 290-0878
Fax (847) 566-4580

Flower Essences

Flower Essence Society
P.O. Box 459
Nevada City, CA 95959
(520) 634-9298

Light

Environmental Health and Light
Research Institute
16057 Tampa Palms Blvd.,
Suite 227
Tampa, FL 33647
(800) 544-4878

Music Therapy

American Music Therapy
Association
8455 Colesville Road, Suite
1000
Silver Spring, MD 20910
(301) 589-3300
Fax (301) 589-5175
www.musictherapy.org

CONVENTIONAL
(ALLOPATHIC) MEDICINE

American Medical Association
515 N. State Street
Chicago, IL 60610-0946
(312) 464-5000
www.am-assn.org

Index